pruuder.

_2012._

CLINICAL PEDIATRIC ANESTHESIA

Clinical Pediatric Anesthesia

A Case-Based Handbook

Edited by
Kenneth R. Goldschneider, MD, FAAP
Associate Professor, Clinical Anesthesia and Pediatrics
Director, Pain Management Center
Cincinnati Children's Hospital Medical Center
University of Cincinnati, College of Medicine
Cincinnati, Ohio

Andrew J. Davidson, MBBS, MD, FANZCA
Associate Professor
Department of Anaesthesia and Pain Management
Director of Clinical Research
Royal Children's Hospital
Victoria, Australia

Eric P. Wittkugel, MD, FAAP
Associate Professor, Clinical Anesthesia and Pediatrics
Cincinnati Children's Hospital Medical Center
University of Cincinnati, College of Medicine
Cincinnati, Ohio

Adam V. Skinner, BSc (Hons), MB, ChB, MRCP (UK), FRCA
Consultant Paediatric Anaesthetist
Royal Children's Hospital
Victoria, Australia

OXFORD
UNIVERSITY PRESS

OXFORD
UNIVERSITY PRESS

Oxford University Press, Inc., publishes works that further
Oxford University's objective of excellence
in research, scholarship, and education.

Oxford New York
Auckland   Cape Town   Dar es Salaam   Hong Kong   Karachi
Kuala Lumpur   Madrid   Melbourne   Mexico City   Nairobi
New Delhi   Shanghai   Taipei   Toronto

With offices in
Argentina   Austria   Brazil   Chile   Czech Republic   France   Greece
Guatemala   Hungary   Italy   Japan   Poland   Portugal   Singapore
South Korea   Switzerland   Thailand   Turkey   Ukraine   Vietnam

Published by Oxford University Press, Inc.
198 Madison Avenue, New York, New York 10016
www.oup.com

Oxford is a registered trademark of Oxford University Press

Library of Congress Cataloging-in-Publication Data

Clinical pediatric anesthesia : a case-based handbook / edited by
Kenneth R. Goldschneider ... [et al.].
      p. ; cm.
Includes bibliographical references and index.
ISBN 978-0-19-976449-5
I. Goldschneider, Kenneth R.
[DNLM: 1. Anesthesia—Case Reports. 2. Child. 3. Infant. WO 440]
617.96—dc23   2011039720

This material is not intended to be, and should not be considered, a substitute for medical
or other professional advice. Treatment for the conditions described in this material is
highly dependent on the individual circumstances. And, while this material is designed to
offer accurate information with respect to the subject matter covered and to be current as
of the time it was written, research and knowledge about medical and health issues is
constantly evolving and dose schedules for medications are being revised continually, with
new side effects recognized and accounted for regularly. Readers must therefore always
check the product information and clinical procedures with the most up-to-date published
product information and data sheets provided by the manufacturers and the most recent
codes of conduct and safety regulation. The publisher and the authors make no representations or warranties to readers, express or implied, as to the accuracy or completeness of
this material. Without limiting the foregoing, the publisher and the authors make no
representations or warranties as to the accuracy or efficacy of the drug dosages mentioned
in the material. The authors and the publisher do not accept, and expressly disclaim, any
responsibility for any liability, loss or risk that may be claimed or incurred as a
consequence of the use and/or application of any of the contents of this material.

9 8 7 6 5 4 3 2 1
Printed in the USA
on acid-free paper

KG: To Toby and Irving Goldschneider—the amount one realizes that he has learned from his parents is proportional to the time lived since adolescence.

EW: To my wife, Kim, and my three children, Andrew, Erica and Ben. Thank you for your steadfast love and the great joy that you bring to life!

AD: To Eliza; and to all my mentors and muses that have inspired and supported me.

AS: To my wife, Gerry. She has supported me throughout and has the patience of a saint.

All: To India Davidson, who made us all hold our breath.

ACKNOWLEDGMENTS

What worthy project is done alone? As for so many ventures, this book would not exist without the support and assistance of others whose role is out of the proverbial limelight.

We would like to acknowledge those people who helped make this book a reality.

Gillian Ormond of the Royal Children's Hospital: Even though you were recruited well into the process, your organizational skills and support were priceless. We are grateful for your help.

Staci Hou of Oxford University Press: Thank you for your support and for putting up with the inevitable but unwanted delays and for taking care of the details.

The authors: You cheerfully contributed your expertise and you represent the best in pediatric anesthesia teaching.

And the most heartfelt acknowledgement goes to. . .

Kim Wittkugel, Jen Goldschneider, Sophie Davidson, and Gerry Skinner, our better halves: Thank you for your patience and your encouragement. We love you.

CONTENTS

PART 6 CHALLENGES IN CONGENITAL HEART DISEASE

PART 7 CHALLENGES IN OPHTHALMOLOGY

PART 8 CHALLENGES IN NEUROSURGICAL CONDITIONS AND NEUROMONITORING

PART 9 CHALLENGES IN PATIENTS WITH HEMATOLOGIC AND ONCOLOGIC DISORDERS

PART 10 CHALLENGES IN METABOLIC AND ENDOCRINOLOGIC CONDITIONS

PART 11 CHALLENGES IN THE PERINATAL PERIOD

PART 12 CHALLENGES IN REGIONAL ANESTHESIA AND PAIN

PART 13 CHALLENGES IN PEDIATRIC SYNDROMES

PART 14 CHALLENGES IN THE POST-ANESTHESIA CARE UNIT

INTRODUCTION: HOW TO USE THIS BOOK

ROBERT McDOUGALL

Case-based learning and teaching have been used in clinical anesthesiology for many years. This book, *Clinical Pediatric Anesthesia: A Case-Based Handbook,* uses case presentations to help the reader learn about the various practical aspects of pediatric anesthesia. This is in contrast to traditional textbooks, which are organized in a content-based format and are often best used as reference tools. The book is aimed at all who have discovered pediatric anesthesia and wish to further their understanding of its practice. This includes, but is not limited to, technicians, nurses, nurse anesthetists, medical students, junior doctors, residents, fellows, and anesthesiologists. It is best used as a primer or a tool for exam preparation. While not designed as a sourcebook or "how-to" guide, it may assist anesthesia providers as they think through their preparation for specific cases.

The notes below explain how this book can be used to help the reader learn about principles and practice of pediatric anesthesia.

Case-based teaching and learning aim to promote the acquisition of knowledge and clinical decision making by encouraging the reader to think about how he or she would manage the case presented. This active involvement in the learning process will encourage higher levels of learning, such as analysis, synthesis, and evaluation, rather than simple "absorption" of the information presented.

Each chapter of this book contains a case presentation relevant to the title of the chapter. Each chapter has learning objectives that drive the discussion that follows each presentation. There are **key words** in boldface throughout the case presentation. Take note of these **key words**: they are intended to relate points within the case to explanation in the text and to help answer the questions posed by the authors. The discussion is in the form of answers to questions that will help the learner meet the objectives. The chapters conclude with some references for important points and suggested further reading.

The reader should think of each case as a "simulation" and, after reading the objectives and case presentation, decide how he or she would manage the case. For the solo learner, it is recommended that ideas be written down. If learning in a group of two or more, discussing the case can be productive. Group members can take turns asking the questions of one another, allowing members to think through an answer prior to sharing the explanations in the text.

WHAT IS THE BEST WAY TO USE THE QUESTIONS IN THE DISCUSSION SECTION?

Before reading the answers to the questions that follow the case, the reader should think about his or her answers or discuss them in a group. The authors' answers are not "the final word" on management. The anesthetic plans described in the chapters are based on evidence in the literature as well as the experience of the authors. There are often several acceptable approaches to the care of children in any given situation. When appropriate, various options are presented and their advantages and disadvantages discussed. Indeed, the more experienced practitioner may disagree with the answers presented. Those who disagree will benefit by thinking about why they disagree and writing down or discussing different approaches or reasoning.

At the end of the chapter ask yourself, "Have I met my learning objectives? If not, why not? Is there a reference that would clarify a point or enhance my understanding?"

This book is intended as a guide to thought and decision making. It is not intended as an exhaustive reference tool. As such a guide, there is a list of helpful references at the end of each chapter. The first few references have been identified by the author as particularly informative and are annotated. A list of other informative references follows for those wishing to pursue specific subtopics. When specific material is cited in the text, the sources will be so identified. Generally, the references provided and the suggestions for further reading will help students to further explore the topics and may help readers achieve objectives that vary from those set out by the authors.

The questions posed by real-life clinical situations call for active thinking, and use of evidence as available. Oral board examiners will ask similar, though hypothetical, questions. In fact, most anesthesia examinations contain case presentations with questions relating to the case. The cases in this book are ideal for assisting with exam preparation.

In summary, think about the cases and try to answer the questions. Enjoy using this book alone or in groups!

CONTRIBUTORS

Lori A. Aronson, MD
Associate Professor, Clinical Anesthesia and Pediatrics
Cincinnati Children's Hospital Medical Center
University of Cincinnati, College of Medicine
Cincinnati, Ohio
*Chapters: 9. Anaphylaxis, 11. Egg and Soy Allergies and Propofol
Use, 27. Liver Transplantation, 47. Diabetic Ketoacidosis During
Appendicitis with Perforation, 48. Hypopituitarism,
49. Mitochondrial Disorder for Muscle Biopsy*

Anne C. Boat, MD
Assistant Professor, Clinical Anesthesia and Pediatrics
Director, Fetal Anesthesia
Cincinnati Children's Hospital Medical Center
University of Cincinnati, College of Medicine
Cincinnati, Ohio
*Chapters: 55. Congenital Diaphragmatic Hernia Repair,
56. Myelomeningocele Repair*

Lindy Cass, MBBS, FANZCA
Department of Anaesthesia and Pain Management
Royal Children's Hospital
Victoria, Australia
Chapter: 20. Intraoperative Wheezing

**George Chalkiadis, MBBS, DA (Lon),
FANZCA, FFPMANZCA**
Department of Anaesthesia and Pain Management
Clinical Associate Professor
Royal Children's Hospital
Victoria, Australia
*Chapters: 59. Acute Pain Management,
67. Cerebral Palsy*

Vidya Chidambaran, MD, MBBS
Assistant Professor, Clinical Anesthesia
and Pediatrics
Cincinnati Children's Hospital Medical Center
University of Cincinnati, College of Medicine
Cincinnati, Ohio
Chapters: 13. Foreign Body in the Airway, 50. Obesity

Jason Chou, MBBS, FANZCA, FFPMANZCA
Department of Anaesthesia and Pain Management
Royal Children's Hospital
Victoria, Australia
Chapter: 59. Acute Pain Management

**Michael Clifford, MBBS (Hons), FJFICM,
FANZCA, Cert Clin Ultrasound**
Department of Anaesthesia and Pain Management
Royal Children's Hospital
Victoria, Australia
*Chapter: 30. Children with Congenital Heart Disease
for Non-cardiac Surgery*

Gillian Derrick, B Med Sci, BM BS, FRCA
Consultant Paediatric Anaesthetist
Clinical Service Director
Directorate of Specialised Services
Birmingham Children's Hospital
Birmingham, UK
Chapter: 27. Liver Transplant

Charles B. Eastwood, MD
Assistant Professor, Clinical Anesthesia and Pediatrics
Cincinnati Children's Hospital Medical Center
University of Cincinnati, College of Medicine
Cincinnati, Ohio
Chapters: 57. Caudal vs. Penile Block, 68. Emergence Agitation

Britt Fraser, MBBS, FANZCA
Department of Anaesthesia and Acute Pain Management
Geelong Hospital
Victoria, Australia
Chapter: 4. Acute Fluid Resuscitation for Intussusception

Geoff Frawley, BSc, MBBS, FANZCA, Dip DHM
Department of Anaesthesia and Pain Management
Clinical Associate Professor
Royal Children's Hospital
Victoria, Australia
*Chapters: 52. Former Premature Infant for Hernia Repair,
64. Mucopolysaccharidoses*

Nancy S. Hagerman, MD
Assistant Professor, Clinical Anesthesia and Pediatrics
Co-Director, Same Day Surgery and Preanesthesia
Consultation Clinic
Cincinnati Children's Hospital Medical Center
University of Cincinnati, College of Medicine
Cincinnati, Ohio
*Chapters: 1. Preoperative Anxiety Management, 7. Preoperative
Fasting in the Pediatric Patient*

Elizabeth A. Hein, MD
Associate Professor, Clinical Anesthesia and Pediatrics
Cincinnati Children's Hospital Medical Center
University of Cincinnati, College of Medicine
Cincinnati, Ohio
Chapters: 15. Tonsillar Bleed, 17. Airway Reconstruction

Liana G. Hosu, MD
Assistant Professor, Clinical Anesthesia and Pediatrics
Cincinnati Children's Hospital Medical Center
University of Cincinnati, College of Medicine
Cincinnati, Ohio
Chapters: 9. Anaphylaxis, 48. Hypopituitarism

Peter Howe, MBBS, FANZCA
Department of Anaesthesia and Pain Management
Royal Children's Hospital
Victoria, Australia
Chapters: 16. Difficult Airway, 28. Craniosynostosis Repair

George K. Istaphanous, MD
Associate Professor, Clinical Anesthesia and Pediatrics
Director, Neurosurgical Anesthesia
Cincinnati Children's Hospital Medical Center
University of Cincinnati, College of Medicine
Cincinnati, Ohio
Chapter: 35. Pulmonary Hypertension

J. Fay Jou, MD
Assistant Professor, Clinical Anesthesia and Pediatrics
Cincinnati Children's Hospital Medical Center
University of Cincinnati, College of Medicine
Cincinnati, Ohio
Chapters: 36. Open Globe Repair, 49. Mitochondrial Disorder for Muscle Biopsy

Michael J. Kibelbek, MD
Associate Professor, Clinical Anesthesia and Pediatrics
Cincinnati Children's Hospital Medical Center
University of Cincinnati, College of Medicine
Cincinnati, Ohio
Chapter: 11. Egg and Soy Allergies and Propofol Use

Matthias W. König, MD
Assistant Professor, Clinical Anesthesia and Pediatrics
Cincinnati Children's Hospital Medical Center
University of Cincinnati, College of Medicine
Cincinnati, Ohio
Chapters: 23. Difficult Ventilation During Laparoscopic Fundoplication, 37. Prone Positioning for Posterior Fossa Tumor Resection, 38. Spinal Surgery

Renee Nierman Kreeger, MD
Assistant Professor, Clinical Anesthesia and Pediatrics
Cincinnati Children's Hospital Medical Center
University of Cincinnati, College of Medicine
Cincinnati, Ohio
Chapters: 32. Tetralogy of Fallot, 63. Muscular Dystrophy

C. Dean Kurth, MD
Chairman, Department of Anesthesiology
Professor, Anesthesia and Pediatrics
Cincinnati Children's Hospital Medical Center
University of Cincinnati, College of Medicine
Cincinnati, Ohio
Chapters: 19. Bacterial Tracheitis Versus Epiglottitis, 69. Stridor After Extubation

Gillian R. Lauder, MBBCh, FRCA, FRCPC
Department of Anesthesia, British Columbia Children's Hospital, Vancouver, British Columbia, Canada
Chapter: 61. Complex Regional Pain Syndrome in the Emergency Department

Jerrold Lerman, BASc, MD, FRCPC, FANZCA
Department of Anesthesiology
Clinical Professor of Anesthesiology
Women and Children's Hospital of Buffalo
Buffalo, New York
Chapter: 70. Postoperative Nausea and Vomiting in Patients with Prolonged QTc

Erica P. Lin, MD
Assistant Professor, Clinical Anesthesia and Pediatrics
Cincinnati Children's Hospital Medical Center
University of Cincinnati, College of Medicine
Cincinnati, Ohio
Chapters: 33. Cardiac Catheterization, 62. Down Syndrome

Andreas W. Loepke, MD, PhD
Associate Professor, Clinical Anesthesia and Pediatrics
Cincinnati Children's Hospital Medical Center
University of Cincinnati, College of Medicine
Cincinnati, Ohio
Chapters: 33. Cardiac Catheterization, 35. Pulmonary Hypertension

Mohamed A. Mahmoud, MD
Associate Professor, Clinical Anesthesia and Pediatrics
Director, Radiology Anesthesia and Sedation
Cincinnati Children's Hospital Medical Center
University of Cincinnati, College of Medicine
Cincinnati, Ohio
Chapters: 10. Anesthesia for MRI, 37. Prone Positioning for Posterior Fossa Tumor Resection, 38. Spinal Surgery, 44. Mediastinal Mass Biopsy

Judith O. Margolis, MD, MPH
Associate Professor, Clinical Anesthesia and Pediatrics
Cincinnati Children's Hospital Medical Center
University of Cincinnati, College of Medicine
Cincinnati, Ohio
Chapters: 15. Tonsillar Bleed, 36. Open Globe Repair

David Martin, MD
Fellow, Pediatric Anesthesia
Cincinnati Children's Hospital Medical Center
University of Cincinnati, College of Medicine
Cincinnati, Ohio
Chapter: 21. Cystic Fibrosis

Nicholas Martin, MBBS, FRCA, FANZCA
Department of Anaesthesia and Pain Management
Royal Children's Hospital
Victoria, Australia
Chapter: 34. Cardiac MRI

Dugald McAdam, MBBS, FANZCA
Department of Anaesthesia and Pain Management
Royal Children's Hospital
Victoria, Australia
*Chapter: 51. Exploratory Laparotomy for
Necrotizing Enterocolitis*

John J. McAuliffe, III, MD, MBA
Associate Professor, Anesthesia and Pediatrics
Director, Division of Neurobiology
Cincinnati Children's Hospital Medical Center
University of Cincinnati, College of Medicine
Cincinnati, Ohio
*Chapters: 10. Anesthesia for MRI, 23. Difficult Ventilation During
Laparoscopic Fundoplication, 37. Prone Positioning for Posterior
Fossa Tumor Resection, 38. Spinal Surgery*

Robert McDougall, MBBS, FANZCA, GradCetHlthProfEd
Department of Anaesthesia and Pain Management
Clinical Associate Professor
Royal Children's Hospital
Victoria, Australia
*Chapters: Introduction: How to Use This Book, 25. Management of
Acutely Burned Children, 26. Management of Burn Patients for
Grafting and Excision*

Rebecca McIntyre, MBBS, FANZCA
Department of Anaesthesia and Pain Management
Royal Children's Hospital
Victoria, Australia
Chapter: 41. Hemophilia

Ian McKenzie, MBBS, Dip RACOG, FANZCA
Department of Anaesthesia and Pain Management
Director, Department of Anaesthesia and Pain Management
Royal Children's Hospital
Victoria, Australia
Chapter: 31. Single Ventricle Physiology

Mark J. Meyer, MD
Associate Professor, Clinical Anesthesia and Pediatrics
Cincinnati Children's Hospital Medical Center
University of Cincinnati, College of Medicine
Cincinnati, Ohio
*Chapters: 6. Do-Not-Resuscitate Orders in the
OR, 42. Oncology Patient, 71. Disclosure After Complication
in the OR*

David L. Moore, MD
Associate Professor, Clinical Anesthesia and Pediatrics
Cincinnati Children's Hospital Medical Center
University of Cincinnati, College of Medicine
Cincinnati, Ohio
Chapters: 22. Pectus Excavatum Repair, 58. Neonatal Epidural

Jacqueline W. Morillo-Delerme, MD
Associate Professor, Clinical Anesthesia and Pediatrics
Anesthesia Director, Liberty Campus
Cincinnati Children's Hospital Medical Center
University of Cincinnati, College of Medicine
Cincinnati, Ohio
Chapter: 49. Mitochondrial Disorder for Muscle Biopsy

Eugene Neo, MBBS, FANZCA
Department of Anaesthesia and Pain Management
Royal Children's Hospital
Victoria, Australia
Chapter: 5. Asthmatic for Adenotonsillectomy

Mario Patino, MD
Assistant Professor, Clinical Anesthesia
and Pediatrics
Cincinnati Children's Hospital Medical Center
University of Cincinnati, College of Medicine
Cincinnati, Ohio
Chapters: 46. Diabetic Patient, 66. Osteogenesis Imperfecta

Elizabeth Prentice, MBBS, FANZCA
Department of Anaesthesia and Pain Management
Royal Children's Hospital
Victoria, Australia
Chapters: 18. Laryngeal Papillomatosis, 60. Peripheral Nerve Block Catheter for Extremity Surgery

Philip Ragg, MBBS, FFARACS, FANZCA, PG DipEcho
Department of Anaesthesia and Pain Management
Clinical Associate Professor
Royal Children's Hospital
Victoria, Australia
Chapter: 8. Malignant Hyperthermia

Lorna Rankin, BSc, FANZCA, MBChB, Dip Paeds
Department of Anaesthesia
Starship Children's Hospital
Auckland, New Zealand
Chapter: 53. Tracheoesophageal Fistula Repair

Shilpa Rao, MBBS, MD
Department of Anesthesiology
Women and Children's Hospital of Buffalo
Buffalo, New York
*Chapter: 70. Postoperative Nausea and Vomiting in
Patients with Prolonged QTc*

Gresham T. Richter, MD
Associate Professor
Department of Otolaryngology-Head and Neck Surgery
University of Arkansas for Medical Sciences
Arkansas Children's Hospital
Little Rock, Arkansas
Chapter: 17. Airway Reconstruction

Stefan Sabato, MBBS (Hons), FANZCA
Department of Anaesthesia and Pain Management
Royal Children's Hospital
Victoria, Australia
*Chapters: 24. Massive Transfusion in a Child,
45. Neuroblastoma Resection*

Senthilkumar Sadhasivam, MD, MPH
Associate Professor, Clinical Anesthesia and Pediatrics
Director, Acute and Perioperative Pain Management
Cincinnati Children's Hospital Medical Center
University of Cincinnati, College of Medicine
Cincinnati, Ohio
*Chapters: 13. Foreign Body in the Airway, 50. Obesity, 55. Congenital
Diaphragmatic Hernia Repair, 56. Myelomeningocele Repair*

Nancy B. Samol, MD
Assistant Professor, Clinical Anesthesia and Pediatrics
Cincinnati Children's Hospital Medical Center
University of Cincinnati, College of Medicine
Cincinnati, Ohio
Chapters: 3. Upper Respiratory Infection, 65. Epidermolysis Bullosa

Paul J. Samuels, MD
Associate Professor, Clinical Anesthesia and Pediatrics
Director, Education for Pediatric Anesthesia
Cincinnati Children's Hospital Medical Center
University of Cincinnati, College of Medicine
Cincinnati, Ohio
Chapter: 68. Emergence Agitation

Ian Smith, MBBS, FANZCA
Department of Anaesthesia and Pain Management
Royal Children's Hospital
Victoria, Australia
Chapter: 29. Kidney Transplant

Ximena Soler, MD
Assistant Professor, Clinical Anesthesia and Pediatrics
Director, Liver Transplantation Anesthesia
Cincinnati Children's Hospital Medical Center
University of Cincinnati, College of Medicine, Cincinnati, Ohio
Chapters: 27. Liver Transplant, 47. Diabetic Ketoacidosis During
Appendicitis with Perforation

James P. Spaeth, MD
Associate Professor, Clinical Anesthesia and Pediatrics
Director, Cardiac Anesthesia
Associate Chief, Division of Clinical Anesthesia
Cincinnati Children's Hospital Medical Center
University of Cincinnati, College of Medicine
Cincinnati, Ohio
Chapters: 32. Tetralogy of Fallot, 44. Mediastinal Mass Biopsy,
62. Down Syndrome, 63. Muscular Dystrophy

Peter Squire, MBBS, FANZCA
Department of Anaesthesia and Pain Management
Royal Children's Hospital
Victoria, Australia
Chapter: 12. Obstructive Sleep Apnea

Peter Stoddart, BSc, FRCA, MRCP(UK)
Bristol Royal Hospital for Children
Senior Clinical Lecturer in Anaesthesia
Bristol, UK
Chapter: 54. Omphalocele/Gastroschisis Repair

Alexandra Szabova, MD
Assistant Professor, Clinical Anesthesia and Pediatrics
Cincinnati Children's Hospital Medical Center
University of Cincinnati, College of Medicine
Cincinnati, Ohio
Chapters: 40. Sickle Cell Disease, 43. Opioid-Tolerant Patient

Jon Tomasson, MD
Assistant Professor, Clinical Anesthesia and Pediatrics
Cincinnati Children's Hospital Medical Center
University of Cincinnati, College of Medicine
Cincinnati, Ohio
Chapter: 44. Mediastinal Mass Biopsy

Ben Turner, MBBS, FANZCA, FCICM
Department of Anaesthesia and Pain Management
Royal Children's Hospital
Victoria, Australia
Chapter: 2. Electrolyte Disturbance in Pyloric Stenosis

Anna M. Varughese, MD, MPH
Associate Professor, Clinical Anesthesia and Pediatrics
Associate Chief, Division of Clinical Anesthesia
Director, Same Day Surgery and Preanesthesia
Consultation Clinic
Cincinnati Children's Hospital Medical Center
University of Cincinnati, College of Medicine
Cincinnati, Ohio
Chapters: 1. Preoperative Anxiety Management, 46. Diabetic Patient, 66. Osteogenesis Imperfecta

Norbert J. Weidner, MD
Associate Professor, Clinical Anesthesia and Pediatrics
Medical Director, StarShine Hospice
Director, Pediatric Palliative and Comfort Care Team
Cincinnati Children's Hospital Medical Center
University of Cincinnati, College of Medicine
Cincinnati, Ohio
Chapters: 6. Do-Not-Resuscitate Orders in the OR,
42. Oncology Patient, 71. Disclosure After Complication in the OR

Junzheng Wu, MD
Associate Professor, Clinical Anesthesia and Pediatrics
Cincinnati Children's Hospital Medical Center
University of Cincinnati, College of Medicine
Cincinnati, Ohio
Chapters: 19. Bacterial Tracheitis Versus Epiglottitis,
21. Cystic Fibrosis, 69. Stridor After Extubation

PART 1

CHALLENGES IN PREOPERATIVE CONSULTATION AND PREPARATION

1

Preoperative Anxiety Management

NANCY S. HAGERMAN AND
ANNA M. VARUGHESE

INTRODUCTION

Up to 65% of pediatric patients experience anxiety and fear in the preoperative period, especially during anesthesia induction. Reasons for this anxiety include the child's perception of the threat of pain, being separated from parents, a strange environment, and losing control. Anxiety and poor behavioral compliance associated with inhalation inductions have been related to adverse outcomes including emergence delirium and maladaptive postoperative behaviors such as general and separation anxiety, eating difficulties, and sleep disturbances. Fortunately, there are behavioral and pharmacological interventions that anesthesiologists can use to improve compliance during induction.

LEARNING OBJECTIVES

1. **Identify patients at risk for emotional distress and poor behavioral compliance during induction of anesthesia.**
2. **Understand adverse outcomes associated with "stormy inductions."**
3. **Be familiar with behavioral and pharmacological preoperative anxiolytic interventions and their advantages and undesirable effects.**

CASE PRESENTATION

A 5-year-old healthy boy presents to outpatient surgery for orchidopexy. His past medical history is significant only for a single hospitalization 6 months ago for a stomach virus. His past surgical history consists of placement of bilateral ear tubes at age 4 with an unremarkable anesthetic. He did not attend the preoperative tour and, unfortunately, his parents got lost on the way to the hospital and arrive late. Because the child appears shy, the anesthesiologist considers premedication with an anxiolytic medication, but decides against it as she doesn't want the operating room to start late.

The parents accompany the child to the operating room, but upon introduction of the mask, he pushes it away and says "no." His tearful mother, the anesthesiologist, anesthesia resident, and nurse all attempt simultaneously to reassure him. As he begins to scream, the anesthesiologist places a mask with 8% sevoflurane and oxygen over the child's face. The rest of his anesthetic and surgery are unremarkable.

In the PACU, the patient has emergence delirium, and his discharge is delayed as a result. One week later, a routine postoperative phone call reveals he has increased separation anxiety and general anxiety and has not been sleeping well since the surgery.

DISCUSSION

1. **Which child is at risk for emotional distress and poor behavioral compliance during the induction of anesthesia?**
   Demographic and personality-related variables identified as risk factors for preoperative anxiety in children include the child's age, a history of previous surgery/anesthesia, behavioral problems with previous healthcare attendances, time spent waiting in the preoperative clinic, the child's temperament and social adaptability, and parent anxiety.

   Behavioral compliance with induction improves with age. Children between the ages of 1 and 4 years appear to be at high risk for distress on induction. A history of surgery, anesthesia, or hospitalization also correlates with preoperative anxiety and poor behavioral compliance in children. Varughese et al. (2008) found that this was modified by both age and the use of a preoperative tour. **Previous anesthesia** can have a negative impact on behavioral compliance in school-age children because they can associate previous anesthetic inductions with unpleasant experiences related to hospitalization and surgery. However, school-age children with previous anesthetic experience may have an internal model of the preoperative experience that can be fruitfully modified by the preoperative tour. Davidson et al. (2006) found that children with a history of behavioral problems with previous healthcare attendances, and children who have had more than five **hospital admissions** were more anxious at induction.

Compliance with induction of anesthesia has been observed to improve as time spent in the preoperative clinic increases. Faster preparation may increase anxiety due to a sensory overload from rapid interactions with numerous providers, and the child may not have adequate time to integrate information and receive assurance.

More personality-related variables include a *child's temperament.* Children who are "**shy** and inhibited" tend to become more nervous in novel settings, as are children who have poor social adaptive abilities. It has also been shown that **parents who are** more **anxious** before their child's surgery have children who are more anxious in the perioperative period. Kain explains this by two mechanisms. First, parents act as stress reducers for their children. When parents are more anxious, they are less available to respond to their child's needs. Secondly, a parent may offer a genetic contribution to a child's tendency to be overanxious (Kain et al., 2000). However, others speculate that although parental anxiety may be a causal link to child anxiety, the reverse can also be true: parental anxiety could be a response to child anxiety.

Factors *not* associated with emotional distress or poor behavioral compliance during induction include mother's age, child's gender, child's ethnicity, number of siblings and sibling order, marital status of parents, parental social status, type of surgical procedure, ASA physical status, and the number of hours fasted.

2. What are the adverse outcomes associated with "stormy inductions"?

Poor behavioral compliance with inhalation induction may be associated with **emergence delirium** and maladaptive postoperative behaviors, including **separation and general anxiety**, eating difficulties, **sleep disturbances**, apathy, withdrawal, aggression toward authority, and new-onset enuresis. Estimates of the degree and frequency of behavior change vary considerably between studies but some have reported that up to 54% of children may have behavior change at 2 weeks after surgery (Kain et al., 2002).

3. What are some behavioral interventions that can help allay a child's anxiety preoperatively?

Preoperative instruction as a means of attenuating anxiety has been used for decades, but the content of the preparation has changed over the years. In 1997, a panel of psychological experts indicated their consensus on behavioral preparation programs (Kain et al., 2002). Coping skills instruction, or preparation by child-life specialists, was ranked the most effective preoperative intervention, followed by modeling, play therapy, operating room tours, and finally printed materials. Since coping skills instruction utilizes more resources and therefore is considerably more expensive than **preoperative tours**, Kain directly compared the anxiety level in children who underwent these different preparation programs. They found that children who received child-life preparation (coping skills) showed less anxiety than children and parents who did not receive the preparation. However, anxiety in these children was no different than the children who attended the preoperative tour. School-age children gain more from preoperative programs if they participate in them more than 5 to 7 days prior to surgery, as opposed to 1 day prior to surgery.

It appears that the children benefit from time to process new information and rehearse newly learned coping skills.

The use of **parental presence** during the induction of anesthesia continues to be controversial. It can reduce the need for premedication and one can avoid the screaming and struggle that can occur with separation from parents. Potential benefits include decreased patient anxiety and decreased long-term adverse behavioral effects. Those who object to parental presence commonly point to the potential breech in sterility of the operating room environment, disruption of routine, overcrowding, and potential for adverse reaction by a parent. Although there have been several reports of disruption by parents, the frequency of these occurrences appears to be quite low. Randomized controlled trials do not always support a benefit of parental presence. This is likely due to the fact that parents cannot be instructed on how to promote coping behaviors during randomized controlled trials. Parental behaviors that include *criticism*, *excessive reassurance*, and *commands* have been associated with greater distress in children. Conversely, parents who engage in *nonprocedural talk* have been shown to reduce child distress (Kain et al., 2002).

4. What are the properties, effects, and limitations of midazolam?

Midazolam is one of the most popular preoperative sedative used and is most commonly given orally to pediatric patients (Kain et al., 2004). It is associated with reduced anxiety in children undergoing surgery and possibly reduced postoperative behavioral changes. Additionally, the parents of children who receive it are less anxious and more satisfied with the surgical experience (Rosenbaum et al., 2009).

Midazolam is a short-acting benzodiazepine that can be administered orally, intravenously, nasally, rectally, or intramuscularly, and has a relatively quick onset. It has been shown to reduce anxiety with separation from parents and in the induction of anesthesia. Recovery times are not significantly delayed with midazolam, and there is no conclusive evidence to suggest that it decreases the incidence of emergence delirium. Evidence that its use can improve behavioral outcomes at home postoperatively is inconsistent.

Midazolam's limitations include a bitter taste when given orally. Nasal administration is associated with burning and stinging sensations. Both oral and rectal administrations can result in low and unpredictable absorption. It is not short-acting when used in infants and adolescents due to its intermediate terminal half-life in these age groups and its active metabolite. Adverse effects include a risk of paradoxical reactions and hiccups. When administered with opioids, it can decrease the patient's respiratory drive. Although it causes anterograde amnesia and loss of explicit memory, implicit memory is preserved (Rosenbaum et al., 2009). This amnestic effect is very troubling to some children as they find the lack of recall even more anxiety-provoking when faced with a similar event in the future. Children who have received midazolam preoperatively have been found to be significantly more anxious when they return for subsequent surgeries (Kain et al., 2003).

5. What other pharmacological options are available for anxiolysis?

Although midazolam is considered by some to be the "gold standard" for children requiring premedication, others argue that different drugs are preferable. The use of alpha-2 agonists is gaining in popularity. Alpha-2 agonists do not affect memory and the sedation they provide is similar to normal tiredness and sleep, while midazolam produces sedation similar to an alcohol-induced stupor. Additionally, alpha-2 agonists have no or minimal effects on respiratory drive. They reduce the dose required for an induction agent and are associated with a decreased stress response from intubation.

Intraoperatively, they decrease anesthetic requirements by approximately 50% (both volatile agents and opioids) and are

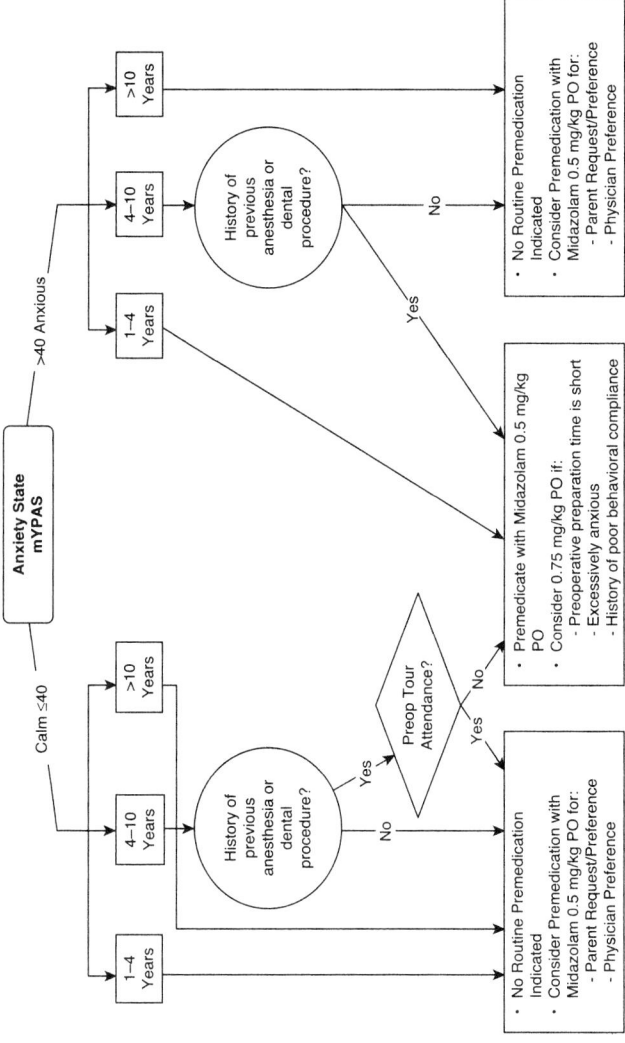

FIGURE 1.1 Premedication Clinical Algorithm.

associated with hemodynamic stability. In the postoperative setting, these drugs are associated with reduced postoperative pain and a lower risk for sevoflurane-associated postoperative delirium (Rosenbaum et al., 2009). Oral clonidine takes considerably longer to reach its effect than midazolam (45 minutes vs. 20 minutes) and can also be associated with slightly prolonged postoperative sedation. The more selective alpha-2 agonist dexmedetomidine may be an even more attractive alternative to clonidine. While it has a shorter onset time and a faster elimination half-life, it cannot be given orally due to limited absorption from the gastrointestinal tract; instead, it must be administered nasally or transmucosally. Unlike midazolam, it is not associated with a stinging sensation when administered nasally. Nasal sufentanil is a useful premedication if rapid onset is desired and close supervision is available. Although it has been associated with respiratory depression, it offers identical anxiety scores and facemask acceptance as midazolam (Rosenbaum et al., 2009).

6. Which children benefit from receiving sedative premedication?

Premedication of selected patients appears to be a better approach than routine premedication of all patients. A study conducted at our institution (Varughese et al., 2008) found that factors predictive of distress and poor behavioral compliance on induction include the patient's anxiety level in the preoperative clinic, age, previous anesthesia experience, preoperative tour attendance, and preoperative preparation time. These significant factors are bundled into a predictive clinical algorithm to help guide premedication (Fig. 1.1).

SUMMARY

1. Risk factors for emotional distress and poor behavioral compliance during the induction of anesthesia

include young age, shy temperament, poor social adaptive abilities, anxiety on part of the child and the parent, and previous anesthesia and hospitalization.

2. Adverse outcomes associated with stormy inductions may include emergence delirium and maladaptive postoperative behaviors such as anxiety, separation anxiety, and sleep disturbances.

3. Valuable behavioral interventions include coping skills instruction and preparation by child-life specialists and preoperative tours.

4. Premedication with midazolam of selected patients based on an assessment of their preoperative anxiety is an effective strategy. Newer agents such as alpha-2 agonists can also be used for preoperative anxiolysis.

ANNOTATED REFERENCES

- Kain ZN, Caldwell-Andrews A, Shu-Ming W. Psychological preparation of the parent and pediatric surgical patient. *Anesth Clin North Am* 2002; 20(1): 29–44.

This comprehensive review article of behavioral preoperative anxiolytic interventions details the risks of not treating preoperative anxiety and reviews studies on the usefulness of nonpharmacological interventions, including preoperative preparation programs for children, parental preparation programs, parental presence during anesthesia induction, the use of perioperative music and sensory stimuli, and the preoperative interview process.

- Rosenbaum A, Kain ZN, Larsson P, Lonnqvist P. Pro-Con Debate: The place of premedication in pediatric practice. *Pediatr Anesth* 2009; 19: 817–828.

This is an interesting international discussion of both pharmacological and nonpharmacological anxiolytic interventions in the preoperative pediatric patient.

Further Reading

Cox RG, Nemish U, Ewen A. Evidence-based clinical update: Does premedication with oral midazolam lead to improved behavioural outcomes in children? *Can J Anaesth* 2006; 53(12): 1213–1219.

Davidson AJ, Shrivastava PP, Jamsen K, Huang GH, Czarnecki C, Gibson M, Stewart S, Stargatt R. Risk factors for anxiety at induction of anesthesia in children: A prospective cohort study. *Pediatr Anesth* 2006; 16(9): 919–927.

Kain ZN, Mayes LC, Weisman SJ, Hofstadter MB. Social adaptability, cognitive abilities, and other predictors for children's reactions to surgery. *J Clin Anesth* 2000; 12(7): 549–554.

Kain ZN, Caldwell-Andrews AA, Wang SM, Krivutza DM, Weinberg ME, Mayes LC. Parental intervention choices for children undergoing repeated surgeries. *Anesth Analg* 2003; 96(4): 970–975.

Kain ZN, Caldwell-Andrews AA, Krivutza DM. Trends in the practice of parental presence during induction of anesthesia and the use of preoperative sedative premedication in the United States, 1995–2002: Results of a follow-up national survey. *Anesth Analg* 2004; 98(5): 1252–1259.

Sadhasivam S, Cohen LL, Szabova A, Varughese A, Kurth CD, Willging P Wang Y, Nick TG, Gunter J. Real-time assessment of perioperative behaviors and prediction of perioperative outcomes. *Anesth Analg* 2009; 108(3): 822–826.

Varughese AM, Nick TG, Gunter J, Wang Y, Kurth CD. Factors predictive of poor behavioral compliance during inhaled induction in children. *Anesth Analg* 2008; 107(2): 413–421.

2

Electrolyte Disturbance in Pyloric Stenosis

BEN TURNER

INTRODUCTION

Pyloric stenosis is a common condition that represents a challenge to the pediatric anesthesiologist. Managing these children requires an understanding of fluid, electrolyte, and acid–base abnormalities, induction techniques where there is potential for a full stomach, and postoperative pain-management choices in small babies. The key perioperative message is to realize this is a *medical* rather than a *surgical* emergency. Preoperative correction of the fluid, electrolyte, and acid–base abnormalities is vital in reducing perioperative morbidity. The anesthesiologist needs to be able to accurately assess when a baby's condition is adequately optimized before proceeding to pyloromyotomy.

LEARNING OBJECTIVES

1. Understand the acid–base and electrolyte disturbances associated with pyloric stenosis, and how to correct them.
2. Evaluate the alternative anesthetic techniques.
3. Develop a post-anesthetic management plan.

CASE PRESENTATION

A 3.6-kg 5-week-old boy presents to the emergency department with failure to gain weight and **non-bilious projectile vomiting** *after breast feeds. He was born at term and there is no history suggestive of cardiac, respiratory, or renal disease. The child takes no regular medications. There is a maternal history of pyloric stenosis. On examination, the baby has a sunken fontanel and a capillary refill time of 3 seconds. He is pale and mildly lethargic, with a pulse of 120 bpm. He had not had a wet diaper for 10 hours. His pre-illness weight is unknown; however, he is estimated to be 5% to 10% dehydrated. A* **palpable olive-sized mass at the upper right costal margin** *is noted. His chest is clear and there are no murmurs. There is no jaundice. Capillary blood gas (CBG) analysis reveals pH 7.57, PCO² 58 mmHg,* **Na⁺ 131 mmol/L,** K⁺ *4.6 mmol/L,* **Cl⁻ 87 mmol/L, HCO₃⁻ 32 mmol/L,** *BE +10.1 mEq/L. The diagnosis of pyloric stenosis is confirmed on ultrasound. He is kept nil by mouth. His* **volume, Na⁺, and Cl⁻ deficit is corrected with IV fluid replacement** *(Table 2.1). A nasogastric tube is put on free drainage. After 2 days his CBG reveals pH 7.44, pCO² 46 mmHg,* **Na⁺ 134 mmol/L,** K⁺ *4.2 mmol/L,* **Cl⁻ 106 mmol/L, HCO₃⁻ 26 mmol/L,** *BE +1 mEq/L. The child is assessed as being adequately fluid-resuscitated, and he is scheduled for an open pyloromyotomy.*

In a warmed operating room, the nasogastric tube is suctioned and a **large-bore orogastric tube** *is inserted and suctioned with the baby supine, in left and right lateral and prone positions (four-quadrant suction). After monitoring, the baby is induced with atropine 20 mcg/kg, propofol 3 mg/kg, and succinylcholine (suxamethonium) 2 mg/kg followed by a 5-mL saline flush. Cricoid pressure is applied. Anesthesia is maintained with sevoflurane 3% in oxygen/nitrous oxide. IV acetaminophen (paracetamol) 15 mg/kg is given on incision. No opiates are given. At the end of the operation, the surgeon* **infiltrates the wound with 2 mL 0.25% bupivacaine.**

The baby is extubated once awake, demonstrating regular spontaneous breathing. He is transferred to recovery to remain nil orally on maintenance fluids for a further 12 hours.

DISCUSSION

1. What is pyloric stenosis and how is it diagnosed?

Pyloric stenosis is a condition of pyloric outflow tract obstruction caused by hypertrophy of the circular muscularis layer of the pylorus. The incidence is approximately 1 in 400 to 500 live births and is the most common surgical cause of vomiting in babies (Table 2.1). It affects males more than females in a ratio of approximately 4:1. It generally presents 3 to 6 weeks after birth. In pyloric stenosis the **vomiting is non-bilious**, which often differentiates the condition from other causes of vomiting. Reviewing recent radiological and surgical literature reveals that the pyloric "olive" may only be palpable in one quarter of patients (Reid, 2009). To avoid an unnecessary laparotomy, ultrasonography is recommended, as the specificity and sensitivity is nearly 100% (Hernanz-Schulman et al., 1994).

2. What is the underlying acid–base disturbance?

Hypochloremic metabolic alkalosis. Vomiting in the presence of pyloric obstruction causes *unopposed loss of gastric acid (HCl), water, Na^+*, and *K^+*. The patient therefore develops a metabolic alkalosis. Under physiological conditions, gastric acid entering the duodenum is neutralized by pancreatic secreted bicarbonate. In pyloric stenosis, pancreatic HCO_3^- is absorbed, contributing to the alkalosis. The net raised bicarbonate concentration overwhelms the resorptive capacity of the proximal convoluted tubule of the kidney, causing an initial alkaline urine pH (Fell & Chelliah, 2001).

The fluid loss and reduced oral intake causes extracellular **fluid volume depletion**. This stimulates the renin-angiotensin-aldosterone system; Na^+ is therefore retained at the expense of K^+ loss in the urine. Total body potassium falls for two other reasons: alkalosis causes a shift of K^+ into the intracellular space and a small amount of K^+ is lost in the vomitus. Thus, the anesthetic implication of the potassium level (which may be low, normal, or high) must be taken in context of the overall acid–base and electrolyte pattern (Schwartz et al., 2003).

Table 2.1

A PREOPERATIVE MAINTENANCE FLUID REGIMEN FOR PYLORIC STENOSIS

Assessed Fluid Deficit	Fluid Regimen (Note: K^+ is added only if baby is passing urine)
Less than 5% (well, reduced urine output)	No bolus required. 0.45% NaCl and 5% dextrose with 20 mmol/L KCl at 150% of normal. maintenance rate for 12 hours.
5–10% (mildly lethargic, pale, dry mouth, poor urine output)	Bolus 0.9% saline 20 mL/kg in 30 minutes; then 0.45% NaCl and 5% dextrose with 30 mmol/L KCl at 200% of normal maintenance rate for 12 hours
Greater than 10% (lethargic, pale, mottled, anuria, tachycardia)	Bolus 0.9% saline 20 mL/kg in 30 minutes; then 0.45% NaCl and 5% dextrose with 30 mmol/L KCl at 200% of normal maintenance rate for 16 hours or more

Glucose, urea, electrolytes, and creatinine should be monitored q4–6h if >10% dehydrated and q6–12h if <10% dehydrated.

Reproduced and modified with permission from Thompson K, Tey D, Marks M. *Paediatric Handbook*, 8th ed. Wiley-Blackwell, 2009.

The expected renal response to metabolic alkalosis is to reduce H^+ ion secretion; this causes a net loss of bicarbonate. In pyloric stenosis, elevated aldosterone levels prevent this. Aldosterone stimulates sodium reabsorption in exchange for K^+ and H^+. Paradoxically, this will cause a more acidic urine and worsen the alkalosis.

Cl^- is lost with H^+ during vomiting. This results in **hypochloremia**. Normally, the kidneys attempt to reabsorb Cl^- (with Na^+) in exchange for the secretion of HCO_3^-; however there is insufficient Cl^- in the glomerular filtrate for this process to occur. Hence, there is complete bicarbonate reabsorption, acidic urine, and maintenance of alkalosis. Urine [Cl^-] is thus very low or zero in metabolic alkalosis with a contracted volume state. Correction of the alkalosis therefore cannot occur until the serum [Cl⁻] is restored. Therefore, by giving volume, Na⁺, and Cl⁻, the homeostasis will be restored.

In extreme uncorrected cases, profound hypovolemia may lead to reduced tissue oxygen delivery and a metabolic acidosis; hemoconcentration may result in polycythemia.

3. **What are the principles of preoperative fluid and electrolyte management and subsequent timing of surgery?**
    a) **Correction of volume deficit**
    b) **Replenish sodium and chloride** to enable the kidney to correct the alkalosis by excreting bicarbonate.

One regimen is outlined in Table 2.2. Targets for resuscitation are **a normal volume state, serum [HCO$_3^-$] <30 mmol/L**, and **serum [Cl⁻] >105 mmol/L**. Although not commonly measured in practice, a urine [Cl⁻] >20 mmol/L provides evidence in pyloric stenosis that volume state has been corrected and the kidney is no longer maximally reabsorbing sodium chloride (Goh et al., 1990).

Table 2.2

DIFFERENTIAL DIAGNOSIS OF VOMITING IN A 1-MONTH-OLD

Category	Example
Sepsis	Septicemia
	Urinary tract infection
	Meningitis
Mechanical	**Pyloric Stenosis**
	Malrotation with volvulus
	Strangulated inguinal hernia
	Gastroesophageal reflux
Others	Overfeeding
	Congenital adrenal hyperplasia

In the absence of adequate resuscitation, perioperative risks include *central respiratory depression due to alkalosis, dysrhythmias* due to electrolyte imbalance, and *hypotension due to hypovolemia.*

4. What anesthetic techniques are appropriate?

The principal goals of anesthesia for pyloromyotomy are to safely secure the airway in a patient with a recognized increased risk of aspiration and to discharge the patient to recovery with adequate analgesia but minimal risk of postoperative apnea. The nasogastric tube inserted on the ward will not reliably reduce gastric volumes. A **large-bore orogastric tube** inserted immediately prior to induction will greatly reduce residual gastric volumes in most patients (Cook-Sather et al., 1997).

General anesthesia following an intravenous induction and intubation with cricoid pressure has been described as the "standard" technique (MacDonald et al., 1987). Preoxygenation is advised before induction, and occasionally mask ventilation is required before intubation. Cricoid pressure may need to be removed to improve ventilating or intubating conditions. If succinylcholine is used, atropine 20 mcg/kg IV before intubation should be given to avoid bradycardia. This may be followed by a nondepolarizing neuromuscular blocker (NDNMB) such as atracurium 0.5 mg/kg, but in my experience this is rarely necessary.

Stenosis of the pylorus reduces the risk of aspiration if the stomach has been emptied. Some clinicians therefore prefer other induction techniques, including inhalational induction with or without NDNMB, IV induction with (or without) NDNMB, or spinal anesthesia alone (Mostafa et al., 2003). One potential advantage would be the avoidance of succinylcholine. The question remains, however, whether the anesthetist can reliably assume the stomach is empty following a four-quadrant aspiration as described above. Cook-Sather et al. (1986) concluded that while blind aspiration reliably removes total gastric contents, it cannot exclude a small amount of residual fluid. The clinical significance of this is uncertain. Awake intubation is used by some but generally not recommended. If a NDNMB is used, reversal must be administered before extubation.

Maintenance with shorter-acting volatile agents such as sevoflurane or desflurane is increasingly being used due to a faster wake-up and theoretical reduced incidence of postoperative apneas. Maintenance using remifentanil and N_2O has also been described (Davis et al., 2001).

Analgesia is frequently provided by **infiltration of the wound with bupivacaine** and intravenous acetaminophen. The rate and extent of absorption of rectal acetaminophen is variable, so if available, the IV form is more reliable. Although a low-dose opioid can be used, it may delay emergence and increase the incidence of postoperative apnea.

5. What is an appropriate postoperative management plan?

Postoperative anesthetic issues include analgesia, maintenance fluids, and monitoring for post-anesthesia apnea. For analgesia, acetaminophen 15 mg/kg IV or oral (maximum 60 mg/kg/day) is usually sufficient. Postoperative hypoglycemia is a risk due to hepatic glycogen depletion. Intravenous 0.45% NaCl with 5% dextrose should continue at 100 mL/kg/day until feeding is re-established; oral intake is often started between 6 and 12 hours postoperatively. For term babies, postoperative apnea monitoring and line-of-sight nursing is required until a 12-hour apnea-free period has elapsed (Andropoulos et al., 1994). Ex-premature infants are often managed on the neonatal intensive care unit in some institutions.

SUMMARY

1. The vomiting of pyloric stenosis causes loss of water, HCl, Na^+, and K^+. This causes dehydration and a hypochloremic metabolic alkalosis; these metabolic abnormalities must be corrected before surgery.

2. Pre-induction precautions to avoid aspiration of gastric contents include drainage of the stomach with a large-bore orogastric tube.
3. Adequate analgesia is usually achieved without opioids using a combination of local anesthetic infiltration and acetaminophen.
4. The risk of postoperative apneas should be considered.

ANNOTATED REFERENCES

- **Bissonnette B, Sullivan PJ. Pyloric Stenosis. *Can J Anesth* 1991; 38(5): 668–676.**
  An excellent overview of the pathophysiology and management of pyloric stenosis.
- **Eaton DC, Pooler JP. Regulation of hydrogen ion balance. In *Vander's Renal Physiology*, 6th ed. New York: McGraw Hill, 2004: 174–176.**
  A clear explanation of renal mechanisms during metabolic alkalosis.

Further Reading

Andropoulos DB, Heard MB, Johnson KL, Clarke JT, Rowe RW. Postanesthetic apnea in full-term infants after pyloromyotomy. *Anesthesiology* 1994; 80: 216–219.

Cook-Sather SD, Tulloch HV, Cnaan A, Nicolson SC, Cubina ML, Gallagher PR, Schreiner MS. A comparison of awake vs paralysed tracheal intubation for infants with pyloric stenosis. *Anesth Analg* 1986; 86: 945–51.

Cook-Sather SD, Tulloch HV, Liacouras CA, Schreiner MS. Gastric fluid volume in infants for pyloromyotomy. *Can J Anesth* 1997; 44(3): 278–283.

Davis PJ, Galinkin J, McGowan F, et al. A randomised multicenter study of remifentanil compared with halothane in neonates and infants undergoing pyloromyotomy. I. Emergence and recovery profiles. *Anesth Analg* 2001; 93: 1380–6.

Fell D, Chelliah S. Infantile pyloric stenosis. *Contin Ed Anesth, Crit Care Pain* 2001; 1: 85–88.

Goh D, Hall S, Gornall P, BuickR, Green A, Corkery J. Plasma chloride and alkalaemia in pyloric stenosis. *Br J Surg* 1990; 77: 922–923.

Hernanz-Schulman M, Sells LL, Ambrosino MM, et al. Hypertrophic pyloric stenosis in the infant without a palpable olive: accuracy of sonographic diagnosis. *Radiology* 1994; 193 (3): 771–776.

MacDonald NJ, Fitzpatrick GJ, Moore KP, Wren WS, Keenan M. Anaesthesia for congenital hypertrophic pyloric stenosis. A review of 350 patients. *Br J Anaesth* 1987; 59: 672–677.

Mostafa S, Gaitini LA, Vaida SJ, Malatzkey S, Sabo E, Yudashkin M, Tome R. The effectiveness and safety of spinal anaesthesia in the pyloromyotomy procedure. *Paed Anaesth* 2003; 13: 32–37.

Reid JR. 2009. *Imaging in hypertrophic pyloric stenosis.* Accessed Feb. 21, 2011. http://emedicine.medscape.com/article/409621-overview.

Schwartz D, Connelly NR, Manikantan P, Nichols JH. Hyperkalemia and pyloric stenosis. *Anesth Analg* 2003; 97: 355–357.

3

Upper Respiratory Infection

NANCY B. SAMOL AND ERIC P. WITTKUGEL

INTRODUCTION

Upper respiratory tract infections (URIs) are common in children, with most children experiencing six to eight episodes per year. Some evidence suggests that the airway reactivity associated with these infections persists for several weeks after resolution of symptoms and increases the risk of perioperative adverse events. Other data indicate that these complications are easily managed and seldom associated with any adverse sequelae. Unfortunately, cancellation of patients harboring URIs is not without economic and emotional implications for the patient, the family, and the operating suite as a whole. Understanding the risk factors associated with administering anesthesia to the child with a URI is important in identifying elements of the preoperative assessment that merit attention and in optimizing the anesthetic plan as a means to limit perioperative complications.

LEARNING OBJECTIVES

1. Review the pathology and clinical presentation of the URI, particularly as it affects the decision to proceed with elective anesthesia.
2. Define and stratify adverse respiratory events during anesthesia.
3. Identify factors evident in the preoperative evaluation that may predict adverse respiratory events during and after anesthesia.

4. Develop evidence-based practice guidelines to optimize perioperative management and reduce risk in the child with a URI who undergoes general anesthesia.

CASE PRESENTATION

A 2-year-old girl with a history of recurrent adenotonsillitis, adenotonsillar hypertrophy, and chronic otitis media presents to the operating room for elective adenotonsillectomy and placement of pressure-equalizing tubes (PETs). She is an otherwise healthy, former full-term baby with a history significant for recurrent **upper respiratory tract infections (URIs)** *concurrent with her adenotonsillitis and recurrent otitis media.*

On review of systems, the patient has near-constant URIs and a **chronic cough** *that is "at baseline" today. Though febrile last week, she has been* **afebrile** *for 5 days. The patient* **snores** *loudly at night, with 1- to 2-second* **pauses**. *The mother is quick to remind the staff that the surgery has been cancelled previously due to URI and that the family drove 2 hours to the hospital this morning. The exam room smells of cigarette smoke; both parents smoke, but deny smoking in the house.*

On physical exam, the girl is alert but fussy, 12.2 kg in weight and in no distress. She is afebrile with normal vital signs and a room air oxygen saturation of 98%. She is a mouth-breather with very large tonsils that are nearly touching and a small amount of **clear rhinorrhea**. *Her pulmonary exam demonstrates* **coarse upper airway sounds**, *a* **wet cough**, *and mild supraclavicular* **retractions** *but no* **rales, rhonchi,** *or* **wheezing.**

The **risks of anesthesia** *are discussed with the family, including* **exacerbation of cough, airway obstruction, postoperative oxygen requirement, prolonged intubation,** *and* **hospital admission.** *During induction of anesthesia with oxygen, nitrous oxide, and sevoflurane by mask, the child coughs, holds her breath, becomes difficult* *to ventilate, and begins to* **desaturate***. While an IV is being placed, the* **laryngospasm** *is broken by positive-pressure mask ventilation.*

After intubation, the remainder of the procedure goes forward uneventfully. Upon emergence, the child begins to **cough** *and* **desaturate** *with* **wheezing** *audible bilaterally. The wheezing improves with albuterol (salbutamol) administration per endotracheal tube. Moderate* **secretions** *are suctioned from her nose and endotracheal tube before awake extubation. She proceeds to the PACU, where she* **requires inhaled albuterol by nebulizer and supplemental oxygen** *for 3 hours. She is discharged uneventfully the next day.*

DISCUSSION

1. What is the pathophysiology of a URI and how is it recognized and defined?

URIs are frequent in children, especially during the winter months and in children attending daycare or school. Studies show that anywhere from 3–33% of children coming for anesthesia and surgery present with active URIs. (Elwood et al., 2005) Approximately 95% of these infections are of viral etiology, representing a spectrum of viral species, most notably rhinovirus. The differential diagnosis of a URI is complicated as URI-like symptoms characterize many illnesses. Infections such as croup, influenza, bronchiolitis, pneumonia, epiglottitis, and strep throat may mimic a URI. Even noninfectious diseases such as allergic or vasomotor rhinitis can masquerade as a URI.

At the tissue level, viral invasion of the respiratory mucosa may increase airway sensitivity to secretions or noxious anesthetic gases. Additionally, growing evidence indicates that chemical mediators and neurological reflexes play an important role in the etiology of bronchoconstriction and that these factors are altered by viral infections. Furthermore, while the designation of URI implies pathology only in the upper airways, several studies have proven the URI to adversely affect pulmonary function studies, including decreases in forced vital capacity, forced expired volume, and peak expiratory flow, as well as decreases in diffusion capacity. Animal studies indicate that the decrease in functional residual capacity and increased intrapulmonary shunting brought on by anesthesia are worsened during a viral URI (Dueck et al., 1991). Although most viral URIs are self-limited, the airway hyperreactivity they produce persists for up to 6 weeks after apparent resolution of clinical symptoms.

Typical symptoms of an uncomplicated URI include some combination of the following: rhinorrhea, sneezing, congestion, nonproductive cough, fever less than 38.5°C, sore or scratchy throat, and laryngitis. Subclinical manifestations include upper and lower airway edema, increased respiratory tract secretions, and bronchial irritability.

Patients with **fever** greater than 38.5°C and constitutional symptoms such as lethargy or signs of lower respiratory tract involvement such as **wheezing**, mucopurulent secretions, **rales**, **rhonchi**, or productive cough do not have a simple URI. Their pathology extends beyond the upper respiratory tract or the infection may be bacterial in nature, requiring a longer convalescence and possible antibiotic administration. Unless the need for surgery is urgent, it is best not to proceed in the face of a lower respiratory tract infection or a bacterial infection.

2. What perioperative adverse respiratory events may occur in a child with a URI? What are the consequences?

Recent large-scale studies have identified active or recent URI as a statistically significant risk factor for adverse respiratory events associated with anesthesia. These studies defined adverse events as breath holding, major arterial oxygen desaturation (<90%), severe coughing, airway obstruction, laryngospasm, bronchospasm, post-extubation croup/stridor, reintubation, pneumonia, copious secretions, and unanticipated admission. It should be noted that while URIs do appear to be associated with a higher incidence of *respiratory* complications, most sequelae are easily managed and there appears to be very little residual morbidity. Indeed, there are no cases in the pediatric or adult anesthesia closed-claims literature implicating URIs with serious adverse events. In fact, increased mortality has not been demonstrated in any controlled study.

Current literature is limited by study design shortcomings, which hamper the clinician in drawing definitive conclusions regarding the risk/benefit ratio of anesthetizing the child with a URI. These include mostly retrospective data acquisition, inconsistent definition criteria for URI, heterogeneity in type of patient, surgery and anesthetic technique, and lack of uniform definition of adverse patient outcomes coupled with underreporting of those incidents.

3. What factors identified in the preoperative history and physical exam may predict adverse respiratory events during and after anesthesia?

The window of opportunity for providing anesthesia to a symptom-free young child is extremely small, in some cases nonexistent. Therefore, it is helpful to assess these children for elective surgery armed with criteria that help the clinician to logically weigh the risks and benefits of proceeding with surgery versus cancellation. To this end, recent studies have identified nine criteria in the history and physical assessment that are useful predictors of adverse respiratory outcomes (Parnis et al., 2001). Active or recent (<4 weeks since diagnosis) URI alone is a statistically significant risk factor for adverse respiratory events. Additionally, eight independent criteria have surfaced as harbingers of perioperative respiratory complications: planned airway surgery, history of prematurity (<37 weeks at birth), reactive airway disease, **parental smoking**, copious secretions, nasal congestion, history of **snoring**, and parent's statement that the child has a "cold." Of note, confirmation of URI by a parent was consistently found to be a reliable predictor and, in one study (Schreiner et al., 1996), a better predictor of laryngospasm than symptom criteria alone.

4. Why not cancel the pediatric patient with a URI if the procedure is elective?

Cancellation or postponement of surgery due to URI was once common practice in anesthesia. But in today's healthcare environment, the decision to cancel a surgical procedure cannot be made lightly. Parents may take time off from work, arrange childcare, and often go to great lengths preparing a child both mentally and physically for surgery. The economic consequences of cancellation are significant for both the family and the surgical facility, while the emotional consequences are shouldered mainly by the child. Most children with mild URIs can be safely managed without the need to postpone surgery. To put it in perspective, one study demonstrated that 2,000 procedures would have to be canceled to prevent 15 cases of laryngospasm, a potentially manageable complication (Schreiner et al., 1996). If the data demonstrate that delaying a procedure will not markedly change the incidence of adverse respiratory events, then cancellation gains little except to create inconvenience for the family, the surgeon, and the surgical schedule.

5. What evidence-based practice guidelines exist to optimize perioperative management and reduce risk in the child with a URI who undergoes general anesthesia?

Management of the patient with a URI should be directed at minimizing stimulation of a potentially irritable airway. In terms of preoperative preparation, benzodiazepine administration appears to increase the risk of respiratory events. Premedication with a bronchodilator such as albuterol or ipratropium showed no decrease in adverse airway events in children with symptoms of URI. Pretreatment with anticholinergic agents such as glycopyrrolate, in hopes of decreasing secretions and attenuating airway hyperreactivity, did not result in fewer complications (Parnis et al., 2001).

Intraoperatively, the risk for complications increased with intubation (up to 11-fold in some studies) and decreased with LMA or facemask use (Tait et al., 2000). Additionally, propofol is

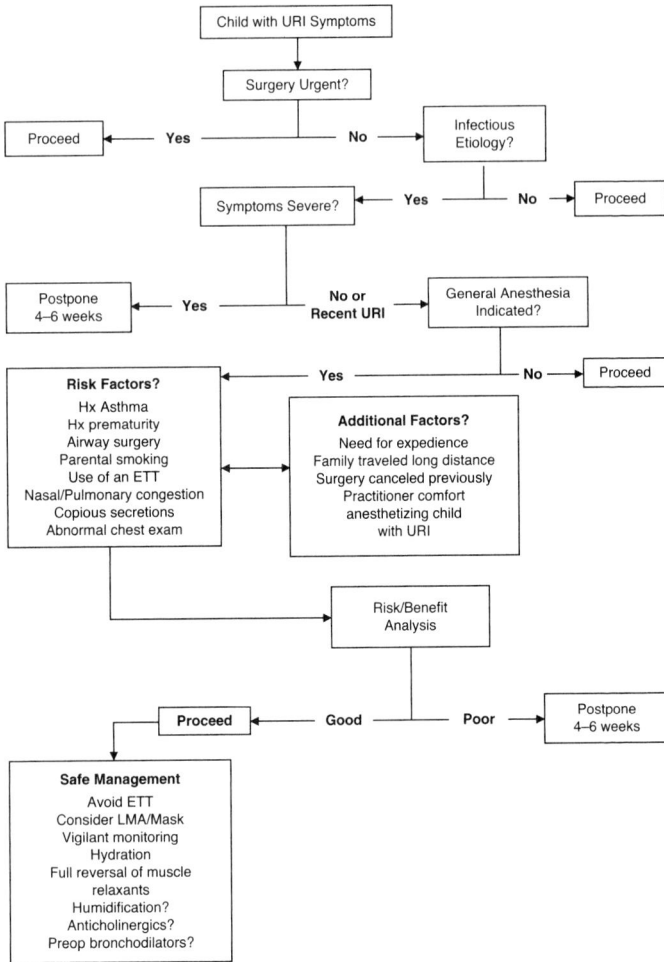

FIGURE 3.1 Suggested algorithm for the assessment and anesthetic management of the child with an upper respiratory tract infection. Reprinted with permission from Tait AR. Anesthetic management of the child with an upper respiratory tract infection. *Curr Opin Anesthesiol* 2005; 18(6): 603–607.

the safest induction agent, ahead of thiopental and inhalation agents. If inhalation induction is necessary, halothane and sevoflurane are less irritating to the airway than isoflurane. For intraoperative maintenance, sevoflurane appears to impair airway mechanics less than desflurane in children with susceptible airways. Instrumentation and suctioning of the airway should be attempted only after a deep plane of anesthesia has been attained. Any muscle relaxant administered should be fully reversed. For long procedures, humidification of inhaled agents avoids drying and inspissation of secretions. An assessment and treatment algorithm appears in Fig. 3.1.

SUMMARY

1. Cancellation of patients harboring URIs has economic and emotional implications for the patient, the family, and the operating room as a whole.
2. The airway hyperreactivity associated with URIs may persist for up to 6 weeks after apparent resolution of clinical symptoms.
3. Although URIs do appear to be associated with a higher incidence of respiratory complications, most sequelae are easily managed, and there appears to be very little residual morbidity and no increased mortality.
4. The following nine factors predict perioperative respiratory complications in children with URI: history of asthma, history of prematurity, airway surgery, parental smoking, intubation, nasal/pulmonary congestion, copious secretions, abnormal chest exam, and parental admission of "illness" in the child.
5. Safe management of a pediatric patient with a URI includes using a mask or LMA instead of an ETT when

possible, vigilant monitoring, hydration, full reversal of muscle relaxants, humidification of gases, and consideration of anticholinergics and preoperative bronchodilators if appropriate.

ANNOTATED REFERENCES

- Elwood T, Bailey K. The pediatric patient and upper respiratory infections. *Best Pract Res Clin Anaesthesiol* 2005; 19(1): 35–46.

  A thorough overview of anesthetic management in the child with a URI. It examines patient, anesthetic, and surgical risk factors, with an emphasis on prediction and prevention of complications. It highlights shortcomings in the current data and suggests future areas of research.
- Parnis SJ, Barker DS, Van Der Walt JH. Clinical predictors of anaesthetic complications in children with respiratory tract infections. *Pediatr Anesth* 2001; 11(1): 29–40.

  This Australian study uses statistical analysis to create discrete checklists used in the preoperative and intraoperative setting that may predict adverse respiratory outcomes based on history and physical exam findings. The authors use logistic regression to stratify risk numerically, allowing clinicians to better predict outcomes.
- Tait AR, Malviya S. Anesthesia for the child with an upper respiratory tract infection: still a dilemma? *Anesth Analg* 2005; 100(1): 59–65.
- This concise and generously referenced review is written by Alan Tait, a pioneer and prolific author on the subject of anesthesia in the child with a URI. In this article, he synthesizes over 50 years of observational and clinical research, much of it his own, to offer a useful algorithm for the assessment and

management of these patients as well as to suggest future research directions to minimize anesthetic risk.

Further Reading

Dueck R, Prutow R, Richman D. Effect of parainfluenza infection on gas exchange and FRC response to anesthesia in sheep. *Anesthesiology* 1991; 74: 1044–1051.

Mamie C, Habre W, Delhumeau C, Argiroffo CB, Morabia A. Incidence and risk factors of perioperative respiratory adverse events in children undergoing elective surgery. *Pediatr Anesth* 2004; 14(3): 218–224.

Schreiner MS, O'Hara I, Markakis DA, Politis GD: Do children who experience laryngospasm have an increased risk of upper respiratory tract infection? *Anesthesiology* 1996; **85**: 475–480.

Tait AR. Anesthetic management of the child with an upper respiratory tract infection. *Curr Opin Anesthesiol* 2005; 18(6): 603–607.

Tait AR, Malviya S, Voepel-Lewis T, Munro HM, Seiwert M, Pandit UA. Risk factors for perioperative adverse respiratory events in children with upper respiratory tract infections. *Anesthesiology* 2001; 95(2): 299–306.

Tait AR, Voepel-Lewis T, Malviya S. Perioperative considerations for the child with an upper respiratory tract infection. *J Perianesth Nurs* 2000; 15(6): 392–396.

Tait AR, Voepel-Lewis T, Munro HM, Gutstein HB, Reynolds PI. Cancellation of pediatric outpatient surgery: economic and emotional implications for patients and their families. *J Clin Anesth* 1997; 9(3): 213–219.

von Ungern-Sternberg B, Boda K, Chambers N, Rebmann C, Johnson C, Sly P, Habre W. Risk assessment for respiratory complications in paediatric anaesthesia: a prospective cohort study. *Lancet* 2010; 376: 773–783.

von Ungern-Sternberg B, Saudan S, Petak F, Hantos Z, Habre W. Desflurane but not sevoflurane impairs airway and respiratory tissue mechanics in children with susceptible airways. *Anesthesiology* 2008; 108: 216–224.

4

Acute Fluid Resuscitation for Intussusception

BRITT FRASER

INTRODUCTION

Intussusception occurs when a proximal section of bowel invaginates into more distal bowel and is then advanced by peristalsis. It is the most common cause of intestinal obstruction in infants, and untreated can lead to bowel ischemia and perforation. Early recognition and treatment can prevent the need for surgical intervention and complications. Intussusception can also result in significant dehydration due to vomiting and diarrhea. An essential aspect of the perioperative management is to identify and treat dehydration.

LEARNING OBJECTIVES

1. Identify signs of dehydration in an infant, and use them to quantify the degree of dehydration.
2. Know the principles of resuscitation of a dehydrated infant.
3. Understand the principles of fluid management therapy in children in the perioperative period.
4. Identify the key management issues and anesthetic implications of a bowel obstruction in an infant.

CASE PRESENTATION

A 6-month-old, previously healthy boy weighing 6 kg presents to the emergency department with a 2-day history of vomiting and lethargy. His vomiting is becoming increasingly frequent, and he is now unable to tolerate any oral intake. He has had loose bowel movements (the most recent was blood-stained) but few wet diapers during the past 24 hours. **He appears pale but mottled, lethargic, and miserable.** *His* **heart rate is 182 and blood pressure 85/45, with O_2 saturations of 98%.** *His* **capillary refill time is 4 seconds.** *Abdominal examination reveals tenderness but no mass.*

He is given a bolus of **120 mL (20 mL/kg) of 0.9% NaCl (normal saline)** *IV, then an infusion of Hartmann's solution (similar to lactated Ringer's solution) with 1% dextrose at 24 mL/hr. A further bolus of 60 mL 0.9% NaCl is repeated while awaiting surgical review. He receives IV morphine for analgesia and is kept nil orally. His capillary refill improves to 2 seconds, and further investigations are arranged.*

A plain abdominal x-ray shows central air fluid levels but no evidence of perforation. A nasogastric tube (NGT) is sited and free drainage commenced. An ultrasound scan demonstrates an intussusception in the ileocolic region. He begins on intravenous cefazolin and metronidazole. An **air enema** *is attempted but fails to reduce the intussusception. He is transferred to the operating room for laparotomy and surgical reduction.*

On arrival in the operating room he is again noted to have sluggish capillary refill. A bolus of 120 mL of Hartmann's solution is administered, followed by an infusion of the same solution at 24 mL/hr. His NGT is aspirated prior to a rapid-sequence induction with propofol and succinylcholine (suxamethonium), and he is intubated with a 4.0 ETT. Anesthesia is maintained with oxygen, air, and sevoflurane, and a caudal anesthetic. Surgical reduction is performed without complication.

Postoperatively, the baby continues on IV maintenance fluids and nasogastric losses are replaced with 0.9% NaCl. These losses gradually reduce over 24 hours and oral intake is reintroduced as bowel *sounds return. **Electrolytes are monitored every day while receiving IV fluids**, which are gradually reduced as oral intake increases. A morphine infusion and regular acetaminophen (paracetamol) provide analgesia. He is discharged home on day 5 tolerating a full oral intake, with no signs of recurrence.*

DISCUSSION

1. How does one identify and quantify dehydration in an infant?

Preoperative resuscitation of the dehydrated child is imperative, with delayed diagnosis and inadequate resuscitation a significant cause of death in children. Dehydration in this case occurred due to a combination of diarrhea and vomiting, as well as losses into the interstitium (third-space losses), which are not visible and hence are often underestimated. Fever can also contribute to fluid loss.

Recognition of the degree of dehydration is based on clinical assessment (Table 4.1). Mild dehydration (<4% of body weight) is

---

Table 4.1

SIGNS OF DEHYDRATION

Degrees of Dehydration

Mild (<4% body weight)	Moderate (4–6% body weight)	Severe (>7% body weight)
Often no signs	Slowed capillary refill (>2 sec)	Greatly reduced capillary refill (>3–4 sec)
Perhaps dry tongue	Reduced tissue turgor	Mottling, cold
Thirsty	Dry mucous membranes	Acidosis
	Tachypnea	Tachycardia, hypotension
	Restless, lethargic, irritable	Reduced urine output
		Altered conscious state

often not associated with any clinical signs. Signs of moderate dehydration (4–6%) include a reduction in capillary refill time (>2 seconds), reduced tissue turgor, and an increased respiratory rate. With more severe degrees of dehydration (>7%), capillary refill time is further slowed (>3 seconds), skin becomes **mottled**, and breathing becomes deeper with developing acidosis. As the child becomes shocked, **tachycardia** and hypotension develop, and **conscious state** becomes **impaired**. The most reliable measure of the degree of dehydration is comparison with a recent documented weight, but this is often not available. **Lethargy** and sunken eyes are often referred to, but these are unreliable signs. In this case, the child had significantly **slowed capillary refill** and was **tachycardic** and **mottled**, indicating severe dehydration.

2. What are the principles of resuscitation of a dehydrated child and subsequent fluid management?

Resuscitation of the dehydrated child should be considered in three phases. Firstly, the preexisting deficit should be calculated. This will include losses from the GI tract (through vomiting, diarrhea and interstitial losses), as well as other deficits from the renal tract, bleeding, and preoperative fasting if present. This deficit should be replaced with 0.9% NaCl, usually as bolus doses of 10 to 20 mL/kg, repeated as needed to correct hypovolemia. The initial bolus of **20 mL/kg of 0.9% NaCl** in the case presentation resulted in some improvement in the boy's clinical status but not full symptom resolution, so it was repeated.

The second component of fluid replacement is the maintenance fluids, covering ongoing losses through respiration, perspiration, and urine. They are usually calculated over a 24-hour period, and include fluid, electrolytes, and glucose. Halliday's "4–2–1 rule" (4 mL/kg/hr for the first 10 kg of the child's weight, plus 2 mL/kg/hr for the next 10 kg of weight, plus 1 mL/kg/hr for every kg thereafter) was first proposed in 1957 and has been the mainstay of maintenance fluid calculations for many years. However, this has been recently revisited, particularly in sick or perioperative children. In these cases, *elevated ADH levels in response to stress, surgery, and pain, combined with the use of hypotonic solutions, are associated with an increased risk of hyponatremia and cerebral edema.* Children are particularly susceptible to this due to their larger brain:cranium ratio and an immature $Na^+K^+ATPase$ at the blood–brain barrier, meaning that they become symptomatic at lesser degrees of hyponatremia than adults. Maintenance fluid rates should be reduced by up to 50% of the regular 4–2–1 rule if the child is at risk of elevated ADH secretion. Further, the 4–2–1 rule presupposes normal renal function, and patients with anuric renal failure may need their maintenance fluid rates reduced by 60% from calculated.

The final component is the replacement of ongoing losses, such as, in this case, those via an NGT. As this patient's nasogastric losses reduced and oral intake increased, his IV fluid rate was reduced by an equivalent amount.

Given the above considerations, a child's ongoing fluid requirement after major surgery must be carefully considered. Hydration status and ongoing losses must be assessed frequently, along with serum electrolytes. The rate will be determined by any deficit that still needs correcting, any expected ongoing losses, and the maintenance requirement. Note that while the maintenance component will usually be less than the 4–2–1 rule (due to ADH secretion), the total rate given is often initially more than the 4–2–1 rule when there are anticipated ongoing losses.

3. What is the best fluid to use in children?

The fluid used to replace an existing deficit should reflect the composition of the fluid being replaced. In most cases, 0.9% NaCl is an appropriate starting solution.

There has been much discussion recently about the optimal fluid for maintenance therapy in children. Once the mainstay, 4% dextrose with 0.18 NaCl ("4% and a fifth") is now no longer recommended in children, other than in very specialized areas (e.g., ICU). It should not be used for routine maintenance therapy. Four percent dextrose with 0.45 NaCl ("4% and half normal saline") is generally safe for most children; however, there are some instances when only isotonic solutions should be given. These include in the perioperative period, in patients with low initial sodium levels, and in children with CNS infections or head injuries, bronchiolitis, or salt-wasting conditions.

There are several fluid preparations available that are isotonic, or nearly isotonic, but all have potential problems with their use. Hartmann's and Ringer's lactate solutions contain calcium, making them potentially incompatible with certain medications. The high chloride:sodium ratio in 0.9% NaCl can cause a metabolic acidosis when large volumes are infused. After initial resuscitation with 0.9% NaCl it may be advisable to avoid such an acidosis by changing to another solution with less chloride relative to sodium. Lastly, Plasmalyte 148™ contains acetate, which can accumulate and cause hypotension.

Dextrose should be included in maintenance fluids, with solutions of 1% to 2% dextrose proving adequate to meet the needs of most children. Higher concentrations are likely to increase blood sugar levels, resulting in deleterious cerebral effects, and an osmotic diuresis, which can worsen hypovolemia. Most importantly, children receiving prolonged periods of IV hydration should be closely monitored and their treatment individualized. Electrolytes should be checked at the start of therapy and daily thereafter. If sodium levels are low (e.g., <130 mmol/L), they should be monitored up to q6h. Blood glucose levels should also be monitored for the duration of treatment. Children who have alterations in their plasma osmolality (e.g., high blood glucose, or hypernatremic dehydration) will be sensitive to rapid correction, and frequent rechecks of electrolytes and osmolality are advisable.

4. What are the anesthetic implications of a bowel obstruction due to intussusception?

Anesthetic management of an infant requiring surgical intervention for intussusception should be performed in a specialist pediatric center (overall characteristics of intussusception are shown in Table 4.2). Adequate fluid resuscitation is vital *prior* to

Table 4.2

KEY FEATURES OF INTUSSUSCEPTION

Demographics	Age: most common 2 months to 2 years, peak at 5–9 months
	Males > females
History	Intermittent, colicky pain, often severe
	Vomiting, often bilious
	Blood in bowel movements (classically described as red-currant jelly appearance)
	Diarrhea common
	May follow a respiratory viral-like prodrome
Examination	Pallor, lethargy
	Abdominal mass or distention
	Dehydration to hypovolemic shock
Investigations	Abdominal x-ray: often normal unless evidence of obstruction
	Ultrasound: high sensitivity and specificity
	Air enema: both diagnostic and therapeutic
Differential Diagnosis	Gastroenteritis
	Appendicitis or other infections
	Other causes of bowel obstruction
Management	Rehydration
	Analgesia, antibiotics
	Nil orally, nasogastric tube
	Air enema ~80% success rate
	Ultrasound-guided hydrostatic enema
	Surgical reduction
Outcome	May recur after air enema (~9%)
	Low mortality with appropriate management

general anesthesia. This is due to the combined effect of loss of sympathetic tone and direct effects of the anesthetic agents at the time of induction, which result in peripheral vasodilation, hypotension, and even cardiovascular collapse. The child will usually have already had a radiographic attempt at reduction, in this case an **air enema**. The child will continue to lose fluid during this procedure, and thus if the procedure is lengthy it is not uncommon for the child to become significantly dehydrated again. The child's hydration state should be reassessed prior to induction, even if it was deemed adequate earlier.

Prior to induction, the NGT should be aspirated, and even though its use is controversial in some circumstances, rapid-sequence induction is still recognized as the safest form of induction in children with bowel obstruction. Nitrous oxide should be avoided during the procedure as there is potential for further distention of already-threatened bowel. Analgesia may be provided with a caudal injection, and a morphine infusion for postoperative analgesia. IV fluids and nasogastric drainage should be continued postoperatively until bowel function returns to normal. In this case an isotonic solution was chosen as the child was deemed to be at risk of hyponatremia. The rate was based on regular assessment of the child's hydration status and **electrolytes were checked regularly**.

SUMMARY

1. Significant dehydration from any cause in an infant warrants immediate attention.
2. The type of fluid used will depend on the type of fluid lost, but hypotonic solutions (such as 4% dextrose with 0.18 NaCl) should be avoided.
3. Regular monitoring of hydration state, as well as electrolytes and blood glucose levels, is important for the duration of IV fluid therapy.

ANNOTATED REFERENCES

- Justice FA, Auldist AW, Bines JE. Intussusception: Trends in clinical presentation and management. *J Gastroenterol Hepatol* 2006; 21: 842–846.

Reviews all patients with intussusception at a tertiary children's hospital over a 6.5-year period.

- **National Patient Safety Agency (2007)** *Reducing the risk of hyponatraemia when administering intravenous infusions to children.* **Patient Safety Alert 22. Accessed Jan. 24, 2011. http://www.nrls.npsa.nhs.uk/resources/?entryid45=59809**

  Comprehensive recommendations regarding fluid management in children, with background material about hyponatremia and hyponatremic encephalopathy. Compares the most commonly used fluids.

Further Reading

Applegate KE. Intussusception in children: imaging choices. *Semin Roentgenol* 2008; 43(1): 15–21.

Kaiser AD, Applegate KE, Ladd AP. Current success in the treatment of intussusception in children. *Surgery* 2007; 142(4): 469–475.

McClain CD, McManus ML. Fluid management." In Cote CJ, Lerman J, Todres ID, eds. *A Practice of Anesthesia for Infants and Children*. Philadelphia: Saunders Elsevier, 2009: 159–175.

5

Asthmatic for Adenotonsillectomy

EUGENE NEO

INTRODUCTION

Asthma affects up to 20% of children in some countries, although many children have only mild asthma and require only intermittent treatment. Acute exacerbations of asthma usually result from exposure to triggers—commonly pollen, cold air, or viral upper respiratory tract infections. General anesthesia is usually uneventful in asthmatic children; however they are more susceptible to intraoperative bronchospasm. Intraoperative bronchospasm is more common if there has been instrumentation of the airway. In the vast majority of cases, these exacerbations are mild with no major sequelae. However, bronchospasm can on rare occasions be severe and very challenging to manage.

LEARNING OBJECTIVES

1. Know how to identify patients at risk of intraoperative bronchospasm.
2. Develop strategies to prevent intraoperative bronchospasm.
3. Review the acute management of intraoperative bronchospasm.
4. Summarize the ventilatory strategies for patients with severe asthma.

CASE PRESENTATION

*An 18-kg 6-year-old boy with a 3-year history of asthma presents for elective adenotonsillectomy for persistent snoring and failure to gain weight. He has had four presentations to the emergency department within the last 12 months for acute exacerbations of his asthma; on each occasion it was **triggered by a cold** and he was treated with an albuterol (salbutamol) nebulizer and a 3-day course of oral prednisolone. He was not admitted to the hospital. His current maintenance therapy is regular inhaled fluticasone (corticosteroid) 2 puffs BID and albuterol via a spacer as required. On average he uses this two or three times per day. There is **no history of** a recent **upper respiratory tract infection** (URI), although he does have an ongoing history of a dry nocturnal cough. On examination the breath sounds are normal. There are **no features of atopy**. He is afebrile and there are no current coryzal symptoms. A **premedication of 2 puffs of albuterol** is administered as well as oral acetaminophen (paracetamol).*

*Anesthesia is induced and maintained with sevoflurane/O_2/N_2O with a FiO_2 of 0.3. After IV cannulation, he is intubated with a size 5.5 uncuffed oral RAE tube while breathing spontaneously. He is given two fentanyl increments of 1 mcg/kg, dexamethasone 0.15 mg/kg, and tramadol 2 mg/kg. Spontaneous ventilation is maintained. Surgery is started. Towards the end of the procedure, the SpO_2 falls from 98% to 81%. Tidal volumes drop from 150 mL to 70 mL. There is no coughing or straining; however, some intercostal retractions are noted. There is no rash and the blood pressure is unchanged. The **FiO_2 is increased** to 1.0. The Boyle-Davis gag is released with no improvement in tidal volume or saturation. Hand ventilation is attempted; high pressures (35 cmH_2O) are required to inflate the lungs adequately. Auscultation reveals bilateral expiratory wheeze. A suction catheter is passed down the ETT without difficulty and no secretions are found. Laryngoscopy is performed; the ETT position has not changed. He is ventilated with intermittent positive-pressure ventilation with pressures of 35/0. The respiratory **rate is reduced** to 10 breaths per minute with an **I:E ratio** of 1:4. This gives tidal volumes of 115 mL (6 mL/kg). The **sevoflurane is increased** to 5%.*

*Oxygen saturations increase to 93%. The capnography trace shows upsloping of the plateau phase. Evidence of **gas trapping** is seen; the flow-volume loop does not return to zero before the start of the next breath. The **end tidal CO₂ (ETCO₂) rises** to 58 mmHg. Six puffs of **albuterol** are administered down the ETT (Fig. 5.1). Surgery is rapidly completed and hemostasis ensured. The airway resistance normalizes and the inflation pressures, capnography trace, and SpO_2 return to normal on FiO_2 0.4. When spontaneous ventilation is restored, the child is extubated deep. In recovery, the SpO_2 drops to 92% in room air, but responds well to oxygen supplementation via face mask. He has a cough and mild expiratory wheeze. Nebulized albuterol is given every 30 minutes; the boy's condition improves over a period of 2 hours. After a normal chest x-ray, he is discharged to the ward for overnight observation and continuous pulse oximetry. No further O_2 is required and he is discharged home on 3 days oral prednisolone.*

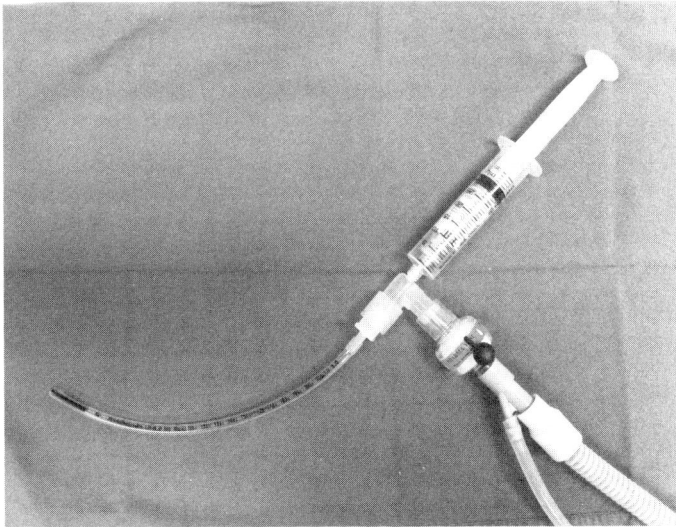

FIGURE 5.1 Albuterol administration via endotracheal tube.

DISCUSSION

1. What are the key features of a pre-anesthetic assessment in an asthmatic patient?

A key aim of preoperative assessment in an asthmatic child is to gauge the severity, control, and "brittleness" of the asthma (Table 5.1). A brittle asthmatic (a patient characterized by intermittent severe asthmatic attacks) is more likely to develop perioperative bronchospasm that is difficult to control. These patients would benefit from a preoperative consultation with their respiratory physician to optimize their asthma control. A short preoperative course of oral steroids may be considered as prophylaxis, although controlled clinical data to substantiate this practice are lacking.

Table 5.1

KEY FACTORS IN DETERMINING SEVERITY OF ASTHMA

Number of acute exacerbations, hospital presentations, and admissions in a year

Recent asthma symptoms, medical interventions, and hospital visits

Usual level of maintenance "preventer" therapy

Usual albuterol frequency, recent use, and especially recent escalation of therapy

Number of episodes of oral corticosteroid use for acute exacerbations within the past year

Previous intensive care admission and invasive ventilation

Any specific triggers for bronchospasm (including previous NSAID exposure)

Presence of a recent cold or coryzal symptoms within the last 2 weeks (this would lower the threshold for delaying surgery more than for a non-asthmatic patient)

Functional exercise tolerance (compared with peers) is a useful marker of severity.

The absence of the above features of severity is reasonably reassuring; however, some studies have found a poor correlation between assessment of disease severity and the occurrence of perioperative bronchospasm. Asthma is often undertreated, so the absence of intensive control medication should not lead the anesthesiologist to assume the disease is mild. It should be remembered that many deaths in the community occur in asthmatic patients who have been stratified as having "mild" or "moderate" disease. Perioperative vigilance and preventive measures are required in all children with asthma.

A history of prolonged oral prednisolone or high-dose inhaled corticosteroid administration within the previous 12 months is likely to produce some degree of adrenal suppression, and the child will benefit from an intraoperative dose of IV corticosteroid. It is unknown what length and cumulative dose of corticosteroid is required before perioperative corticosteroid supplementation is required; however, it is commonly thought that the potential benefit obtained from a single intraoperative dose of corticosteroid outweighs the risk of adverse effects.

2. What is the risk in children of worsening asthmatic symptoms with nonsteroidal anti-inflammatory drugs (NSAIDs)?

Some asthmatic adults have an aspirin-sensitive condition in which NSAIDs are relatively contraindicated. This seems to be less of a problem in children. Most children with asthma are able to take NSAIDs with no adverse effect. In general, older children (teenagers) with **atopy** and severe brittle asthma are the group most likely to suffer ill effects of NSAIDs (Palmer, 2005). NSAIDs are still only relatively contraindicated in this group, though alternatives for pain relief exist and should be used in preference to NSAIDs in this group of pediatric patients with asthma.

3. What are the common triggers for childhood asthma?

The most common trigger for a childhood asthma exacerbation is a **URI**. This is usually viral in nature. Other triggers include inhaled irritant gases (e.g., smoke), pollen, and foreign bodies. Crying or coughing (e.g., during uncooperative inhalational induction) may also trigger acute bronchospasm. During anesthesia, instrumentation of the airway is the most common trigger (e.g., placement of an ETT or tracheal suctioning). Carinal irritation in particular may precipitate bronchospasm. Irritant volatile agents such as desflurane may also predispose to bronchospasm. The differential diagnosis of wheezing always needs to be considered (see Chapter 20).

4. How is bronchospasm prevented?
The key strategy is to avoid triggers of bronchospasm.

Delay elective surgery. Delaying surgery should be considered in the presence of poor asthma control, recent or current URI, or lower respiratory tract infection. Airway hyperreactivity related to a viral URI persists for approximately 4 weeks. The threshold for delaying surgery in an asthmatic child with a URI would be lower than for a child who does not have asthma.

ETT versus LMA. This is a controversial issue; although intubation has been associated with an increased incidence of pulmonary complications, causation is not always clear and there are inadequate outcome data to make definitive recommendations. When considering the risks versus benefits of choice of airway device, the ETT should not be avoided "at all costs"; LMA insertion can also produce bronchospasm, and it would be much more difficult to manage the consequent ventilatory requirements without an ETT. If an ETT is inserted, it is important not to place the tube close to the carina.

Preoperative medications. The usual inhaled and oral medications should be given on the day of surgery. In addition, it is suggested that giving patients an inhaled bronchodilator 30 to 60 minutes before induction of anesthesia will reduce the incidence and severity of perioperative bronchospasm. Inhaled β_2-agonists are known to attenuate the increased airway resistance associated with tracheal intubation (Scalfaro et al., 2001). In addition, the use of sedative premedication such as midazolam or clonidine in selected patients can avoid or reduce the child's distress on induction. Crying may in itself induce bronchospasm. Anticholinergic drugs (e.g., glycopyrrolate) have been used to dry secretions but may worsen mucus plugging postoperatively.

Depth of anesthesia. A deep plane of anesthesia reduces airway reactivity associated with intubation. Patience is the key: wait until the child is deep enough, and then wait a little more. If possible, deep extubation is recommended for the same reasons. Topical anesthesia of the airway with local anesthetic seems appealing but may increase bronchomotor tone.

Avoidance of histamine-releasing drugs. This is somewhat controversial because not all histamine-releasing drugs will reliably trigger bronchospasm. However, with alternatives available, it is simple enough to avoid histamine-releasing drugs such as atracurium and morphine.

5. What is the acute management of an intraoperative asthmatic attack?

Acute management is initially supportive, ensuring adequate oxygen delivery and reasonable carbon dioxide clearance. Mechanical causes should be considered (e.g., blocked/kinked ETT, carinal irritation, defective circuit) as well as other causes of raised airway pressures (pneumothorax, abdominal splinting due to light anesthesia, anaphylaxis). Where possible, ventilatory pressures should be limited to reduce the risk of barotrauma and cardiovascular collapse (from high intrathoracic pressure). Simple measures include **increasing FiO$_2$, reducing the respiratory rate,** and **reducing the I:E ratio** (prolonging expiratory time) to avoid gas trapping. Permissive hypercarbia is often employed.

Be aware that patients tend to be hyperventilated (especially during manual ventilation) during an acute respiratory crisis. This runs the risk of increasing **gas trapping**. Placing the patient on a mechanical ventilator reduces this risk. Also consider intermittently reducing the intrathoracic pressure by disconnecting the patient from the breathing circuit and manually compressing the chest to produce a more complete exhalation of trapped gas within the lung.

Concurrent specific treatment of bronchospasm is equally important. This is rapidly achieved by the use of **volatile anesthetic agents**, although this must be balanced against its cardiovascular-depressant effects at higher concentrations. Repeated doses **of inhaled albuterol** (Fig. 5.1) is a simple method of delivering topical bronchodilator quickly. However, it is thought that as little as 3% of the nominal dose if aerosolized drug reaches the airways, though a spacing chamber can increase the delivered dose (Duarte, 2004). Terbutaline is available for subcutaneous injection in circumstance in which inhaled β_2-agonists cannot be delivered dependably. Should the wheezing result from anaphylaxis, epinephrine (adrenaline) is the drug of choice.

Corticosteroids should be given early to those who do not respond promptly to β_2-agonists; although the onset time of the anti-inflammatory effects of corticosteroids take 4 to 6 hours, it does enhance and prolong the effects of β_2-agonists within an hour. It is thought the latter effect occurs due to an increase in the expression of the β-adrenoreceptor, restoring G-protein/β_2-receptor coupling and decreasing desensitization (Johnson, 2004).

Status asthmaticus under anesthesia is extremely uncommon. Ventilatory management of these patients is a very complex area, and early involvement of intensive care should be sought. If the patient does not respond to inhaled albuterol and basic ventilation maneuvers (above), more advanced ventilator and pharmacological management is required. A meta-analysis concluded that IV magnesium sulfate has been shown to probably provide additional benefit in moderate to severe acute asthma in children treated with bronchodilators and steroids (Cheuk et al., 2005). $MgSO_4$ also has the advantage of an apparent paucity of side effects. IV aminophylline has been used in severe asthma, but it is often associated with cardiovascular side effects under anesthesia. Studies have failed to show whether IV albuterol or aminophylline is more effective in children with acute severe asthma (Roberts et al., 2003). The most severe cases may potentially require high-frequency oscillation or even extracorporeal membrane oxygenator (ECMO) support.

SUMMARY

1. Assessment is targeted at eliciting the severity, control, and brittleness of disease.
2. Prevention is the key in ALL patients with asthma: patients should take their usual drugs preoperatively and inhaled β_2-agonists before induction. Avoid bronchospasm triggers.
3. Intraoperative management involves excluding mechanical causes of wheezing, considering alternative diagnoses, and simple ventilator measures. Volatile anesthetic agents and inhaled β_2-agonists can rapidly reverse the bronchospasm in most cases.

ANNOTATED REFERENCES

- Doherty G, Chisakuta A, Crean P, Shields M. Anesthesia and the child with asthma. *Pediatr Anesth* 2005; 15:446–454.

  A comprehensive review article covering many aspects of anesthetizing a child with asthma.

Further Reading

Cheuk DKL, Chau TCH, Lee SL. A meta-analysis on intravenous magnesium sulphate for treating acute asthma. *Arch Dis Child* 2005; 90: 74–77.

Duarte AG. Inhaled bronchodilator administration during mechanical ventilation. *Respir Care* 2004; 49(6): 623-34.

Mitra A, Bassler D, Ducharme FM. Intravenous aminophylline for acute severe asthma in children over 2 years using inhaled bronchodilators. *Cochrane Database Syst Rev* 2001; (4): CD001276.

Roberts G, Newsom D, Gomez K, et al. Intravenous salbutamol bolus compared with an aminophylline infusion in children with severe asthma: a randomized controlled trial. *Thorax* 2003; 58: 306–310.

Johnson M. Interactions between corticosteroids and ß$_2$-agonists in asthma and chronic obstructive pulmonary disease. *Proc Am Thorac Soc* 2004; 1: 200–206.

Palmer GM. A teenager with severe asthma exacerbation following ibuprofen. *Anaesth Inten Care* 2005; 33(2): 261–265.

Scalfaro P, Sly P, Sims C, Habre W. Salbutamol prevents the increase of respiratory resistance caused by tracheal intubation during sevoflurane anesthesia in asthmatic children. *Anesth Analg* 2001; 93: 898–902.

von Ungern-Sternberg B, Habre W, Erb T, Heaney M. Salbutamol premedication in children with a recent respiratory tract infection. *Pediatr Anesth* 2009; 19: 1064–1069.

Tait A, Pandit U, Voepel-Lewis T, Munro H, Malviya S. Use of the laryngeal mask airway in children with upper respiratory tract infections: a comparison with endotracheal intubation. *Anesth Analg* 1998; 86: 706–711.

6

Do-Not-Resuscitate Orders in the OR

MARK J. MEYER AND NORBERT J. WEIDNER

INTRODUCTION

A physician signs a do-not-resuscitate order (DNR) when aggressive resuscitation measures will not benefit the patient in the presence of a life-threatening illness. Many children living with a life-threatening illness derive benefit from invasive diagnostic and therapeutic procedures such as tracheostomies, peripherally inserted central lines, gastrostomy tubes, and tumor debulking procedures. These procedures are considered palliative rather than curative in that they improve or preserve quality of life but do not prevent progression of the underlying condition. In children, the presence of a DNR order may not be a harbinger that death is imminent and can be consistent with pursuing life-prolonging interventions aimed at improving quality of life. However, these orders confound pediatric anesthesiologists who, during the conduct of a routine anesthetic, can cause cardiovascular and respiratory compromise.

LEARNING OBJECTIVES

1. Distinguish between a goal-directed and intervention-directed approach to the management of the patient with a DNR in the perioperative period.

2. Outline the roles of the surgeon, the anesthesiologist, and other members of the team in caring for a patient with a perioperative DNR.
3. Discuss the key components of the anesthesia consent for the patient with regard to interventions and goals. Include the importance of accurate documentation.
4. Know the responsibility of the physician team in supporting the OR personnel in this instance.

CASE PRESENTATION

A 14-year-old boy with Duchenne's muscular dystrophy presents for gastrostomy tube placement under general anesthesia. His history is notable for cardiomyopathy with moderate systolic dysfunction and resting tachycardia. He has been wheelchair-dependent since 11 years of age. He uses BiPAP at night and intermittently through the day. In the past 2 years, he has had several admissions to the intensive care unit for respiratory failure associated with pneumonia and pulmonary congestion. The admissions required intubation, mechanical ventilation, and lengthy periods of convalescence.

In the past year, he experienced difficulty swallowing, decreased appetite, and weight loss of 12 kg accompanied by fatigue. Last month, a nasogastric feeding tube was placed and he began to regain weight; his energy level and endurance have improved. With this experience, he believes that nutrition will be important to preserve his quality of life now that his respiratory status has stabilized with BiPAP.

Previously, he and his family had been unwilling to undergo any procedures. They could not accept the anesthetic risk posed by his cardiac and pulmonary dysfunction. After discussions with his pulmonologists and cardiologists, as well as anesthesia and surgical consultations, he decides for a surgically placed gastrostomy tube under general anesthesia. He presents to the operating room with a DNR signed by his pediatrician.

*The anesthesiologist **reconsiders** the DNR order and works with the patient to develop a **goal-directed plan** for the conduct of his anesthetic: general anesthesia with endotracheal intubation, followed by postoperative monitoring in the intensive care unit. During the **informed consent** discussion, the patient elaborates on his goals. The **family and patient establish the goal** that if he arrests, any interventions, including chest compressions, inotropes, and defibrillation, are acceptable. Postoperatively, he does not want to be on the ventilator for a lengthy period of time. "If things are not going well for me after a few days, I want to be made comfortable, removed from the ventilator and extubated. My parents will know when enough is enough." Further, if he will not be able to return home and enjoy a similar quality of life as before, then he wants the interventions to stop. He explains that he wants to get home as soon as possible and does not want a tracheostomy under any circumstance. His parents are supportive of his goals.*

Following an uneventful induction, the patient becomes hypotensive and inotropes are started with good effect. Upon completion of the gastrostomy, he is transferred to the intensive care unit. His inotropes are discontinued within hours of completion of the procedure. Shortly thereafter, he is successfully extubated to BiPAP. He is discharged the next day.

DISCUSSION

1. What are the advantages and limitations of a policy that rescinds the DNR in the perioperative period?

Historically, institutional policies for the pediatric patient with a DNR order have been to suspend the DNR order for the duration of the perioperative period and to reinstate the order afterward. The rationale is that the administration of anesthesia causes cardiovascular compromise, apnea, and loss of airway reflexes necessitating "resuscitative" efforts, though these efforts are routine in the course of an anesthetic. Therefore, the DNR order is rescinded to allow these efforts. For the perioperative team, it eliminates ambiguities and allows for aggressive measures to be used without discretion. However, this policy presents some limitations and challenges to parent and patient autonomy. It does not consider the unique clinical status of each patient, nor does it permit individualizing the surgical and anesthetic plan that respects patient goals. For the anesthesiologist, it requires aggressive resuscitation to be pursued even in scenarios of medical futility.

The duration of the perioperative period is not stipulated in these policies. The perioperative period could be limited to the intraoperative portion and terminate at the immediate conclusion of the post-anesthesia care unit (PACU) stay, or include time for recovery spent in the critical care unit, or until the first postoperative visit. In all cases the duration of the perioperative period should be determined by the perioperative team and documented.

2. What is "required reconsideration"?

The American Society of Anesthesiologists (ASA), the American College of Surgeons, and the American Academy of Pediatrics (AAP) have endorsed an approach called "**required reconsideration**." (American College of Surgeons, 1994) This is a review of the **patient's goals** in light of the surgical procedure to be performed as **part of the informed consent** for surgery and anesthesia. There are three options under required reconsideration: full resuscitation, goal-directed approach, and procedure-directed approach. These options include the rescind order but also include two options that individualize and respect patient autonomy (Table 6.1).

3. How does the goal-directed and procedure-directed approach challenge the perioperative team?

The **goal-directed approach** benefits from an established relationship between the perioperative team, the patient, and the family. Few anesthesiologists have established relationships with their patients. The anesthesiologist is challenged to make

Table 6.1

DNR IN THE OR: THREE APPROACHES TO REQUIRED CONSIDERATION AND CARE PLANNING

All DNR Patients		
Required Reconsideration		

Approach		
Full Resuscitation	Goal-Directed Plan	Procedure-Directed Plan

Underlying steps of approach		
All procedures, with a goal of maximizing chances for immediate survival from a cardiac or respiratory event	Full, modified, or no resuscitation, based on overall goal. **Components:** __Patient's/family's general goals __Spiritual goals __Respiratory goals __Cardiac goals __Comfort goals __Care team's ability to help achieve these goals	Procedures based on invasiveness, likely benefit, complexity. **Checklist:** __Supplemental oxygen __Bag and mask ventilation __Intubation __Mechanical ventilation __Arterial puncture __Needle thoracentesis __Chest tube insertion __Blood product transfusion __Invasive monitoring __Chest compressions __Vasoactive drugs __Defibrillation __Cardiac pacing

judgments about which resuscitative interventions support the goals of the patient. This creates discomfort in the event of an arrest or if aggressive action is required, as the anesthesiologist must decided how aggressive to be based upon the patient's goals. In the absence of a prior relationship, few anesthesiologists are comfortable making such decisions. However, this approach does not prevent the anesthesiologist from performing interventions that address iatrogenic complications (e.g., transient hypotension on induction) as long as the overall focus remains on the patient's goals.

The procedure-directed approach individualizes the resuscitative interventions based upon the patient's physiologic status. This allows for patients or their surrogates to refuse certain resuscitative procedures. The benefit of each intervention is considered individually with regard to the patient's condition. The anesthesiologist must inform the patient which interventions are necessary to conduct the anesthetic and which interventions can be refused. This removes the anesthesiologist from interpreting the wishes and goals of the patient during the conduct of the anesthetic.

As in the case above, the informed consent discussion should include a detailed review of the components of a standard resuscitation, with an emphasis on which ones are also part of a routine anesthetic. This case illustrates that inotropic support would be part and parcel of standard supportive care for this patient, without which the procedure could not be done. Therefore, the goal-directed approach allowed for inotropic support as a planned event, rather than as a rescue. The same holds true for intubating the patient, which is a planned part of the anesthetic, but would be otherwise resuscitative. Due to the nuances and variety of combinations that could arise as reasonable outcomes of the consent discussion, it is imperative to document the plan carefully in the chart.

The American College of Surgeons strongly supports the policy of required reconsideration. The surgeon's role as recommended by the American College of Surgeons (1994) is to advise the family about the risks and benefits of the operative procedure.

Ideally, both the anesthesiologist and the surgeon, as physician leaders, would together document the overall plan as made with the patient and family.

4. Who should inform the operating staff of the patient's DNR status?

From the patient's and family's perspective, all parties—the anesthesiologist, the surgeon, and the OR staff—are responsible for their care, so all participants in perioperative care should be considered. The OR personnel may be uncomfortable caring for a patient with an active, rescinded, or modified DNR, and they may be apprehensive about procedure-directed measures or the nuances of a goal-directed plan. The perioperative physician team should inform and direct the OR staff with regards to the patient's medical condition, expected problems, and any limits of intervention. They will need clarification about the plan for resuscitation, contingencies, and support. That way, in the event that the patient dies in the OR, the staff will understand that the lack of resuscitative efforts was not a failure of care, but an active endorsement of the patient's right to self-determination. This may help avoid feelings of doubt or guilt that might otherwise accompany withholding of what would traditionally be thought of as standard care for a cardiopulmonary arrest.

5. Can one refuse to comply with a DNR order in providing perioperative care?

There may be times when the anesthesiologist is morally unable to comply with a specific plan. If there is another attending anesthesiologist available, it is ethically permissible to recuse oneself from the case and transfer care to the other attending. However, in the case of an urgent or emergent procedure, where no timely alternative exists, "then in accordance with the American Medical Association's Principles of Medical Ethics, care should proceed with reasonable adherence to the patient's directives, being mindful of the patient's goals and values" in order to preserve the patient's right to self-determination (ASA, 2008) (Table 6.2).

Table 6.2

OBJECTIVES AND DISCUSSION PROMPTS FOR THE
ANESTHESIOLOGIST FOR PERIOPERATIVE DNR WITH
PATIENT AND FAMILIES

Goal: Clarify patient's goals for care.
Example:
"How did you decide to have a DNR?"
"When you made this decision with your pediatrician, what was important to you?
What are your goals for medical care? What are your goals for this procedure?"

Goal: Discuss the risks of the present anesthetic specific to the patient and the procedure.
Example:
"The anesthetic for this procedure causes breathing to stop.
A ventilator and breathing tube are needed. I am concerned that your son will need the ventilator for several hours after the procedure until he can breathe on his own. What are your thoughts about that? Is that consistent with your goals?"

Goal: Consider contingency planning for the unexpected or unlikely.
Example:
"If his heart were to stop in the operating room during the procedure, we could start CPR with chest compressions and give medications to restart the heart. In my judgment, it is unlikely that his heart would restart. We should talk about how we should handle that if it occurs."

SUMMARY

1. Pediatric patients with life-threatening conditions can benefit from surgical interventions that may not be curative but can improve quality of life.

2. The American Society of Anesthesiologists and the American College of Surgeons endorse "required reconsideration" for patients presenting for surgery. As part of required reconsideration, the DNR is reviewed prior to surgery. The options for the perioperative period include full resuscitation, goal-directed approach, or procedure-directed approach.
3. As part of the informed consent, the individualized plan must be documented, including the duration of the perioperative period.

ANNOTATED REFERENCES

- Fallat ME, Deshpande JK. Do-not-resuscitate orders for pediatric patients who require anesthesia and surgery. *Pediatrics* 2004; 114(6): 1686–1692.

  This clinical report specific to pediatrics addresses required reconsideration as well as the rights of children and surrogate decision making.
- Margolis JO, McGrath BJ, Kussin PS, Schwinn DA. Do not resuscitate (DNR) orders during surgery: ethical foundations for institutional policies in the United States. *Anesth Analg* 1995; 80: 806–809.

  This special report discusses the unique ethical challenges for the anesthesiologist who cares for patients with perioperative DNR orders.

Further Reading

American College of Surgeons. Statement on advance directives by patients: "Do not resuscitate" in the operating room. Reprinted from: Statement of the American College of Surgeons on advance directives by patients. "Do not resuscitate" in the operating room. *Bull Am Coll Surg* 1994: 79(9): 29. Accessed Jan. 23, 2011. http://www.facs.org/fellows_info/statements/st-19.html.

American Society of Anesthesiologists, Committee on Ethics, 2008. Ethical guidelines for the anesthesia care of patients with do not resuscitate orders or other directives that limit treatment. Accessed on Jan. 23, 2011. http://www.asahq.org/For-Members/Clinical-Information/Standards-Guidelines-and-Statements.aspx

Truog RD, Waisel DB, Burns JP. DNR in the OR. *Anesthesiology* 1999; 90: 289–295.

7

Preoperative Fasting in the Pediatric Patient

NANCY S. HAGERMAN AND
ERIC P. WITTKUGEL

INTRODUCTION

Preoperative fasting guidelines are designed to minimize the risk of pulmonary aspiration of gastric contents. As pulmonary aspiration is a rare occurrence, however, few evidence-based recommendations for ideal fasting intervals exist. An understanding of the research involved in the creation of these guidelines is useful in ensuring the maximum safety of patients while minimizing the disadvantages of prolonged fasting.

LEARNING OBJECTIVES

1. Know the current preoperative fasting guidelines from the American Society of Anesthesiologists.
2. Understand the risk of pulmonary aspiration in the pediatric population, common sequelae, and treatment.
3. Describe implications for overweight/obese pediatric patients.
4. List advantages associated with a liberalized preoperative fast.
5. Name common medical conditions that are associated with an increased risk of pulmonary aspiration.

CASE PRESENTATION

*An 8-year-old girl presents for outpatient **upper endoscopy** to evaluate her eosinophilic esophagitis. She weighs 35 kg, and aside from being **overweight**, she has mild asthma, which is well controlled with daily use of her maintenance inhaler. On arrival, the patient is **chewing gum**, which she is instructed to spit out. She has been fasted for solids since the evening before and drank a cup of **apple juice** just **2 hours ago**. The gastroenterologist informs the team that he is ready to take her to the endoscopy suite.*

DISCUSSION

1. What are the current ASA preoperative fasting guidelines? Who is the intended patient population for these guidelines?

The American Society of Anesthesiologists (ASA) Task Force on Preoperative Fasting published their guidelines in 1999. These guidelines were compiled based on an analysis of current literature, expert opinion, open forum commentary, and clinical feasibility data. The guidelines recommend a fasting interval of *2 or more hours after* the consumption of *clear liquids*, *4 or more hours after breast milk both in neonates and infants, and 6 or more hours after infant formula, a light meal, or non-human milk* ("2–4–6 rule"). The guidelines note that the ingestion of fried or fatty foods or meat may prolong gastric emptying time and recommend that both the amount and type of foods ingested be considered when determining an appropriate fasting period (ASA, 1999). Clear liquids are defined as water, fat-free and protein-free liquids, pulp-free fruit juice, carbonated drinks, clear tea, and black coffee (Kalinowski & Kirsch, 2004). Cow's milk has gastric emptying characteristics similar to those of solids as it separates into liquid and solid (curd) phases once in contact with gastric fluid.

The ASA guidelines are intended only for healthy patients of all ages undergoing elective procedures. The guidelines are not intended for women in labor or patients with coexisting diseases or conditions that may affect gastric emptying or gastric fluid volume such as pregnancy, obesity, diabetes, hiatal hernia, gastroesophageal reflux disease, or bowel obstruction. Additionally, the guidelines are not considered appropriate for patients in whom difficult airway management may be anticipated. Of note, the ASA guidelines do not recommend the routine use of gastrointestinal stimulants (e.g., metoclopramide), medications that block gastric acid secretion (e.g., omeprazole, ranitidine), antacids, and/or antiemetics to decrease the risk of pulmonary aspiration in patients who have no apparent increased risk.

Other countries carry similar guidelines regarding the preoperative fast. Guidelines published by the Royal College of Nursing in 2005 and the Canadian Anesthesiologists' Society in 2008 also follow the ASA "2–4–6 rule." Additionally, the Canadian Anesthesiologists' Society recommends an 8-hour fast after a meal that includes meat or fried or fatty foods. The Scandinavian Guidelines (2005) are different only in that they include infant formula in the 4-hour rule, along with breast milk (Brady et al., 2009). Summary guidelines are given in Table 7.1.

The determination of what constitutes a safe preoperative fasting duration is difficult, as the incidence of pulmonary aspiration is very low and sample sizes in studies are often too small. Because of this, surrogate markers for aspiration, usually gastric fluid volume, are used throughout the anesthesia literature to determine safe practice.

2. What is the risk of pulmonary aspiration in the pediatric population?

Fortunately, the incidence of perioperative pulmonary aspiration is rare—it is estimated to be between 1 in 10,000 and 10 in 10,000 depending upon the methods used. The majority of these events occur upon induction of anesthesia, usually associated with patients who cough or gag during airway manipulation (Cook-Sather & Litman, 2006).

A large prospective study showed a greater frequency of aspiration in emergency procedures versus elective procedures.

Table 7.1

GUIDELINES FOR PEDIATRIC PREOPERATIVE FASTING

Age Group	Solids	Clear Fluids	Breast Milk	Non-Human Milk + Formula
Neonates <6 months	N/A	2 hrs (a,b,c)	4 hrs (a,b,c); (d) milk type not specified	6 hrs (a,b); 4 hrs (d: milk type not specified); 4 hrs formula milk (c)
Infants 6–36 months, <12 months (e)	6 hrs (b,c,d,e)	2 hrs (a,b,c,d,e)	4 hrs (a,b,c,e); 6 hrs (d: milk not specified)	6 hrs (a,b,e), (d: milk type not specified); 4 hrs formula milk (c)
Children >36 months, >12 months (e)	6 hrs (a,c,e); 8 hrs (d); 6 hrs for light meal & 8 hrs for meal that includes meat, fried or fatty foods (b)	2 hrs (a,b,c,d,e)	4 hrs (a,b,c,e); 8 hrs (d: milk type not specified)	6 hrs (a,b,e); 8 hrs (d); 4 hrs formula milk (c)

Key:

a = American Society of Anesthesiologists. 1999

b = Canadian Anesthesiologists' Society. 2008, ages not specified

c = Scandinavian Guidelines (Task Force). 2005, ages not specified

d = American Academy of Pediatrics. 1992

e = Royal College of Nursing. 2005

From Brady MC, Kinn S, Ness V, et al. Preoperative fasting for preventing perioperative complications in children. *Cochrane Database Syst Rev.* Oct 2009; (4): CD005285. Copyright Cochrane Collaboration, reproduced with permission.

Furthermore, the majority of infants and children younger than 3 years of age who aspirated had ileus or bowel obstruction. The authors also found that most children who have mild to moderate aspiration events have no significant medical sequelae. In fact, based on their experience, Warner and colleagues would discharge a child from the recovery room after 2 hours of observation after an episode of mild aspiration as long as the child does not present with new symptoms such as coughing and wheezing, new hypoxia while breathing room air, or radiological abnormalities (Warner et al., 1999).

Severe aspiration classically presents with bronchospasm, tachypnea, wheezing, cyanosis, and fever and requires supportive care that may escalate to include tracheal intubation, pulmonary lavage, and admission to intensive care for mechanical ventilation. An infiltrate in the right middle lobe on chest x-ray is consistent with aspiration pneumonia. Radiographic changes usually occur within a few hours and show gradual improvement over the next 48 to 72 hours. With appropriate treatment, mortality from perioperative pulmonary aspiration is very rare—estimated at 1 in over 70,000 patients.

3. How do these guidelines apply to children with obesity?

Childhood obesity in the United States has become very common, increasing from an incidence of 5% in the 1960s to approximately 16% in the early 2000s. In fact, it has been estimated that nearly one third of children presenting for surgery are overweight or obese. **Overweight** children tend to be older, probably related to the fact that obesity is a cumulative disease that begins in early childhood. The Preoperative Fasting Guidelines published by the ASA were specifically noted by the Taskforce as not applicable for obese patients, as obesity could affect gastric emptying and fluid volumes (ASA, 1999). However, since the publication of those guidelines, Cook-Sather et al. (2009) found that although BMI percentile positively correlates with increased gastric fluid volumes, the correlations are exceedingly small and not helpful to the clinician in assessing the potential risk of aspiration.

Additionally, they found no difference in fasting duration between those obese patients who vomited during anesthesia and those who did not, suggesting that prolonged fasting (>2 hours for clear liquids) does not diminish risk in obese patients. As such, they advocate extending the 2-hour clear liquid ASA fasting guideline to include overweight and obese children who present for day surgery. Similarly, Warner et al. (1993) found in a review of 172,334 adult patients that BMI of >35 was not an independent risk factor for perioperative aspiration.

4. How should one manage the patient who is chewing gum?

Although adult studies do not demonstrate a change in gastric fluid volumes or pH in patients who chew gum prior to anesthesia, gum chewed for 30 minutes immediately before surgery in pediatric patients is associated with significantly increased gastric fluid volumes and higher pH (Schoenfelder et al., 2006). Because of this, many practitioners treat gum that has not been swallowed as a clear liquid, allowing 2 to 3 hours to pass prior to the start of the anesthetic. Because the use of **chewing gum** preoperatively could indicate other fasting violations, the child and parent should be carefully questioned about any other NPO violations (Cook-Sather & Litman, 2006).

5. What are the advantages associated with a more liberal preoperative fasting policy?

Preoperative fasting guidelines have become more liberal in the past 20 to 25 years. Large studies that would definitively show no increase in the risk of pulmonary aspiration with even further liberalization (beyond the current "2–4–6 rule") have not been performed. Encouraging healthy patients who present for elective surgery to consume clear liquids up until 2 hours prior to their anesthetic may be associated with several advantages. Specifically, these patients would be less dehydrated with improved hemodynamic stability upon induction of anesthesia (particularly with inhalational inductions in small children), easier intravenous access, and improved glucose homeostasis.

They may also have reduced irritability, improved child and parent satisfaction, and a decreased risk of postoperative nausea and vomiting (Cook-Sather & Litman, 2006).

6. What common medical conditions are associated with an increased risk of pulmonary aspiration?

Gastric emptying of liquids and solids is delayed by 40% to 50% in adults with type 1 and type 2 diabetes. The adult literature has shown that this reduced gastric emptying is most likely secondary to diabetic autonomic neuropathy and not related to HbA1C, preprandial blood glucose, or age. Renal failure has also been shown to be associated with delayed gastric emptying in patients who are on hemodialysis or peritoneal dialysis. Patients with both diabetes and renal failure have a further delay in gastric emptying (Kalinowski & Kirsch, 2004)

Infants and toddlers may have an increased risk of pulmonary aspiration compared to older children. In a large prospective study of pulmonary aspiration in children, the majority of children who aspirated had bowel obstruction or ileus (Warner et al., 1999). Of this subpopulation, the majority of those children were under the age of 3 years. This was thought to occur because infants and toddlers are known to have reduced lower esophageal sphincter tone compared to older children and adults. The frequency of gastroesophageal reflux decreases to a rate similar to that seen in adulthood by the time a child reaches his or her third birthday. Additionally, young children frequently swallow moderate amounts of air while crying or sucking on a pacifier, which can contribute to higher intragastric pressures.

Interestingly, the presence of gastrointestinal disorders such as chronic intermittent vomiting, abdominal pain, and gastroesophageal reflux has *not* been found to be associated with an increased risk of pulmonary aspiration of gastric contents. It has been demonstrated that children who fasted for at least 6 to 8 hours presenting for **upper endoscopy** had similar gastric fluid volumes and pH levels compared to historical groups of healthy children without gastrointestinal symptoms who were fasted for the same length of time (Schwartz et al., 1998). The authors concluded that their study does not support the argument that children with gastrointestinal symptoms are a greater risk of pulmonary aspiration during sedation or anesthesia. However, they did acknowledge that the safety of shortening the fasting interval in these patients to less than 6 hours would be questionable. It should be noted, however, that children with esophageal dysmotility conditions, such as achalasia, may have very large volumes of food in their esophagus even with prolonged fasting.

SUMMARY

1. ASA Guidelines are as follows: 2 hours for clear liquids, 4 hours for breast milk, 6 hours for infant formula, nonhuman milk, or a light meal.
2. The risk of pulmonary aspiration is very low. Most children who do aspirate have no significant medical sequelae. If a patient aspirates, consider discharging him or her from the PACU after 2 hours if there are no new symptoms such as hypoxia, cough, or wheezing.
3. In obese children, restricting oral intake beyond the ASA guidelines may not be of any benefit.
4. Treat unswallowed chewing gum as a clear liquid.
5. Conditions with an increased risk of aspiration are type 1 and type 2 diabetes, renal failure, bowel obstruction, ileus, pregnancy, hiatal hernia, gastroesophageal reflux disease, and patients in whom difficult airway management is anticipated.

ANNOTATED REFERENCES

· Cook-Sather SD, Litman RS. Modern fasting guidelines in children. *Best Pract Res Clin Anaesthesiol* 2006; 20(3): 471–481.

This is a comprehensive review of fasting guidelines for children. It is easy to read and provides a nice discussion of the evidence supporting current guidelines, the management of pulmonary aspiration, and how NPO status affects the patient intraoperatively, as well as its impact on family-centered care.

- Practice guidelines for preoperative fasting and the use of pharmacologic agents to reduce the risk of pulmonary aspiration: application to healthy patients undergoing elective procedures: A report by the American Society of Anesthesiologist Task Force on Preoperative Fasting. *Anesthesiology* 1999; 90(3): 896–905.

This is the ASA's 1999 guidelines for the preoperative fast. It is useful to read these guidelines and the analysis on which they were created to gain a greater understanding of NPO policies.

- Warner MA, Warner ME, Warner DO, Warner LO, Warner DJ. Perioperative pulmonary aspiration in infants and children. *Anesthesiology* 1999; 90(1): 66–71.

This amazing prospective study of 56,138 consecutive patients under the age of 18 who underwent 63,180 general anesthetics at the Mayo Clinic identified 24 cases of pulmonary aspiration. It gives great insight into the incidence and outcomes of this rare complication.

Further Reading

Brady MC, Kinn S, Ness V, O'Rourke K, Randhawa N, Stuart P. Preoperative fasting for preventing perioperative complications in children. *Cochrane Database Syst Rev* 2009; (4): CD005285.

Cook-Sather SD, Gallagher PR, Kruge LE, Beus JM, Ciampa BP, Welch KC, Shah-Hosseini S, Choi JS, Pachikara R, Minger K, Litman RS, Schreiner MS. Overweight/obesity and gastric fluid characteristics in pediatric day surgery: Implications for fasting guidelines and pulmonary aspiration risk. *Anesth Analg* 2009; 109(3): 727–736.

Kalinowski CPH, Kirsch JR. Strategies for prophylaxis and treatment for aspiration. *Best Pract Res Clin Anaesthesiol* 2004; 18(4): 719–737.

Schoenfelder RC, Ponnamma CM, Freyle D, Wang SM, Kain ZN. Residual gastric fluid volume and chewing gum before surgery. *Anesth Analg* 2006; 102(2): 415–417.

Schwartz DA, Connelly NR, Theroux CA, Gibson CS, Ostrom DN, Dunn SM, Hirsch BZ, Angelides AG. Gastric contents in children presenting for upper endoscopy. *Anesth Analg* 1998; 87(4): 757–760.

Warner MA, Warner ME, Weber JG. Clinical significance of pulmonary aspiration during the perioperative period. *Anesthesiology* 1993; 78(1): 56–62.

PART 2

CHALLENGES IN PEDIATRIC

PHARMACOLOGY

8

Malignant Hyperthermia

PHILIP RAGG

INTRODUCTION

Malignant hyperthermia, or malignant hyperpyrexia (MH), is a rare but frightening condition that occurs with an incidence of between 1:6,000 and 1:50,000 general anesthetics. To put this in context, a full-time anesthesiologist is likely to see one case in his or her working lifetime, and a major children's hospital may expect to see one case every 2 to 3 years. Its presentation is nonspecific and the course of MH can be insidious or rapidly progressive.

LEARNING OBJECTIVES

1. Know the clinical features of MH.
2. Understand the pharmacogenetic disturbance of skeletal and cardiac muscle in MH and know how to practically make a diagnosis of MH while considering the differential diagnoses.
3. Know the emergency treatment of MH in a team environment.
4. Know how to follow up a suspected case of MH and evaluate the implications for the patient and family.

CASE PRESENTATION

*A 40-kg 11-year-old boy is booked for a laparoscopic appendectomy. He presents with a 24-hour history of fever, abdominal pain, and anorexia. He has no past medical history and is taking no medication. He has had one previous (uneventful) general anesthetic for a fractured radius 3 years earlier. There is **no family history** of problems with anesthesia. On examination the child looks unwell, with pulse 110 bpm, BP 100/50 mmHg, respiratory rate 20/min, temperature 38.4°C. He has tenderness of his right iliac fossa with guarding; heart and lung sounds are normal. Investigations reveal white count 18 × 10^6/L (80% neutrophils), Hb 130 g/L, and platelets 420 × 10^9/L. He is intubated following a rapid-sequence induction with propofol (3 mg/kg) and **succinylcholine** (suxamethonium) 2 mg/kg, followed by **sevoflurane** 3% in oxygen/air (FiO_2 0.5). The following IV drugs are given: fentanyl 2.5 mcg/kg, granisetron 1 mg, atracurium 0.5 mg/kg, cephalexin 250 mg, metronidazole 400 mg, 0.9% saline 500 mL.*

*Fifteen minutes into the procedure, the heart rate increases to **140 bpm** (sinus). The end-tidal (ET) CO_2 has increased from 35 to 55 mmHg despite tidal volumes of 400 mL and no increase in airway pressure. Other observations are SpO_2 97%, BP 90/40, esophageal temperature 39°C. He is ventilated at RR 20/min. Sevoflurane concentration is increased to 5%. No abnormality is seen in the machine, soda lime, or ventilation circuit. A suction catheter is passed down the ETT without obstruction and chest expansion remains normal. The pupils are small and symmetrical. A provisional diagnosis of CO_2 absorption from the laparoscopy is made and the surgeons are asked to stop the surgery; FiO_2 is increased to 1.0 and the patient is hyperventilated with tidal volumes of 15 mL/kg (600 mL) and a rate of 35 breaths per minute. The patient continues to deteriorate: **$ETCO_2$ 70 mmHg, HR 160** (sinus), BP 80/40, **temperature 39.2°C,** ABG pH 7.05, pO_2 300 mmHg, **pCO_2 75 mmHg**, base excess–8.6. The diagnosis of MH is made. The surgical ports are removed, and the **local MH protocol** is instituted with specific roles for all members of the surgical care team (Tables 8.1a and 8.1b). A bolus of 3 mg/kg **dantrolene** is given; the patient's heart rate, $ETCO_2$, and temperature rapidly*

Table 8.1a and 8.1b

PROTOCOL FOR THE ROLES OF OR PERSONNEL IN THE MANAGEMENT OF MH

Table 8.1a

ANESTHESIOLOGIST

---

1. *Call for help* and *stop volatile/triggering agent.*
2. Ask the surgeon to stop *or rapidly complete the surgery.*
3. Change the anesthetic circuit to a clean one (e.g., a bag-valve-mask with O_2 reservoir). If this wastes too much time, increase flows to 15 L/min using the original machine.
4. *Hyperventilate* the patient in 100% oxygen (e.g., 3 times minute ventilation)
5. Administer IV *dantrolene* (see Question 6) *2 to 3 mg/kg* as a bolus and repeat every 5 to 10 minutes (up to 10 mg/kg) until $ETCO_2$ and temperature decrease.
6. *Cool the patient.* Switch off warming devices and expose the patient. Switch convection blower to ambient temperature. Administer cold IV solutions. Ice packs to vascular plexuses (axilla and groin); consider cold lavage of stomach or bladder.
7. Insert an *arterial line* for monitoring and *arterial blood gases,* electrolytes (especially potassium and calcium), complete blood count (CBC), and coagulation studies.
8. Place urinary catheter; *consider diuretics* if urine output is <0.5 mL/kg/hr.
9. Insert *central venous catheter* to monitor central venous pressure, and administer inotropes if necessary.
10. When under control, transfer to the *intensive care unit.* Potassium, lactate, and myoglobin abnormalities can occur for a number of hours or days. Further dantrolene may need to be given several hours later if symptoms or signs of increased metabolic activity recur.

Care must be appropriate, timely, and organized.

(continued)

Table 8.1b *(continued)*
OTHER OR PERSONNEL

Surgeon: Cease surgery temporarily until some control is obtained, then complete surgery ASAP; following this, assist the anesthesiologist.

Anesthetic Assistant: Send for MH trolley; mix dantrolene in the vial or pour into a burette or sterile container. Organize blood gases, monitoring, and ice packs.

OR Nurse: Call for assistance and help mix dantrolene. Notify PICU and help prepare additional monitoring.

Surgical Technician: Collect ice, cool fluids, drugs, and blood specimens.

return to normal within 5 minutes. The surgery is quickly completed and the patient is transferred (ventilated) to the pediatric intensive care unit. Over the next 12 hours of ventilation and fluid therapy, the patient develops mild hyperkalemia (K^+ 5.9 mmol/L) and a rise in serum creatinine kinase to 500 U/L. His ECG shows a few ventricular ectopic beats. No further dantrolene is required. The patient is extubated the following morning and discharged to the ward after 24 hours.

DISCUSSION

1. What is the pathophysiology of MH? What are the clinical features?

MH is a pharmacogenetic disease or syndrome characterized by a potentially life-threatening hypermetabolic state in susceptible individuals. It was first described by Denborough et al. (1962). In most cases, the abnormality is a mutation in the *ryanodine receptor*. This receptor is located on the sarcoplasmic reticulum within skeletal muscle cells and, if abnormal, opens and releases calcium into the cell in response to certain anesthetic *triggers*, namely the

volatile anesthetic agents and the depolarizing muscle relaxant **succinylcholine**. Early suggestions that nitrous oxide, phenothiazines, tubocurarine, amide local anesthetics (lidocaine and bupivacaine), and anticholinergics may be triggers in susceptible patients have been disproven (Hopkins, 2000). In susceptible individuals, these triggers result in *an increase in the intramyoplasmic calcium* levels either from the sarcoplasmic reticulum stores or from the extracellular milieu. This causes a sustained contracture of the muscle and stimulation of the enzyme calcium-ATPase, which leads to a *hypermetabolic state* involving increased aerobic (oxygen consumptive) and anaerobic (glycogen breakdown) metabolic pathways. Heat is generated, CO_2 production is increased, and O_2 is consumed. The clinical signs are **tachycardia**, hyperventilation, **rising arterial and ETCO$_2$**, **hyperthermia**, and muscle rigidity. If undiagnosed this may progress to renal failure, disseminated intravascular coagulopathy, progressive acidosis, and death. If unrecognized and untreated, MH has a mortality rate up to 90%. Early detection and treatment can *decrease this mortality risk to <5%*.

2. What are the molecular genetics of MH?

MH is usually inherited as autosomal dominant with variable penetrance, however the genetics is not simple and because more than one genetic locus has recently been identified , it appears that both hetero- and homozygote forms exist. The abnormality in more than 50% of cases is a mutation of the ryanodine receptor subtype RYR1. This receptor subtype is encoded by a gene on the 19th chromosomes (Zhou et al., 2010). Five other loci associated with MH have been identified on chromosomes 17, 1, 3, 7, and 5 but the only other known causative gene for MH is CACNA1S, which encodes a voltage-gated calcium channel on the α subunit of the cell membrane.

3. What are the conditions associated with MH?

Although there has been a suggested association with various myopathies, dystonias, exertional stress, and enzymopathies, clear linkage with other pathologies exists for only a few. The conditions for which there is an association with MH are *King Denborough syndrome*, *central core disease*, and possibly *hypokalemic periodic paralysis*.

4. How is MH diagnosed?

There is no single clinical sign, monitored variable, or biochemical finding specific to MH, and the course can be insidious or rapidly progressive. There may not be a family history. The most frequent early signs are related to increased oxygen consumption and **increased carbon dioxide** and lactate production. This is usually followed by signs of autonomic sympathetic stimulation. The key early features of increased muscle metabolism are **unexpected tachycardia,** increased respiratory rate, **increased ETCO$_2$** (despite adequate ventilation), and **raised temperature** (which may increase by up to 2°C per hour or be delayed for several hours).

Muscle rigidity commonly occurs and is prolonged and nonpropagated. In the unparalyzed patient rigidity may help differentiate the diagnosis from septicemia. Muscle rigidity of the jaw (spasm of the masseter and lateral pterygoid muscles) is commonly seen after **succinylcholine** administration. If this is severe or prolonged ("jaws of steel") and is associated with contracture of skeletal muscle elsewhere, there is a very high likelihood of MH.

If any of these signs develop, MH should be considered but they should also prompt further investigation to exclude other causes (Table 8.2).

Other features that may develop in an MH event include *cardiovascular collapse* with decreased cardiac output, *arrhythmias* including *hyperkalemic cardiac arrest* (peaked T-waves and ventricular ectopy may be seen on ECG preceding this), *neurological collapse, coma and fixed dilated pupils* (hyperthermia, acidosis, and fluid shifts can cause acute cerebral edema), *disseminated intravascular coagulopathy* (may occur with thromboembolism due to release of tissue thromboplastin), *rhabdomyolysis and myoglobinuria* (this may cause renal failure), and *desaturation or cyanosis, sweating, and being hot to the touch.*

Table 8.2

DIFFERENTIAL DIAGNOSIS OF MH

Inadequate depth of anesthesia

Ventilation delivery problem: defective or inappropriate breathing circuit, inadequate gas flow, inadequate ventilation settings (low minute volume), ventilator mechanical fault, exhausted soda lime, blocked ETT/LMA

Anaphylaxis

Tourniquet ischemia

Endocrine causes: pheochromocytoma, thyroid storm

Neuroleptic malignant syndrome (e.g., if on neuroleptic medication, antidopaminergic drugs)

Drugs (e.g., Ecstasy)

Cerebral ischemia

Other muscular diseases (e.g., isolated masseter spasm in patients with Duchenne's)

Other (e.g., overzealous active heating where the patient has reduced ability to lose heat, such as bilateral leg tourniquets)

In some clinical situations, patients are treated for MH empirically without definite diagnosis.

In classic MH, the arterial blood gas analysis will confirm a *mixed respiratory and metabolic acidosis,* an increased serum lactate, and possible hyperkalemia. Later tests may show an *increased creatinine kinase level, continued hyperkalemia, and abnormal renal function.*

5. What is the practical treatment of MH?

Early diagnosis of MH is arguably the most important step. Any delay in treatment increases the risk of morbidity and mortality. Even if subsequent follow-up demonstrates another diagnosis, there are few disadvantages in treating a patient with possible signs of MH early; it is better to overtreat than delay treatment.

A **local protocol** should allocate tasks to individual members of the operating room staff (see Tables 8.1a and 1b). The Malignant Hyperthermia Australia and New Zealand group has developed a MH Resource Kit (MHANZ, 2007). This kit contains information and aids in the management of patients suspected of an MH diagnosis, including "task cards" for members of the team and OR education posters.

6. What is dantrolene?

Dantrolene is the most important agent in the management of MH. The dose is *2 to 3 mg/kg* as a bolus, which is repeated every 15 minutes (up to 10 mg/kg) until $ETCO_2$ and temperature decrease. Dantrolene sodium is a hydantoin derivative that acts as a muscle relaxant but not a paralyzing agent. It appears to work directly on the ryanodine receptor to prevent the release of calcium from the sarcoplasmic reticulum. Each ampoule provides 20 mg of dantrolene. This drug should be kept in every hospital providing general anesthesia along with an MH treatment box. Due to the rarity of this condition, the cost of dantrolene, and its short shelf life, most hospitals have an arrangement with a sister hospital to provide backup supplies of the drug in the event of an MH crisis. Dantrolene comes as a powder and is notoriously difficult to mix with water—it does not dissolve easily, so more than one person should help with this task.

7. How are patients and families managed after the event?

The history should be re-reviewed in detail; information regarding triggering agents, previous anesthesia, and family history of incidents during anesthesia should be documented. Some centers measure serum creatinine kinase levels at rest and fasting in the patient and family members. If these are elevated, there is a good correlation with MH susceptibility and biopsy may be unnecessary. However, this is controversial, and many centers will still require a biopsy for diagnosis. Normal levels of CK are not predictive. Muscle (quadriceps) biopsy contracture studies are the definitive test for MH susceptibility; they are offered to the family but cannot be performed on the patient until several months after the event. These are performed at many designated centers around the world.

Many of these centers will not perform biopsies on prepubertal children, and Australian centers have a minimum age of 12 years. North American centers require children to have a lean body mass of at least 20 kg. The reason for age and weight limitation is to ensure standardization of the test, which requires a relatively large piece of vastus lateralis muscle. The muscle sample is calculated for cross-sectional area using a formula of weight and length and usually measures 3 to 5 cm long and up to 1 cm wide. If a child is too young or small for biopsy, the parents should be offered testing. Only one parent need be biopsied if the first parent is found to be positive; the child would then be considered MH sensitive. If both parents are found to be MH negative, the child should be considered MH susceptible until old enough for a definitive diagnosis with biopsy.

Two biopsy protocols exist: European and North American. The European Protocol (in vitro contracture test [IVCT]) uses incremental concentrations of caffeine (0.5–32 mM) and halothane (0.5–3%). The result yields three potential diagnoses: *MH sensitive* if halothane and caffeine are abnormal, *MH negative* if halothane and caffeine are normal, and *MH equivocal* (and therefore considered "sensitive") if one result is abnormal. The North American Protocol (caffeine halothane contracture test [CHCT]) uses graded caffeine (0.5–32 mM) and a halothane bolus of 3%. This yields only two possible diagnoses; normal or sensitive.

If the result is sensitive or equivocal, the patient and family are usually DNA tested for mutation of the ryanodine gene. Family members found to have 1 of 15 known RYR1 mutations are considered sensitive. The patient/family should be supplied with written information of their MH susceptibility, which they should carry with them at all times. This might also include the wearing of a Medic-Alert bracelet.

8. **Who are the patients at risk for MH and how should they be approached?**

Patients should be considered susceptible if:

a) *Previous MH reaction or*

b) *A relative* has had either *positive IVCT, positive DNA, or previous MH reaction.*

The key is to identify the above patients and avoid the triggering agents. The anesthesia machine should be "cleansed" of volatile agent by removing vaporizers, previous circuits, and soda lime and flushing at 10 L/min with 100% oxygen for 20 minutes. Informed consent should include discussion of risks with the patient. Core temperature should be measured in addition to standard monitoring. Dantrolene should be available but not given prophylactically.

SUMMARY

1. MH is an uncommon, potentially fatal pharmacogenetic condition that results in a hypermetabolic state after exposure to volatile anesthetic agents or depolarizing muscle relaxants.
2. It is usually related to the ryanodine receptor RYR1 gene mutation on skeletal muscle endoplasmic reticulum.
3. There is no single feature that is pathognomonic for MH.
4. The important step in management is to first consider the diagnosis; treatment can reduce mortality from 90% to 5%.

ANNOTATED REFERENCES

• Davis PJ, Brandom BW. The association of malignant hyperthermia and unusual disease: when you're hot you're hot or maybe not. *Anesth Analg* 2009; 109(4): 1001–1069.

A thought-provoking editorial discussing various MH issues, including the limitations of our knowledge concerning its pathophysiology, the difficulty in testing for the disease, and the risk stratification of MH with various myopathies.

- **Hopkins PM. Malignant hyperthermia: advances in clinical management and diagnosis.** *Br J Anaesth* 2000; 85(1): 118–128.

  Good overview of the topic.

- **MHANZ. Malignant Hyperthermia Australia and New Zealand. ANZCA Publication 2007. Accessed Oct. 15, 2010. http://www.anaesthesia.mh.org.au/mh-resource-kit/w1/ i1002692/%3E**

  An excellent website containing a "kit" with advice on the contents of a MH emergency box, OR posters, and task cards for individual members of the team in the event of a MH crisis.

Further Reading

Denborough MA, Forster JF, Lovell RR, Maplestone PA, Villiers JD. Anaesthetic deaths in a family. *Br J Anaesth* 1962; 34: 395–396.

Larach MG for the North American Malignant Hyperthermia Group. Standardization of the caffeine halothane muscle contracture test. *Anesth Analg* 1989; 69: 511–515.

Malignant Hyperthermia Association of the United States of America. Accessed Nov. 30, 2010. http://www.mhaus.org/.

Pollock N, Langton E, Macdonell N, Tiemessen J, Stowell K. Malignant hyperthermia and day stay anaesthesia. *Anaesth Intens Care* 2006; 34: 40–45.

Xiao B, Masumiya H, Jiang D, et al. Isoform dependent formation of heteromeric calcium release channels (ryanodine receptors). *J Biol Chem* 2002; 277(44): 41778–41785.

Zhou J, Allen PD, Pessah IN, Naguib M. Neuromuscular disorders and malignant hyperthermia. In RD Miller, LI Eriksson, LA Fleisher, JP Wiener-Kronish, WL Young, eds. *Miller's anesthesia, 7th Ed.* Philadelphia: Elsevier, 2010: 1181–1195.

9

Anaphylaxis

LIANA G. HOSU AND LORI A. ARONSON

INTRODUCTION

Anaphylaxis has been defined as a "severe, life-threatening generalized or systemic hypersensitivity reaction" (Johansson et al., 2004). It is rapid in onset and may cause death or permanent disability. Early recognition and optimal management are critical. During anesthesia, recognition of anaphylaxis is often delayed because the clinical presentation can mimic other conditions. Epinephrine is the drug of choice in the treatment of anaphylaxis and should be given as early as possible.

LEARNING OBJECTIVES

1. Understand the pathophysiology of anaphylaxis.
2. Learn the prevalence, etiology, and risk factors of anaphylaxis.
3. Be able to recognize perioperative anaphylaxis.
4. Know basic therapies of perioperative anaphylaxis, including prevention.

CASE PRESENTATION

*A 10-year-old boy is scheduled for surgical repair of a dislocated hip. His past medical history is significant for **meningomyelocele** that was repaired at 2 days of age. This was associated with hydrocephalus,* *for which he required a ventriculoperitoneal (VP) shunt at 3 months of age. This subsequently required three VP shunt revisions. At age 5, he had a release of his tethered spinal cord.* He has a neurogenic bladder requiring scheduled bladder catheterization and is wheelchair-bound. He has no known drug allergies but is on **latex precautions** due to his diagnosis of meningomyelocele and neurogenic bladder. There is no history of anesthetic complications.

The boy has an unremarkable inhalational induction with intubation aided by propofol, fentanyl, and cisatracurium. A dose of cefazolin is administered before incision. Twenty minutes after incision there is **profound hypotension, desaturation, increased peak airway pressures, and decreased ETCO$_2$**. Anesthetics are discontinued and the patient is aggressively resuscitated with 100% **oxygen, epinephrine (adrenaline), albuterol (salbutamol), diphenhydramine, hydrocortisone,** and **crystalloid infusion**. Blood is taken for **tryptase** and **histamine** levels. After the hemodynamics are stabilized, the patient is transferred to the intensive care unit on an epinephrine infusion. Before his discharge, an **allergy consult** is obtained to investigate the cause of his intraoperative anaphylaxis and to make recommendations for future anesthetics.

DISCUSSION

1. What is the pathophysiology of anaphylaxis?

Perioperative anaphylaxis is an acute, potentially lethal, multisystem process resulting from the *sudden release of mediators from mast cells and basophils* into the circulation. The World Allergy Organization categorizes anaphylaxis as either *allergic or nonallergic* (Johansson et al., 2004). Allergic anaphylaxis includes IgE-, IgG-, and immune complex/complement–mediated reactions. Nonallergic anaphylaxis (formerly called anaphylactoid reaction) is caused by agents that induce sudden, massive mast cell or basophil degranulation in the absence of immunoglobulins. Regardless of type, the *immediate treatment is identical* but subsequent evaluation, testing, and recommendations may vary.

Multiple substances and mediators are released, with *histamine* and *tryptase* being the most readily measurable. Histamine H_1 receptor stimulation initiates nitric oxide synthesis and has been implicated in the hypotension of sepsis and anaphylaxis. The predominantly affected organs are the skin, mucous membranes, cardiovascular and respiratory systems, and the gastrointestinal tract. Fatalities are divided between circulatory collapse and respiratory arrest. Anaphylaxis has characteristics of both *distributive shock*, characterized by a profound reduction in venous tone, and *hypovolemic shock*, with increased vascular permeability causing massive fluid shifts and reduced venous return. Up to 35% of intravascular volume can shift to the extravascular space within 10 minutes during anaphylaxis. In addition, myocardial function is depressed. Clinical signs of *erythema, edema, urticaria, arterial hypotension, tachycardia, bronchoconstriction,* and gastrointestinal smooth muscle constriction are described by the Ring and Messmer clinical severity scale (Table 9.1), which was created to describe immediate perioperative reactions and help guide care. Biphasic anaphylaxis (recrudescence) occurs in up to 20% of cases. It is of unclear etiology and may occur as early as 1 hour or as late as 72 hours after the initial symptoms.

2. What is the incidence and etiology of anaphylaxis? What are the risk factors?

Perioperative anaphylaxis is estimated to occur in 1 in 10,000 to 20,000 general anesthetic administrations with a mortality rate of a few percent, though data are probably incomplete, precluding exact estimates of prevalence (DeWachter et al., 2009). In adults, neuromuscular blocking agents (*NMBAs*) are the most common cause of intraoperative anaphylaxis, being responsible for 50% to 70% of cases. All NMBAs can elicit immune-mediated or non-immune-mediated anaphylaxis. Anaphylaxis usually occurs shortly after induction with NMBAs or antibiotics, but may occur at any time with all potentially allergenic agents. Many over-the-counter drugs, cosmetics, and food products contain quaternary or tertiary ammonium ions (also part of the structure

Table 9.1

CLINICAL SEVERITY SCALE OF IMMEDIATE HYPERSENSITIVITY REACTIONS

Grades	Clinical Signs
I	Cutaneous-mucous signs:
	Erythema
	Urticaria with or without angioedema
II	Moderate multivisceral signs: cutaneous-mucous signs
	+/– hypotension
	+/– tachycardia
	+/– dyspnea
	+/– gastrointestinal disturbances
III	Life-threatening mono- or multivisceral signs:
	Cardiovascular collapse:
	Tachycardia or bradycardia, +/– cardiac arrhythmia
	+/– bronchospasm
	+/– cutaneous–mucosal signs
	+/– gastrointestinal disturbances
IV	Cardiac arrest

Reprinted with permission from Dewachter P, Mouton-Faivre C, Emala C. Anaphylaxis and anesthesia: controversies and new insights. *Anesthesiology* 2009; 111: 1141–1150.

of NMBAs), resulting in sensitization, thus explaining first-exposure reactions. Succinylcholine (suxamethonium) is more likely to cause anaphylaxis than nondepolarizing muscle relaxants. Because cross-reactivity between NMBAs is common (approximately 60–70%), safe alternative NMBAs should be identified during allergy testing.

In adults, the second most common cause of perioperative anaphylaxis is natural rubber **latex** sensitivity; it is responsible for 20% of cases. In children, latex allergy is the leading cause of intraoperative anaphylaxis. Latex-induced anaphylaxis usually occurs 30 to 60 minutes after the beginning of the surgery but may be immediate or considerably delayed. Children at increased risk include patients with **myelomeningocele** and congenital urogenital malformations, children who have had repeated operations (especially in the first year of life), patients who require daily intermittent urinary catheterization, and children with atopic conditions (eczema, asthma, allergic rhinitis). While there may be a genetic component to latex allergy in patients with myelomeningocele, environmental exposure to latex from repeated operations and urinary catheterization appears more likely. Since the 1990s, the incidence of latex allergy in children seems to be decreasing due to removal of latex materials from healthcare settings and increased awareness and improved diagnosis of latex allergy. Latex anaphylaxis is most likely with parenteral or mucous membrane exposure. The only effective treatment is complete avoidance of latex in the healthcare setting, including the use of latex-free gloves.

Anaphylaxis triggered by antibiotics involves primarily *penicillin* and *cephalosporins,* which share the beta-lactam ring. Diagnosis is performed with prick and intradermal skin testing. Cross-reactivity between penicillins and cephalosporins seems to be low (10%) and is attributed to the common beta-lactam ring. IV drugs used for anesthetic induction are the fourth most common cause of perioperative anaphylaxis. Anaphylaxis to thiopental and propofol (see Chapter 11 for discussion of egg and soy allergies and propofol administration) is rare and even less likely with etomidate and ketamine. Opioids, especially morphine, commonly cause flushing and urticaria via direct histamine release following peripheral IV administration; however, the risk of anaphylaxis is very low.

3. How can one recognize perioperative anaphylaxis?
The initial diagnosis of perioperative anaphylaxis is *clinical*, based on history and physical examination, and the retrospective diagnosis relies on serologic and skin tests.

A survey of anaphylaxis during anesthesia demonstrated that cardiovascular symptoms (73.6%), cutaneous symptoms (69.6%), and bronchospasm (44.2%) are the most common clinical features (Laxenaire et al., 2001). Anaphylaxis may be mild and resolve spontaneously due to endogenous production of compensatory mediators, or it may be severe and progress within minutes to respiratory or cardiovascular compromise and death. During anesthesia the initial symptoms often go unnoticed because the patient is unconscious and draped for surgery. As a result, the reaction may be detected only when dramatic respiratory and cardiovascular changes develop. This explains why cardiovascular collapse is the first detected manifestation in up to 50% of cases.

In addition to the Ring and Messmer clinical grading scale, three criteria that predict severe anaphylaxis are (1) *rapid onset,* (2) *absent cutaneous signs,* and (3) *paradoxical bradycardia.* Paradoxical bradycardia is considered an adaptive mechanism that allows maximal ventricular filling in the face of massive hypovolemia. Atropine is contraindicated. Resuscitation should include **oxygen**, aggressive **volume resuscitation**, and inotropic support with **epinephrine** or vasopressin.

The *differential diagnosis* of an anaphylactic reaction during general anesthesia includes (1) other causes of respiratory symptoms: asthma, post-extubation stridor, pulmonary edema, pulmonary embolus, tension pneumothorax; (2) other causes of hypotension: arrhythmia, cardiogenic shock, hemorrhage, hypoglycemia, overdosage of vasoactive drug, pericardial tamponade, sepsis, vasovagal reaction, venous air embolism; and (3) other causes of angioedema: hereditary or acquired angioedema, treatment with ACE inhibitors.

The clinical diagnosis can be supported by documentation of elevated concentrations of plasma **histamine** and total **tryptase**. It is critical to obtain blood samples as soon as possible after the onset of symptoms, as elevations are transient. Skin testing based on the likely offending causes remains the gold standard for the detection of IgE-mediated reactions. This should be performed 4 to 6 weeks after an anaphylactic reaction to avoid false-negative results because of mast cell depletion.

4. What is the treatment of perioperative anaphylaxis?

The management of anaphylaxis consists of immediately removing the offending drug or latex gloves, immediate reduction or discontinuation of anesthetic drugs, intubation if not already performed, ventilation with 100% **oxygen**, early administration of **epinephrine** and expansion of the intravascular **volume**, placing the patient in the Trendelenburg position, and abbreviating the surgical procedure if possible. **Epinephrine** is the drug of choice in the treatment of anaphylaxis, because its alpha-1 effects help to support the blood pressure while its beta-2 effects provide bronchial smooth muscle relaxation.

For the treatment of bronchospasm not responsive to epinephrine, inhaled beta-2 agonists (**albuterol**) should be administered as needed. **Corticosteroids** are given on an empiric basis in the treatment of anaphylaxis, with the rationale that they may help to prevent the biphasic or protracted reactions that occur in up to 20% of patients and are useful for angioedema. Although H_1 and H_2 receptor antagonists are often recommended, there is minimal evidence to support the use of these medications in the emergency treatment of anaphylaxis.

Patients receiving beta-blockers may be resistant to treatment with epinephrine and can develop hypotension and bradycardia requiring glucagon for its inotropic and chronotropic effects that are not mediated through beta-receptors. Epinephrine-resistant anaphylaxis may require norepinephrine (noradrenaline), metaraminol, or arginine vasopressin (AVP). AVP may be preferred because it does not rely on adrenergic receptors (Table 9.2).

5. How can one prevent perioperative anaphylaxis?

A careful history regarding adverse drug reactions and allergies, including latex allergy or **latex precautions,** should be obtained before every anesthetic. Premedication with steroids, antihistamines, and beta-agonists is not recommended because this may blunt the early signs of anaphylaxis. The safest approach for managing future anesthetics in a patient who suffered perioperative

Table 9.2

CHECKLIST FOR SUSPECTED ANAPHYLAXIS

Treatment	Laboratory testing	Consultations
Oxygen	Immediate:	Critical care
Epinephrine	Tryptase,	Allergy
Fluids	histamine	Skin testing in
Corticosteroids	Delayed: Tryptase	4–6 weeks
H$_1$ & H$_2$ blockers	24 hours	
Arginine vasopressin (AVP)		

anaphylaxis is identification and complete avoidance of the offending drug.

SUMMARY

1. Anaphylaxis can have a variable presentation, from mild cutaneous signs to cardiopulmonary collapse. Prompt recognition and treatment with epinephrine, fluids, oxygen, and supportive care are crucial. Steroids and antihistamines may also be beneficial. ICU care is necessary for continued resuscitation and monitoring for recrudescence.

2. Blood histamine and tryptase levels should be obtained soon after the event. Allergy consultation and testing will help determine the causative agent and guide future anesthesia care.

3. The three most common causes of intraoperative anaphylaxis are neuromuscular drugs, latex, and antibiotics. Latex reactions may be delayed and difficult to recognize. A high index of suspicion is required.

ANNOTATED REFERENCES

- Dewachter P, Mouton-Faivre C, Emala C. Anaphylaxis and anesthesia: controversies and new insights. *Anesthesiology* 2009; 111: 1141–1150.

  A recent European review of the etiology, diagnosis, and treatment of intraoperative anaphylaxis.

- Hepner DL, Castells MC. Anaphylaxis during the perioperative period. *Anesth Analg* 2003; 97: 1381–1395.

  A detailed review of perioperative anaphylaxis concentrating on pathophysiology, diagnosis, management, prevention, and specific drugs involved in perioperative anaphylaxis.

- Sampathi V, Lerman J. Case scenario: perioperative latex allergy in children. *Anesthesiology* 2011; 114: 673–680.

  An excellent case study and discussion of perioperative pediatric latex allergy.

Further Reading

Chacko T, Ledford D. Peri-anesthetic anaphylaxis. *Immunol Allergy Clin North Am* 2007; 27(2): 213–230.

Gueant JL, Aimone-Gastin I, Namour F, Laroche D, Bellou A, Laxenaire MC. Diagnosis and pathogenesis of the anaphylactic and anaphylactoid reactions to anaesthetics. *Clin Exp Allergy* 1998; 28 Suppl 4: 65–70.

Harper NJ, Dixon T, Dugué P, et al. Suspected anaphylactic reactions associated with anaesthesia. *Anaesthesia* 2009; 64(2): 199–211.

Johansson SGO, Bieber T, Dahl R, et al. Revised nomenclature for allergy for global use: Report of the Nomenclature Review Committee of the World Allergy Organization, October 2003. *J Allergy Clin Immunol* 2004; 113(5): 832–836.

Karila C, Brunet-Langot D, Labbez F, Jacqmarcq O, Ponvert C, Paupe J, Scheinmann P, de Blic J. Anaphylaxis during anesthesia: results of a 12-year survey at a French pediatric center. *Allergy* 2005; 60(6): 828–834.

Laxenaire MC, Mertes PM; Groupe d'Etudes des Réactions Anaphylactoïdes Peranesthésiques. Anaphylaxis during anaesthesia: results of a two-year survey in France. *Br J Anaesth* 2001; 87: 549–558.

10

Anesthesia for MRI

**MOHAMED A. MAHMOUD AND
JOHN J. McAULIFFE, III**

INTRODUCTION

Choosing an appropriate anesthetic or sedative technique for children undergoing diagnostic procedures can be a challenge. Children presenting for MRI may have significant coexisting medical problems, including airway obstruction, a difficult airway, and sleep apnea. The MRI environment poses a unique set of constraints and potential risks. Therefore, a thoughtful and carefully implemented plan is essential to ensure safety and high-quality imaging.

LEARNING OBJECTIVES

1. Discuss the recognition and management of the difficult airway in the MRI environment.
2. Recognize the risks and challenges of using general anesthesia versus sedation for MRI.
3. Identify suitable sedative and anesthetic choices for children with obstructive sleep apnea presenting for MRI.

CASE PRESENTATION

A 3-year-old, 21-kg boy born at 32 weeks' gestation is scheduled for an MRI of the brain. The MRI is being done as part of the workup for recurrent seizures. **On pre-imaging evaluation**, the child's exam reveals **micrognathia** and a **cleft palate**. His mother reports that he "snores a lot" and seems to obstruct at night. A look through the medical records shows that the patient recently underwent an **overnight sleep study (polysomnography)**, which demonstrated a moderate degree of **obstructive sleep apnea** (OSA) with a minimum oxygen saturation of 86%. Upon inhalation induction with sevoflurane/nitrous oxide in oxygen, mask ventilation is difficult despite placement of an oral airway and the patient's oxygen saturation drops to 83%. Direct laryngoscopy is performed but no laryngeal strictures are seen and the boy desaturates rapidly. A laryngeal mask airway (LMA) is placed successfully and the boy is now adequately ventilated. Anesthesia is then maintained with oxygen/air/sevoflurane. At the end of the MRI scan, the LMA is removed in the MRI suite when the patient is **awake**. The patient recovers uneventfully and is discharged home.

He returns 6 months later for a follow-up MRI evaluation. This time, sedation is planned using **dexmedetomidine**. An intravenous catheter is inserted after inhalation of 70% nitrous oxide in oxygen. A **loading dose** of dexmedetomidine (2 mcg/kg over 10 minutes) is given. A significant increase in blood pressure and a decrease in heart rate are noticed after the loading dose. A dose of atropine (0.01 mg/kg) corrects the **bradycardia**. Sedation is maintained with a **dexmedetomidine infusion** (2 mcg/kg/hour). The patient breathes spontaneously throughout the scan, **upper airway patency** is aided by the placement of a **shoulder roll**, and supplemental oxygen is administered via nasal cannula. The minimum oxygen saturation recorded during imaging was 94%. At the completion of imaging, the dexmedetomidine infusion is discontinued and the patient recovers uneventfully.

DISCUSSION

1. What is the role of pre-imaging evaluation and why is it important?

Evaluation of children presenting for imaging studies is very similar to the evaluation of children requiring surgery. There are, however, special challenges relating to the off-site environment.

In the MRI environment, the powerful magnetic field constrains the type of anesthesia and monitoring equipment that can be used. Help in the case of an emergency may be less readily available than in the operating room environment. As in this case, it is especially important to carefully evaluate the airway prior to beginning anesthesia or sedation in the MRI environment. It may be prudent in some cases to start the anesthetic in the more controlled environment of the operating room, secure the airway with an endotracheal tube, and then transport the patient to radiology. The operating room provides a safe, secure, and familiar environment in which the anesthesiologist has access to emergency airway equipment and assistance from colleagues who can assist with airway management.

Most imaging studies require only immobilization and are not stimulating. Intubation is frequently not necessary. In a child with a difficult airway, avoiding instrumentation of the airway is a prudent course as long as emergency backup is immediately available. The child in this case did not have a prior procedure requiring intubation; his micrognathia was first recognized on the day of his MRI.

Evaluation of the pediatric airway can be challenging as the patient may be uncooperative and the history given by parents may be misleading. The **overnight polysomnography** provides clues to the severity of the airway obstruction during sleep by providing the lowest oxygen saturation observed, as well as the types of apnea (obstructive, central, or mixed) and the frequency of apnea events. During the second MRI study, a supplemental airway was not necessary. In all cases, it is critical to have MRI-compatible airway devices readily available in the event of an unanticipated airway emergency. Oral pharyngeal airways, nasal trumpets, and appropriate-size LMAs should be immediately available.

2. **General anesthesia versus sedation? The dilemma still exists.**
Anesthesiologists tend to prefer general anesthesia for diagnostic procedures, rather than sedation, because **general anesthesia** is regarded as safe, controllable, and relatively easy to perform.

One commonly used general anesthetic technique is an inhalation induction for placement of an intravenous line, which is then followed by a propofol infusion. Supplemental oxygen is provided with a nasal cannula. Placement of a shoulder roll and/or an oral airway is helpful in maintaining patency of the airway. If the airway remains obstructed, a LMA or endotracheal tube can then be placed.

In contrast, the effects of drugs commonly used for **sedation** are sometimes unpredictable. The literature suggests that sedation has a relatively high failure rate (15%) and can be associated with morbidity and, rarely, mortality (Malviya et al., 2000). However, the use of general anesthesia for diagnostic imaging has been viewed as costly, impractical, and inefficient. For some complex patients, especially those with a difficult airway, an anesthesiologist may provide the safest and most effective sedation or anesthesia necessary for the imaging studies. If it is deemed essential to secure the airway in a patient like this one, it may be prudent to have additional resources available and to begin the anesthetic in an operating room environment. If one chooses to use sedation without airway intervention to obtain the imaging study, then it is essential to choose a technique that will provide the desired immobility with minimal effects on the integrity of the airway.

MRI studies of the airway present additional challenges. These studies in patients with known airway obstruction are undertaken to examine airway dynamics while asleep and to determine the site and severity of the airway obstruction. To obtain effective imaging studies, the patient's airway is ideally not altered with airway adjuncts. As a result, airway obstruction and subsequent desaturation may well occur during the anesthesia and sedation for these children. To obtain optimal imaging, the anesthesiologist may need to tolerate some airway obstruction and oxygen desaturation. There is no consensus among anesthesiologists on when to interrupt airway imaging studies. Absolute lower limits of oxygen saturation below which artificial airway adjuncts are required may differ from patient to patient depending on the benefits to be gained from the imaging study and the severity of the patient's condition. In the case presented, review of the overnight polysomnography report, noting in particular the severity of oxygen desaturation during natural sleep, provided a guide to acceptable minimal arterial oxygen saturations. Prior to entertaining the question as to whether general anesthesia or sedation is preferred, it is critical to have an understanding of the requirements for completion of the imaging study planned. One can then match the needs for the procedure with the appropriate anesthetic or sedative agent for each patient on an individual basis.

3. What are the challenges associated with safely anesthetizing or sedating a child with a difficult airway and OSA?

Micrognathia in this child most likely contributed to his OSA. Maintaining the **patency of the upper airway** during spontaneous ventilation in sedated or anesthetized children with preexisting sleep-disordered breathing or airway obstruction is a major challenge for anesthesiologists. Anesthetic agents impair the ability of the upper airway muscles to overcome the negative pressures generated during inspiration, resulting in increased upper airway resistance and predisposing the patient to obstructive events, particularly in the retropalatal region. Children with significant OSA are sensitive to all sedative and anesthetic drugs. Upper airway obstruction and/or respiratory depression can occur even with minimal levels of sedation. Pharyngeal airway muscle tone is decreased during sleep; this reduction is even more pronounced during anesthesia or sedation, increasing the likelihood of upper airway obstruction leading to the development of hypoxia and hypercapnia. The genioglossus muscle is sensitive to sedatives and anesthetics, and reduced tone allows the tongue to fall back into an already unfavorable anatomic situation, worsening obstruction. These changes are accentuated in children with OSA, particularly with anesthetic or sedative drugs that exhibit strong respiratory depressant or airway relaxant effects.

4. **What are the suitable sedative and anesthetic choices for children with a difficult airway and OSA presenting for MRI of the airway?**

Sedatives and anesthetics commonly used in children for MRI studies include pentobarbital, propofol, benzodiazepines, ketamine, and dexmedetomidine. Propofol and barbiturates can exacerbate upper airway obstruction and increase the risk of respiratory depression and apnea. Benzodiazepines have relaxant effects on the pharyngeal musculature, causing a reduction of the pharyngeal space. In contrast, ketamine has been shown to preserve hypopharyngeal caliber in adults. A combination of ketamine and dexmedetomidine followed by a dexmedetomidine infusion has also been found to be effective in providing anesthesia without exacerbating respiratory problems during MRI in three children with Down syndrome and OSA (Luscri & Tobias, 2006). **Dexmedetomidine** is an alpha-2 adrenergic agonist with sedative, analgesic, and anxiolytic properties similar to clonidine. Because of its sedative and anxiolytic properties, dexmedetomidine has been shown to be a useful agent for pediatric procedural sedation. In contrast to other sedative agents, dexmedetomidine has been shown to have sedative properties that mimic natural sleep without significant respiratory depression. These advantages make dexmedetomidine an attractive agent for noninvasive procedural sedation in children. A recent retrospective study (Mahmoud et al., 2009) showed that children with OSA anesthetized with dexmedetomidine for MRI sleep studies experienced **fewer episodes of oxygen desaturation** and airway obstruction requiring **airway interventions** than those anesthetized with propofol. The advantages of dexmedetomidine appear particularly dramatic in children with more **severe OSA**.

5. **What side effects should be expected when using dexmedetomidine as a sole sedative agent?**

To use dexmedetomidine as a sole sedative agent for MRI sedation, higher doses are required, as shown in this case. Dexmedetomidine typically causes a decrease in the heart rate and an increase in blood pressure during the loading phase, followed by a decrease in blood pressure during the infusion phase due to a reduction in plasma catecholamine levels. Hemodynamic parameters return to baseline within 1 hour of stopping the infusion. Therefore, careful attention to hemodynamics is essential during administration of the **loading dose**. Dexmedetomidine causes peripheral α_2-receptor stimulation, leading to paradoxical vasoconstriction, transient hypertension, and profound **bradycardia**. Other reported side effects include sinus arrest and cardiac arrhythmias. Current understanding of the complete hemodynamic profile of dexmedetomidine, including its effects on pulmonary vascular resistance, remains incomplete. Dexmedetomidine has a half-life of about 2.5 hours, so full recovery may be delayed in some patients. As a result of its low potential for respiratory depression, dexmedetomidine is seeing widespread off-label use for pediatric sedation, even in children with congenital heart defects, in whom dexmedetomidine administration has been reported during imaging studies, cardiac surgery, and postoperative ICU recovery.

SUMMARY

1. Children scheduled for MRI imaging may have complex medical problems, including airway obstruction; thorough preoperative assessment is essential.
2. Sedation and general anesthesia can be safely used in the MRI suite, but both must be tailored to the individual patient.
3. In the case of a difficult airway, it may be wise to secure the airway in the operating room before proceeding to the MRI suite.
4. Sedation with dexmedetomidine for MRI sleep studies provides sedation that mimics natural sleep without

significant respiratory depression. Dexmedetomidine may be a better choice than propofol for children with significant OSA.

5. Dexmedetomidine can cause hypertension and bradycardia with the loading dose, following by a decrease in blood pressure during the infusion phase. Because of its low potential for respiratory depression, it is being used more commonly for pediatric sedation.

ANNOTATED REFERENCES

- Mahmoud M, Gunter J, Donnelly LF, Wang Y, Nick TG, Sadhasivam S. A comparison of dexmedetomidine with propofol for magnetic resonance imaging sleep studies in children. *Anesth Analg* 2009; 109(3): 745–753.

This article concludes that compared with propofol, dexmedetomidine has less effect on upper airway tone and airway collapsibility, provides more favorable conditions during dynamic MRI airway studies in children with OSA, and requires fewer scan interruptions and less aggressive airway interventions.

- Malviya S, Voepel-Lewis T, Eldevik OP, Rockwell DT, Wong JH, Tait AR. Sedation and general anaesthesia in children undergoing MRI and CT: adverse events and outcomes. *Br J Anaesth* 2000; 84(6): 743–748.

Quality assurance data were collected prospectively in this study for children who were sedated (n = 922) or given general anesthesia (n = 140) for MRI or CT. For preselected high-risk children, MRI scanning was more successful with general anesthesia than with sedation.

- Tobias JD. Dexmedetomidine: applications in pediatric critical care and pediatric anesthesiology. *Pediatr Crit Care Med* 2007; 8(2): 115–131.

This article provides a general descriptive account of the end-organ effects of dexmedetomidine and an evidence-based review of the literature regarding its use in infants and children. Table 3 in this article summarizes the use of dexmedetomidine for non-invasive procedural sedation.

Further Reading

Cravero JP, Beach ML, Blike GT, Gallagher SM, Hertzog JH. The incidence and nature of adverse events during pediatric sedation/anesthesia with propofol for procedures outside the operating room: a report from the Pediatric Sedation Research Consortium. *Anesth Analg* 2009; 108(3): 795–804.

Koroglu A, Demirbilek S, Teksan H, Sagir O, But AK, Ersoy MO. Sedative, haemodynamic and respiratory effects of dexmedetomidine in children undergoing magnetic resonance imaging examination: preliminary results. *Br J Anaesth* 2005; 94(6): 821–824.

Luscri L, Tobias J. Monitored anesthesia care with a combination of ketamine and dexmedetomidine during magnetic resonance imaging in three children with trisomy 21 and obstructive sleep apnea. *Pediatr Anesth* 2006; 16: 782–786.

Mason KP, Zurakowski D, Zgleszewski SE, Robson CD, Carrier M, Hickey PR, Dinardo J. High-dose dexmedetomidine as the sole sedative for pediatric MRI. *Pediatr Anesth* 2008; 18(5): 403–411.

11

Egg and Soy Allergies and Propofol Use

MICHAEL J. KIBELBEK AND LORI A. ARONSON

INTRODUCTION

Pediatric gastroenterologists are increasingly requesting the services of anesthesiologists for the comfort, safety, and peace of mind of their patients and their families. Although outpatient endoscopic procedures are usually brief, these patients often have histories of reflux, multiple drug and food allergies, and delayed gastric emptying.

LEARNING OBJECTIVES

1. Understand the significance of gastroesophageal reflux (GERD) in this population relative to anesthetic management.
2. Know the options for airway management during endoscopy.
3. Appreciate the significance of egg and soy allergy with propofol usage.

CASE PRESENTATION

*A 4-year-old, 14-kg girl presents for repeat surveillance upper endoscopy of her **eosinophilic esophagitis (EoE)** and **gastroesophageal*** *reflux disease (GERD)*. She has a history of **reactive airway disease** *and wheezing, treated with an albuterol (salbutamol) inhaler twice daily. Her last asthma exacerbation was 4 weeks ago, associated with an upper respiratory infection, and it was managed at home with frequent treatments of nebulized albuterol. She has had a previous uneventful anesthetic for endoscopy at another institution, but the records are not available. Since then, radioallergosorbent testing (RAST) has revealed* **allergies to penicillin, wheat, soy, and eggs**. *There is no significant family history. Her physical exam is unremarkable. She has fasted 10 hours after solids and 2 hours after apple juice.*

The patient receives nebulized albuterol before coming to the operating room, where she undergoes an uneventful inhalational induction with her parents present. A peripheral intravenous line is established, and pharyngeal **topical anesthesia** *is provided with* **2 mL of 1% lidocaine**. *The inhalation agent is discontinued and her anesthetic is deepened with 20 mg propofol while maintaining spontaneous respirations.* **Propofol is provided in intermittent boluses** *for maintenance anesthesia. During the procedure, supplemental oxygen is delivered at 2 L/min via nasal prongs. The procedure is completed without evidence of gastric reflux or wheezing. After removal of the endoscope and verification of spontaneous respirations and a patent airway, the patient proceeds to the recovery room.*

DISCUSSION

1. What is the significance of GERD to this anesthetic?
Although many pediatric GI patients are being evaluated for **GERD** or are already carrying this diagnosis, regurgitation during induction is a relatively rare event. In general, fasted children presenting for upper endoscopy have gastric volumes and pHs similar to those found in fasted children presenting for other surgeries. The standard pediatric NPO guidelines (8 hours solids, 6 hours milk or formula, 4 hours breast milk, 2 hours clears) appear to be effective in reducing passive regurgitation for GI endoscopy patients (see also chapter 7). It should be noted,

however, that children with esophageal dysmotility conditions, such as achalasia, may have very large volumes of food in their esophagus even with prolonged fasting.

2. Does the history of egg and soy allergy preclude the use of propofol?

GI patients frequently present with a history of multiple food intolerance and allergies. They may have been experiencing abdominal pain, vomiting, malabsorption, loose stools, or **eosinophilic esophagitis (EoE)**. Adverse immune reactions to various foods are thought to cause EoE through *delayed cell-mediated immunity*. Some children with EoE will also have a history of food allergy capable of producing histamine-mediated systemic reactions, including rash, urticaria, wheezing, and even anaphylaxis. GI exposure to food allergens in EoE patients and in others who have immune-mediated GI disorders causes changes in the GI mucosa resulting in vomiting, malabsorption, abdominal pain, or diarrhea. An empiric "six-food elimination diet," avoiding milk, **egg, soy, wheat**, shellfish, and nuts, allows improvement in about 75% of these children (Putnam & Rothenberg, 2009). Parents often report their child to be "allergic" to all foods on the elimination diet, and all foods identified by RAST or skin prick tests. Although foods associated with oral adverse immune reactions have the potential to re-produce esophageal disease, anaphylaxis to **propofol** is rare in EoE patients, even among patients who report being **egg** and **soy allergies**.

The anesthetic induction agent **propofol** is poorly soluble in water and must be formulated in an oil–water emulsion. Propofol's active ingredient, 2, 6-diisopropylphenol, is dissolved in an emulsion of highly purified soy oil identical to parenteral lipid infusion. Lecithin, a mixture of phosphatidylcholine and phosphatidylethanolamine, helps prevent the oil emulsion from separating into oil and water layers after manufacturing. The lecithin used is a highly purified extract of egg yolk. The lipid emulsion used in propofol contains 10% soy oil, 2.25% glycerol, and 1.2% egg yolk lecithin.

Patients who report allergy or intolerance to either egg or soy are almost always intolerant to the *egg* or *soy protein*, not egg yolk or soy oil. The manufacturing and purification processes remove all but trace amounts of soy protein and ovalbumin, the strongest allergens. Patients who develop anaphylaxis to soy protein may cross-react with other allergens in the legume family, especially peanuts; this is the genesis of the warnings in the various package inserts. The Diprovan® insert reads, "Diprovan Injectable Emulsion is contraindicated in patients with a known hypersensitivity to Diprovan Injectable Emulsion or its components. . ." In late 2009 and early 2010, the United States experienced a critical shortage of domestically produced propofol, necessitating importation of an alternate preparation, Propoven®. The package insert for Fresenius Propoven 1%®, manufactured in Italy, contains the following warning: "Fresenius Propoven 1% (propofol 1%) is contraindicated in patients who are allergic to soy or peanut." Personal communication with AAP Pharmaceuticals, LLC, the supplier of Propoven®, explains that this warns against the possibility of residual soy allergen in the soy oil. It is also theoretically possible for cross-contamination of the soy oil with residual peanut allergen to occur at the pressing plants, where processing equipment may have been used to press both soy and peanut oils, before it is purified. Reaction to soy allergen as a result of exposure to soy oil is rare. Both the U.S. Food Labeling and Consumer Protection Act of 2004 and the European Food Safety Authority exempt highly refined vegetable oils, including soy oil, from being explicitly listed as ingredients in food products. Instead, the manufacturers are permitted to include a listing of the different oils the product *may* contain.

The incidence of propofol anaphylaxis has been reported as 1 in 60,000, and it accounts for 1.2% to 2.1% of perioperative anaphylaxis cases in France, but the specific allergen in the propofol emulsion was not identified (Hepner & Castells, 2003). Propofol injectable emulsion has also been tested by skin prick and intradermal injection with negative results in adult, egg-allergic patients.

The literature has only very rare reports of allergic reactions to parenteral infusion of oil emulsion (Intralipid®). Our gastroenterology colleagues do not consider a history of egg or soy allergy to be a contraindication to the use of Intralipid® parenteral alimentation. Yet, propofol and parenteral Intralipid® differ only in the addition of the active ingredient. It seems that the recommendation for contraindication of soy lipid emulsion in egg- and soy-allergic patients occurs most strongly within the anesthesia community. Propofol should *not* be considered to be contraindicated in pediatric or adult patients with ingestible **egg or soy intolerance**.

3. Is intubation required for most upper endoscopy patients?

Endoscopies in adults are commonly performed under conscious sedation, relying upon **topical local anesthesia** of the esophagus and anxiolysis with benzodiazepine or propofol infusion. Pediatric endoscopies are often thought to require general anesthesia with endotracheal intubation for airway control. In a randomized controlled study of children ages 1 to 12 years, insufflation with sevoflurane during upper endoscopy was associated with a higher incidence of adverse airway events, including desaturation and laryngospasm, than patients who received sevoflurane via endotracheal tube (ETT) (Hoffman et al., 2010). Intubation was associated with more frequent complaints of sore throat. Therefore, they recommended endotracheal intubation over insufflation during upper endoscopy, especially in patients who are younger or obese or who have received midazolam premedication. However, the minimum alveolar concentration level required for intubation of the trachea and tolerance of the ETT likely exceeds the stimulation produced by the endoscope in the esophagus, with biopsies being essentially painless.

To improve patient comfort and facilitate turnover, many anesthesiologists choose not to intubate uncomplicated pediatric endoscopy patients aged 4 and older. In addition, tracheal instrumentation of patients with **reactive airways** may precipitate bronchospasm. The oropharynx of these patients is ordinarily large enough to accommodate the endoscope and still allow sufficient room for air exchange. An oral airway or a bite block will protect the scope from the patient's teeth and vice versa, given that many children are in the process of losing deciduous teeth. Several specifically designed products are available that allow the scope to pass through the center of the bite block rather than alongside it.

If necessary to improve the airway with a bite apparatus in place, a jaw lift will usually relieve a partial obstruction. Supplemental oxygen can be provided by **nasal prongs** directed into the nares or the mouth, with blow-by oxygen from a circuit directed toward the nose and mouth, or via a nasal trumpet with an ETT adapter inserted. Practically, airway patency often improves once the scope is inserted beyond the oropharynx. Anesthetic maintenance can then be maintained with volatile anesthetic insufflation (with caution, as noted above) or with total intravenous anesthesia (TIVA). When a longer or more involved endoscopic procedure is planned, it is preferable to secure the airway with an ETT. Some institutions use laryngeal mask airways (LMAs) to maintain the airway during upper endoscopy. This works very well, though the endoscopist has to become accustomed to the slightly greater resistance to passing the scope and the anesthesiologist must remain vigilant that the LMA is not dislodged.

Effective **topical anesthesia** of the oropharynx and the esophagus is beneficial to reduce the stimulation of scope insertion and to reduce the amount of anesthesia necessary to produce patient compliance. Patients old enough to be cooperative can gargle and swallow several milliliters of lidocaine (lignocaine) slurry (2% lidocaine mixed with a sweetener to reduce the bitter taste), or permit their oropharyx to be sprayed with topical anesthetic. Asking older patients to suck on two sodium benzonatate vesicles (Tessalon Perles®) 10 minutes before the procedure produces extremely effective anesthesia of the esophagus and oropharynx. Unfortunately, all effective topical oral anesthetic agents have a noxious, bitter, metallic taste, even the flavored ones. Younger patients may not be willing to cooperate with awake application of local anesthetic, due to the taste. The sticky, glutinous consistency of lidocaine jelly will cause many patients to gag when asked to swallow it, and is best avoided. Remember that flavored topical oral spray Hurricane® (prilocaine) can cause methemoglobinemia in infants and other susceptible patients.

Younger, noncooperative patients can be given a conventional inhalation induction. After IV access is achieved, 2 to 3 mL of **1% or 2% lidocaine** (both work equally well) is trickled into the oropharynx. Following a jaw thrust, the topical agent can be instilled behind the tongue. Next, the inhalation agent is discontinued and 20 seconds of spontaneous or controlled ventilation distributes the topical agent and usually permits the return of spontaneous ventilation. Before allowing the endoscopist to insert the scope, a 1- to 1.5-mg/kg **bolus of propofol** will keep the patient still while usually preserving spontaneous respirations. Additional similar **bolus** doses of **propofol** are given **intermittently** as necessary for the remainder of the procedure.

Upper endoscopy can be performed with the patient either supine or in the lateral decubitus position without compromising the airway, according to the preference of the endoscopist. Most diagnostic upper endoscopies take about 15 minutes or less. Ask the endoscopist to suction liquid stomach contents through the scope upon entering the stomach and before withdrawing the scope to remove insufflated air, if this is not his or her routine practice. These steps will aid patient comfort during recovery. Emergence is generally smooth and rapid, with discomfort limited to a sore throat from friction of the endoscope against the mucosa.

SUMMARY

1. Children who present with GI symptoms for GI endoscopy have gastric contents with similar volumes and

pHs compared to other children who fasted for similar times. Special precautions are rarely indicated for these patients with GERD.

2. Reports of egg and soy allergy are not contraindications to receiving propofol. Propofol may be used in patients with nonsystemic allergic reactions such as GI symptoms of food intolerance and positive skin and RAST tests.

3. Monitored anesthesia care/sedation with pharyngeal local anesthesia is an appropriate alternate technique to endotracheal intubation for routine diagnostic pediatric upper endoscopy. Endotracheal intubation for upper endoscopy is associated with fewer adverse respiratory events in young children and obese children and may be better for longer endoscopies.

ANNOTATED REFERENCES

- Furuta GT, Liacouras CA, Collins MH, Gupta SK, Justinich C, Putnam PE, Bonis P, Hassall E, Straumann A, Rothenberg ME. First International Gastrointestinal Eosinophil Research Symposium (FIGERS) Subcommittees. Eosinophilic esophagitis in children and adults: a systemic review and consensus recommendations for diagnosis and treatment. *Gastroenterology* 2007; 133: 1342–1363.

  An excellent review of the symptoms, pathophysiology, and treatment of EoE.
- Hepner DL, Castells MC. Anaphylaxis during the perioperative period. *Anesth Analg* 2003; 97: 1381–1395.

  This extensive review summarizes the literature experience with anaphylaxis from anesthetic and non-anesthetic drugs commonly given in the perioperative period.

Further Reading

Alalami AA, Ayoub CM, Baraka AW. Laryngospasm: review of different prevention and treatment modalities. *Pediatr Anesth* 2008; 18: 281–288.

Hefle S, Taylor S. "Refined soybean oil not an allergen, say food scientists." Accessed Oct. 13, 2010. http://www.foodnavigator-usa.com/Science-Nutrition/Refined-soybean-oil-not-an-allergen-say-food-scientists.

Hoffmann CO, Samuels PJ, Beckman E, Hein EA, Shackleford TM, Overbey E, Berlin RE, Wang Y, Nick TG, Gunter JB. Insufflation versus intubation during esophagogastroduodenoscopy in children. *Pediatr Anesth* 2010; 20(9): 821–830.

Package insert for Diprivan® 1% (Propofol), APP Pharmaceuticals, LLC, Revision, July 2009. (Includes discussion of Fresenius Propoven 1%).

Package insert for Diprivan® 1% (Propofol), Abraxis Pharmaceutical Products, Issued January 2007.

Putnam PE, Rothenberg ME. Eosinophilic esophagitis: concepts, controversies, and evidence. *Curr Gastroenterol Reports* 2009; 11: 220–225.

PART 3

CHALLENGES IN AIRWAY

MANAGEMENT

12

Obstructive Sleep Apnea

PETER SQUIRE

INTRODUCTION

Adenotonsillectomy has become first-line treatment for obstructive sleep apnea (OSA) and it is increasingly performed as a day-case procedure. A diagnosis of OSA increases the risk for postoperative respiratory morbidity from 1% to approximately 20% and unfortunately, the clinical history may be unreliable at distinguishing which children are at greatest risk. The gold standard investigation is overnight polysomnography (PSG), but this is a scarce resource considering the number of procedures performed. Fortunately, overnight home pulse oximetry also provides a useful stratification of severity and may predict postoperative problems. Children with OSA have a respiratory drive and airway tone that may be exquisitely sensitive to anesthetic and analgesic agents. Accordingly, the anesthesiologist needs to identify which patients are most at risk, and therefore which patients can be managed as "day cases," what is an appropriate anesthetic regimen, and how best to monitor these patients postoperatively.

LEARNING OBJECTIVES

1. Know how to assess the severity of obstructive sleep apnea and decide if ambulatory surgery is appropriate.
2. Know the anesthetic principles for and complications of adenotonsillectomy.

CASE PRESENTATION

*A 2-year-old boy is booked for adenotonsillectomy. His parents give a history that he has labored breathing with **snoring**, **pauses** in breathing, and "**heroic gasping**" at night. He is also noted to be very restless and occasionally sweaty. He is "slow to get going" in the morning, **struggles to keep up with his siblings** in the playground, and **routinely falls asleep** as a car passenger. His past history is otherwise unremarkable.*

*On examination he weighs only 11 kg and exhibits mouth breathing with hyponasal speech, and his SaO_2 is 96% on air. He has no added chest or cardiac sounds on auscultation. Results of the **polysomnogram (PSG)** demonstrate an SaO_2 nadir of 44%, an obstructive apnea hypopnea index (OAHI) of 35.4/hr, an REM respiratory disturbance index (REM RDI) of 80.5/hr, and an average transcutaneous CO_2 in total sleep time (TST) of 46.1 mmHg (with increase in average $TcCO_2$ in REM sleep of 11 mmHg).*

*Anesthesia is induced intravenously with propofol 50 mg and fentanyl 7.5 mcg after premedication with 220 mg oral acetaminophen (paracetamol). Immediate airway obstruction is noted on induction, though easy bag–mask ventilation can be performed with a Guedel airway. He is intubated with a size 4.5 RAE endotracheal tube (ETT) without muscle relaxants. 150 mL 0.9% saline is administered along with tramadol 20 mg, dexamethasone 2 mg, and granisetron 0.4 mg. Anesthesia is maintained with sevoflurane/oxygen/air. After proper positioning, the surgeon inserts a **Boyle-Davis gag, which is checked to ensure** no **ETT kinking**, and the child is allowed to breathe spontaneously with pressure support of 10 cmH_2O. Aliquots of **fentanyl** are **titrated** to keep the respiratory rate approximately 15–20 breaths min^{-1} and the ETCO$_2$ 40–50 mmHg. At the end of the procedure, a lubricated **nasal airway** is carefully inserted under vision by the surgeon, and then silk ties around the airway are taped to the face. After residual secretions are suctioned, the child is turned to the left lateral position and **extubated "deep."** The boy is taken to the post-anesthesia care unit (PACU) with oxygen and continuous positive airway pressure (CPAP) applied via mask. With no intensive care bed available, a* *longer stay in recovery is* arranged. *Arrangements are made for an overnight stay on the ward with pulse oximetry, "line-of-sight" nursing, and instructions regarding oxygen application, managing airway, and MET (medical emergency team) criteria.* **Analgesia** *is provided with regular acetaminophen q6h, and oxycodone syrup 0.1 mg/kg q4h prn. The first dose of oxycodone is given 1 hour prior to discharge from the PACU to observe for any effects on respiration. IV fluids (0.9% saline with 5% dextrose) are run at half-maintenance rate until adequate oral fluid intake. Metoclopramide serves as* **anti-emetic** *coverage when needed. Overnight, only two desaturations to 90% are noted during sleep; both are easily relieved by turning the boy to the left lateral position, applying oxygen, and mouth opening. The patient is discharged the next day.*

DISCUSSION

1. What is obstructive sleep apnea?

Obstructive sleep apnea (OSA) is a disorder of breathing during sleep characterized by prolonged partial upper airway obstruction and/or intermittent complete obstruction that disrupts normal ventilation. It is associated with symptoms of habitual **snoring** (with **pauses**, snorts, and "**gasps**"), daytime behavioral problems, **disturbed sleep**, and **daytime somnolence**. It may result in a significant degree of hypercarbia and hypoxemia leading to cognitive impairment, failure to thrive, dyspnea, systemic or pulmonary hypertension, and even death from cor pulmonale or arrhythmias.

OSA is distinguished from primary snoring, which is snoring without apnea, arousals, or gas-exchange abnormalities. OSA is a subset of sleep-disordered breathing: a spectrum of conditions that includes OSA, upper airway resistance syndrome and obstructive hypopnea. The peak in incidence between 2 and 6 years of age relates to when a physiological enlargement of tonsils and adenoids has occurred relative to the mid-facial skeleton (which significantly expands only from 6 years of age). Indeed, a susceptibility to OSA relates to the propensity for upper airway collapse, and in any given person this is determined by anatomic and neuromuscular factors influencing upper airway size and function. Accordingly, the condition has a wide spectrum of severity. There is an increased incidence among children with syndromes affecting their upper airway (mandibular hypoplasia in Treacher-Collins or Pierre-Robin; maxillary hypoplasia in Crouzon's, Apert's, or Pfeiffer's; relative macroglossia in Down syndrome) and among children of Asian or African origin. Neuromuscular conditions can also predispose to OSA due to reduced pharyngeal tone (Schwengel et al., 2009)

2. Which OSA patients need to be monitored in the hospital postoperatively, and where?

This much-discussed issue reflects concern that patients with more severe OSA are at greater risk of postoperative respiratory problems. It is preferable that patients identified as having severe OSA be referred to a tertiary hospital, but in practice, children with OSA respond variably to adenotonsillectomy, and it is difficult to know exactly which children need high-dependency units postoperatively, especially if there is no PSG or oximetry. Often how the patient behaves in the recovery room may well determine where the overnight stay should be.

It is reasonable to expect that a pediatric surgical ward should be equipped to monitor SaO_2 effectively and deliver supplemental oxygen and should be able to reposition the patient and summon assistance if necessary. If a ward cannot do this, then young OSA patients should be monitored in a high-dependency or intensive care facility. A well-secured **nasopharyngeal airway** is a sensible precaution in patients with moderate to severe OSA who are not sent to a high-dependency unit postoperatively.

Patients with mild or moderate OSA who have their surgery in smaller hospitals should be monitored with caution and should preferably have surgery scheduled in the morning. The rationale for this is that the onset of respiratory compromise may be delayed for several hours until a sleep pattern is achieved, and a morning procedure allows a greater period of postoperative observation in the presence of more medical staff.

When no PSG has been performed, then other clinical factors need to be taken into consideration before deciding on an appropriate place for surgery. Table 12.1 is by no means exhaustive but provides an outline of how to streamline the process and avoid overcrowded intensive care units and unnecessarily cancelled procedures. The anesthesiologist needs to remain flexible

---

Table 12.1

CLINICAL INDICATIONS FOR CONSIDERING WHEN AN INTENSIVE CARE UNIT OR A MONITORED WARD BED IS NEEDED AFTER ADENOTONSILLECTOMY

- Age <24 months
- Weight <3rd centile or morbid obesity
- Any significant neuromuscular disease (e.g., muscular dystrophies, myasthenia, myopathies, spinal cord disorders, mitochondrial and glycogen storage diseases; even severe cerebral palsy—may have associated central apnea)
- Genetic or chromosomal syndromes prone to airway obstruction; e.g.,:
  - Down syndrome
  - Pierre-Robin sequence and Treacher-Collins (mandibular hypoplasia)
  - Mucopolysaccharidoses (Hunter's, Hurler's)
  - Craniofacial syndromes (velocardiofacial, hemifacial microsomia, even major cleft palate repair)
  - Achondroplasia
- Complex or cyanotic congenital heart disease
- Cor pulmonale/right ventricular hypertrophy/pulmonary hypertension (especially if requiring oxygen therapy)
- Significant hematologic disorders/coagulopathies/factor deficiencies (risk of primary hemorrhage)
- Sickle cell disease
- Previous trauma or burns to airway/face/neck

in planning, as some patients deemed fit for a ward stay may actually cause unexpected problems. Severe obstruction at induction, copious nasal secretions, laryngospasm, or a need for CPAP in recovery are all risk factors for later obstructive events.

3. What are the anesthetic principles and management of adenotonsillectomy?

The airway: Anesthesia for adenotonsillectomy involves a *shared airway* with the surgeon. Intubation without muscle relaxants is straightforward up to the age of 8 to 9 years, or a weight of approximately 35 kg. Older children may require muscle relaxants to facilitate intubation. In older children some anesthetists will choose to use a laryngeal mask airway (LMA) and throat pack rather than a tracheal tube; this practice requires a cooperative surgeon and close vigilance to look for airway dislodgement. Always check airways for compliance after the **Boyle-Davis gag** has been applied as the ETT or LMA may be compressed. The RAE or "south-facing" ETT is ideally suited as it sits within the gag neatly.

Positioning for surgery usually necessitates a significant degree of *neck extension* by the surgeon. This needs to be considered in the preoperative assessment of the child, especially in conditions such as achondroplasia, Morquio's syndrome, Klippel-Feil, possibly Down syndrome, or any disease process involving fused cervical vertebrae, atlanto-axial instability, or surrounding soft tissue deposition (for example, the mucopolysaccharidoses). In these cases, it is appropriate to use less neck extension.

Analgesia: Adenotonsillectomy is a painful procedure, and provision of adequate **analgesia** is essential. However, excessive doses of opiates may precipitate postoperative hypoventilation and airway obstruction in OSA patients, especially in young toddlers. Young patients with significant OSA do not have large opiate requirements, and one approach to administering opiates is to carefully titrate fentanyl to their respiratory rate intraoperatively. In older patients morphine is more suitable but harder to titrate given its longer time to peak effect. A dose of oral oxycodone can be given in the PACU and a period of observation allowed prior to discharge to ward or home. Careful titration is the key, and if airway problems postoperatively are thought to be due to the opiate, then naloxone should be considered.

Acetaminophen (paracetamol) (15–20 mg/kg) should be used regularly if not contraindicated. NSAIDs are excellent analgesics, but their use after adenotonsillectomy remains controversial as a possible risk factor for secondary bleeding. Parecoxib or other COX-2 inhibitors have minimal antiplatelet effect and would appear ideally suited as a single dose, where available. Ketamine may also be used in OSA children. A low dose (0.1–0.2 mg/kg) provides added intraoperative analgesia but is not sufficient by itself. Ketamine's respiratory-sparing effect makes it attractive; however, accumulated dosing may still cause some hypoventilation, sedation, and possibly nausea. Tramadol can be a useful adjunct, though the intravenous form is not universally available. Clonidine is occasionally used in school-age children with mild to moderate OSA as it provides a degree of sedation without hypoventilation and has some analgesic effect. It may also help avoid "emergence delirium."

Bupivacaine or ropivacaine injection into the tonsillar fossae may be performed by the surgeon and has variable effectiveness in reducing pain and enabling early oral intake of fluids. Dilute epinephrine (adrenaline) added to the local anesthetic reduces bleeding. Great care must be taken to avoid intravascular injection.

Provision of soothing, cold "icy poles" to suck in recovery can reduce discomfort, and most PACUs in pediatric hospitals have a supply.

Antiemetics: **Antiemetics** are prescribed routinely for most patients. Adenotonsillectomy is one of the most emetogenic of procedures, with an incidence of vomiting up to 70% when no anti-emetic is used. Low-dose dexamethasone (0.125 mg/kg) and a 5-HT$_3$ antagonist are efficacious. Blood in the stomach is a potent cause of vomiting, and often the patient will vomit once postoperatively despite anti-emetics. Ongoing nausea and vomiting warrants the use of another agent such as droperidol, metoclopramide, or promethazine. IV fluids should be continued until there is an adequate oral intake. Hypotonic solutions should be avoided as pain, nausea, opiates, and NSAIDs are all associated with an increased risk of hyponatremia.

Preventing airway complications: Overall, safe management of the airway is the most important principle of adenotonsillectomy. Aspiration is a rare but potential hazard of any airway surgery. It may occur during the procedure but is more a problem in the post-extubation period if there is ongoing ooze from the tonsillar bed and the patient remains excessively sedated. For this reason laryngospasm is also not uncommon after adenotonsillectomy. Patients scheduled for adenotonsillectomy often have concurrent upper respiratory tract infections or hypersalivation, or may have muscle hypotonia related to an underlying medical condition. Some would argue that the risk of aspiration or laryngospasm necessitates extubating patients only when awake, but this may increase the risk of coughing and hence bleeding; thus, many prefer a **"deep" extubation** in the lateral position. Extubating deep relies on an experienced PACU and readily available equipment to recognize and manage airway problems. Choice of anesthetic agent may have some influence on laryngospasm, with sevoflurane being the most popular of the shorter-acting volatiles. Desflurane's potential for airway reactivity discourages some practitioners. Nitrous oxide has lost popularity owing to emetogenesis and environmental concerns. Use of intravenous anesthesia with a propofol infusion and concurrent spontaneous ventilation of 50% N_2O in oxygen may well be a good choice of anesthetic maintenance for these patients as it provides the anti-emetic and pleasant emergence profile of propofol, avoids volatile agents as a source of airway irritation.

Postoperative care: The postoperative environment must be well equipped and staffed to manage the airway in children. Mode of analgesia should consider the risk of respiratory depression versus desirability of a relaxed, comfortable patient who is able to tolerate swallowing liquid. Appropriate prescription of analgesics prior to discharge is vital as these patients often have significant discomfort for up to 2 weeks postoperatively. Bleeding after tonsillectomy ranges from minimal to torrential and is often delayed; further discussion can be found in Chapter 15.

ANNOTATED REFERENCES

- Brown KA, Laferriere A, Lakheeram I. **Recurrent hypoxemia in children is associated with increased analgesic sensitivity to opiates.** *Anesthesiology* 2006; 105: 665–669.
  A good study highlighting the anesthetic principle that titration of opiates is prudent.
- Nixon GM, Kermack AS, McGregor CD, Davis GM, Manoukian JJ, Brown KA, Brouillette RT. **Sleep and breathing on the first night after adenotonsillectomy for obstructive sleep apnea.** *Pediatr Pulmonol* 2005; 39: 332–338.
  Emphasizes that the preoperative SaO_2 nadir is an important and inexpensive way to predict which cases may be problematic.
- Schwengel DA, Sterni LM, Tunkel DE, Heitmiller ES. **Perioperative management of children with obstructive sleep apnea.** *Anesth Analg* 2009; 109: 60–75.
  Excellent and up-to-date review article on diagnosis of OSA, components of polysomnography, and strategies for postoperative care.

Further Reading

Walker P, Whitehead B, Rowley M. Criteria for elective admission to the paediatric intensive care unit following adenotonsillectomy for severe obstructive sleep apnoea. *Anaesth Intens Care* 2004; 32: 43–46.

13

Foreign Body in the Airway

VIDYA CHIDAMBARAN AND
SENTHILKUMAR SADHASIVAM

INTRODUCTION

Airway foreign body aspiration is associated with significant airway distress that can lead to morbidity and mortality, especially in young children. Children who inhale a foreign body into the airway and require bronchoscopy under general anesthesia present the anesthetist with some of the most difficult and demanding cases in pediatric anesthesia.

LEARNING OBJECTIVES

1. Know how to recognize and evaluate a foreign body in the airway.
2. Learn the anesthetic management for rigid bronchoscopy, including pros and cons of controlled versus spontaneous ventilation, and likely perioperative airway complications.
3. Describe the postoperative management of children after airway body removal and what problems to anticipate.

CASE PRESENTATION

*A healthy, 11-kg 2-year-old girl with **suspected foreign body aspiration** presents for diagnostic and therapeutic rigid bronchoscopy.*

She was playing with her doll yesterday and suddenly started choking and had transient cyanosis. This morning, the child develops a **fever** and a **croupy cough** and has intermittent **stridor**. Although a chest x-ray shows no foreign body, the patient has inspiratory stridor, suprasternal and intercostal retractions, and an oxygen requirement. ENT is consulted and schedules her for urgent rigid bronchoscopy. On arrival in the operating room, an IV is placed, **glycopyrrolate** is given, and inhalation induction with sevoflurane begins, maintaining **spontaneous ventilation**. During the prolonged inhalation induction, the airway becomes more obstructed and the oxygen saturation falls into the 80s. As soon as the surgeon inserts the bronchoscope to see if the larynx is obstructed, the child coughs, her partial obstruction becomes complete, and the saturation falls to the 50s. The surgeon sees something yellow in the airway beyond the vocal cords but is not able to intubate the trachea. With the rigid bronchoscope, he pushes the object deeper into the right main bronchus. The patient is bradycardic with a heart rate of 40 due to hypoxia, which is treated immediately with atropine 0.2 mg IV. With the foreign body pushed into the right main bronchus, a 3.5 endotracheal tube (ETT) is passed through the cords. Chest movement and breath sounds are heard on the left side only. With positive-pressure ventilation and deepening of anesthesia with propofol, her saturations improve to 91% and her heart rate increases to 120. The surgeon then removes the ETT, sprays her vocal cords and trachea with 1 mL of 4% lidocaine, and inserts a rigid ventilating bronchoscope. The patient is ventilated by connecting the anesthesia circuit to the side port of the ventilating bronchoscope and a propofol infusion is started. The surgeon is now able to remove the foreign body, a bead, from the right bronchus through the vocal cords. Another look with the rigid bronchoscope reveals modest **airway edema**, which is treated with dexamethasone 4 mg IV. On awakening with a mask airway in the operating room, the patient has mild stridor. In the post-anesthesia care unit (PACU), she is given nebulized **racemic epinephrine** (adrenaline) with good effect before being transferred to the ward for overnight observation.

DISCUSSION

1 How does one recognize and evaluate a foreign body in the airway?

The presenting symptoms of **foreign body aspiration** vary depending on the location of the foreign body, the degree of obstruction, and the duration of the aspiration. Common symptoms include those seen in this case—**cough, dyspnea, and stridor**—as well as *wheezing, fever,* and *pneumonia.* The severity of symptoms may vary from a mild cough to severe respiratory distress. A high degree of suspicion is warranted, especially in young children from 1 to 3 years of age. Findings on physical examination may also vary considerably, from a normal chest exam to decreased breath sounds, wheezing, and rales in the case of pneumonia. Inspiratory and expiratory chest radiographs as well as AP and lateral airway films are usually performed. Since the majority of aspirated foreign bodies are radiolucent (e.g., organic materials such as food), a third of children will have a *normal radiograph.* Lateral decubitus chest films are helpful in the diagnosis of foreign bodies in the lower airway in young children who cannot cooperate for expiratory films. With a lateral decubitus film in a normal child, the mediastinum shifts to the down side. In the case of a foreign body in the right main bronchus, for example, a right lateral decubitus film would show no shift of the mediastinum to the right and would show persistent hyperinflation of the right lung. The history and physical examination cannot exclude the suspicion of an aspirated foreign body, and because radiographic findings may be normal, the diagnosis relies on bronchoscopy. A positive history and clinical symptoms are sufficient to justify bronchoscopy for the diagnosis and retrieval of an airway foreign body.

Peanuts are especially hazardous because they cause *profound inflammation* and *edema* of the airway, necessitating urgent removal. Vegetable matter expands with moisture and may fragment into multiple pieces, making its removal more difficult.

Esophageal foreign bodies, often associated with drooling and dysphagia, may mimic airway foreign bodies by compressing the posterior membranous trachea. Of note, irregularly shaped or sharp esophageal foreign bodies pose a risk for puncturing the posterior trachea and represent a contraindication to cricoid pressure. Ingested disc batteries must be removed promptly to avoid tissue necrosis from sodium hydroxide produced by a local current generated by the battery.

2. What are the principles of anesthetic management for a child with an airway foreign body?

Preoperative assessment of the child's condition, including a review of the radiographs, is important. Discussion with the surgeon about the approach and backup plans cannot be overemphasized. Other preoperative considerations are (1) cautious premedication to avoid worsening airway obstruction, (2) intravenous **anticholinergic** administration (such as the **glycopyrrolate** given here) to decrease secretions and prevent reflex bradycardia during airway instrumentation, and (3) assessment of the risk for aspiration of gastric contents (Fig. 13.1).

Unless the child is moribund, general anesthesia is usually necessary for removal of an airway foreign body. Important factors to consider are (1) the patient's condition (airway, respiratory, and fasting status), (2) size, location, and effects of the foreign body on the airway, and (3) surgical technique. Removal of a foreign body may necessitate laryngoscopy, bronchoscopy, thoracoscopy, thoracotomy, or even a tracheotomy. The following discussion will focus on rigid bronchoscopy, which is the most commonly employed technique.

A peripheral intravenous catheter should be placed prior to bringing the child to the operating room. The surgeon should be present for the induction of anesthesia and should be prepared to address acute airway obstruction. Anesthetic priorities include:

1) Safe sharing of the airway with the endoscopist while maintaining the airway and the ability to ventilate, administering 100% oxygen
2) Adequate depth of anesthesia, use of topical lidocaine on the airway, and judicious doses of opioids such as fentanyl during the procedure to blunt airway reflexes

Condition of the child	Stable Child		Child in respiratory distress	
NPO Status	Ideally fasted	Fasted		Full Stomach
Location/ Degree of Obstruction	Esophageal/Lower airway FB	Upper airway FB or Risk for airway obstruction supersedes aspiration risk		Risk for aspiration more than airway obstruction
Induction/ Intubation	IV/Inhalation Usually intubate for esophageal FB	Inhalation If airway obstruction becomes total, surgeon should try to remove FB or push it distally		Consider RSI first, then bronchoscopy

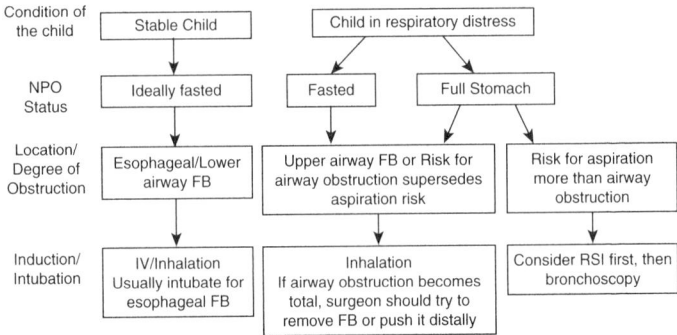

FIGURE 13.1 Anesthetic management options for bronchoscopy for foreign body removal. FB, foreign body; RSI, rapid-sequence induction.

3) Use of steroids to prevent airway **edema**
4) Prevention of pulmonary aspiration. If the patient has a full stomach and immediate bronchoscopy is indicated, consider rapid-sequence induction, immediate intubation, and gastric suctioning. The rigid bronchoscope is then inserted as the endotracheal tube is withdrawn.
5) Meticulous monitoring of the electrocardiogram (ECG), oxygen saturation, end-tidal carbon dioxide, and blood pressure

Ventilation can be effectively provided through the side port of the ventilating bronchoscope. Maintenance of anesthesia can be accomplished with an inhalation technique with supplemental boluses of propofol as needed or a total intravenous anesthesia (TIVA) technique. TIVA provides an uninterrupted anesthetic even in cases of severe airway obstruction and inadequate ventilation and also decreases OR pollution, which occurs through the open proximal port of the bronchoscope.

3. Is spontaneous or controlled ventilation preferred?
It is controversial whether **spontaneous** or controlled ventilation is superior for the maintenance of anesthesia (Table 13.1).

Table 13.1

CONTROLLED VERSUS SPONTANEOUS VENTILATION FOR FOREIGN BODY REMOVAL

Spontaneous Ventilation	*Controlled Ventilation*
Advantages	**Advantages**
1. More effective ventilation as there is less pressure drop across obstruction	1. Patient immobility ensured, especially if using muscle relaxants
2. Ability to ventilate sustained even when proximal port of scope open	2. Quicker emergence with use of short-acting muscle relaxants as less need for anesthetic agents
3. Less air trapping	
4. Less risk for pushing foreign body distally	
PATIENT ALWAYS BREATHING!	
Disadvantages	**Disadvantages**
1. Prolonged emergence due to high concentrations of inhalation agent needed for depth of anesthesia	1. Air trapping due to stacking of breaths
2. Hypercarbia due to low minute ventilation	2. Increased risk of pushing foreign body distally
	3. Inability to ventilate with the proximal port of the bronchoscope open
	4. Risk of converting a compromised airway to "no airway"

Source: Holzman RS, Mancuso TJ. Point Counterpoint: Spontaneous vs. controlled ventilation for suspected airway foreign body. *Soc Pediatr Anesth Newsletter* 2001; 14(3).

While **spontaneous ventilation** has definite theoretical advantages, assisted ventilation often becomes necessary to prevent hypoxia and hypercarbia.

4. What postoperative complications can occur? How should they be treated?

The postoperative course can be associated with various complications related to the procedure, the anesthesia, and the effects of the foreign body having been in the airway. Manipulation of the airway can cause airway bleeding and swelling, resulting in postoperative stridor. **Steroids** are beneficial in preventing post-extubation stridor, due to anti-inflammatory actions that inhibit the release of inflammatory mediators and decrease capillary permeability. Doses vary from four to six doses of dexamethasone (0.25–0.5 mg/kg) given every 6 to 8 hours. The risk of harm from steroid therapy for 24 hours is negligble. **Racemic epinephrine**, a mixture of the D and L isomers of epinephrine, is also used to treat **airway edema**. The alpha-adrenergic effects of racemic epinephrine mediate mucosal vasoconstriction and its beta effects produce smooth muscle relaxation as well as inhibition of mast cell-mediated inflammation. **Racemic epinephrine** 2.25% in 2 mL normal saline can be used in a dose of 0.25, 0.5, and 0.75 mL for a child weighing 0 to 20, 20 to 40, and >40 kg respectively. It has a peak effect in 30 minutes and lasts for 2 hours. ECG monitoring should be used as arrhythmias and myocardial infarction have been reported in children after repeated doses of **racemic epinephrine**. Treatment may cause rebound upper **airway edema**, which usually occurs within 2 hours, and therefore close monitoring is essential for 2 hours after the administration of racemic epinephrine. The child can be discharged if free of resting stridor and otherwise stable at the end of the observation period. Sometimes, postoperative intubation may be required to rest the airway and allow the swelling to subside before extubation.

Other possible complications include pulmonary aspiration, pulmonary edema due to sudden relief of airway obstruction, pneumothorax due to barotrauma from ventilation or mechanical trauma from the procedure, and post-obstructive pneumonia. A chest x-ray is usually taken postoperatively as a routine to rule out these problems.

SUMMARY

1. Recognize the degree, site, type, and duration of airway obstruction preoperatively. Develop a coordinated plan with the surgeon.
2. Expect a slow and prolonged inhalation induction, and maintain spontaneous ventilation until confirmation of the ability to ventilate.
3. Maintain deep planes of anesthesia with minimal airway reflexes via inhalation or intravenous anesthetic technique. Topical lidocaine is important.
4. In case of total airway obstruction due to a tracheal foreign body and difficult removal, the object could be pushed deeper into one of the main bronchi for temporary relief.
5. Postoperative steroids, racemic epinephrine, and intubation/ventilation may be necessary. Obtain a chest x-ray postoperatively.

ANNOTATED REFERENCES

- Holzman RS, Mancuso TJ. Point Counterpoint: Spontaneous vs. controlled ventilation for suspected airway foreign body. *Soc Pediatr Anesth Newsletter* 2001; 14(3).
  Detailed review of pros and cons of spontaneous versus controlled ventilation for maintenance of anesthesia during bronchoscopic removal of airway foreign body in children.
- Kain ZN, O'Connor TZ, Berde CB. Management of tracheobronchial and esophageal foreign bodies in children: a survey study. *J Clin Anesth* 1994; 6(1): 28–32.
  A survey of anesthetic management of airway foreign bodies that showed that practice type, greater percentage of time spent

in pediatric anesthesia, and greater experience are related to a higher likelihood of inhalation induction.

- **Zur KB, Litman RS. Pediatric airway foreign body retrieval: surgical and anesthetic perspectives.** *Pediatr Anesth* **2009; 19 (Suppl 1): 109–117.**

  A comprehensive review of the practical aspects of anesthetic management of foreign bodies in the airway in children.

Further Reading

Chatterji S, Chatterji P. The management of foreign bodies in air passages. *Anaesthesia* 1972; 27(4): 390–395.

Eren S, Balci AE, Dikici B, Doblan M, Eren MN. Foreign body aspiration in children: experience of 1160 cases. *Ann Trop Paediatr* 2003; 23(1): 31–37.

Fidowski CW, Zheng H, Firth PG. The anesthetic considerations of tracheobronchial foreign bodies in children: a literature review of 12,979 cases. *Anesth Analg* 2010; 111: 1016–1025.

Holzman R. Prevention and treatment of life-threatening pediatric emergencies requiring anesthesia. *Semin Anesthesia Periop Med Pain* 1998; 17: 154–163.

Markovitz BP, Randolph AG. Corticosteroids for the prevention of reintubation and postextubation stridor in pediatric patients: A meta-analysis. *Pediatr Crit Care Med* 2002; 3(3): 223–226.

Matsuse H, Shimoda T, Kawano T, Fukushima C, Mitsuta K, Obase Y, Tomari S, Saeki S, Kohno S. Airway foreign body with clinical features mimicking bronchial asthma. *Respiration* 2001; 68(1): 103–105.

Pahade A, Green KM, de Carpentier JP. Non-cardiogenic pulmonary oedema due to foreign body aspiration. *J Laryngol Otol* 1999; 113(12): 1119–1121.

Vardhan V, Singh M, Reddy S, et al. Airway foreign body in pediatric patient: a fishy experience. *J Cardiothorac Vasc Anesth* 2005; 19(1): 90–92.

14

Laryngospasm

KENNETH R. GOLDSCHNEIDER AND
ERIC P. WITTKUGEL

INTRODUCTION

Laryngospasm is one of the most common complications of anesthesia in children. If not recognized immediately and treated promptly, laryngospasm may progress to complete airway obstruction with subsequent hypoxia, hypercarbia, bradycardia, and cardiac arrest. All anesthesiologists who anesthetize children must have a good understanding of when it can occur and how it is managed.

LEARNING OBJECTIVES

1. Know the risk factors for laryngospasm.
2. Identify how laryngospasm presents.
3. Understand how to manage and prevent laryngospasm.

CASE PRESENTATION

A healthy 3-year-old girl presents for adenotonsillectomy (T+A). Both **parents smoke** *cigarettes. The prior several days, the patient had a bit of a* **runny nose** *and a* **mild morning cough***, which has resolved. She presents with a normal examination. She is anxious and cries during inhalational induction with oxygen, nitrous oxide, and sevoflurane. About 60 seconds into the induction, the nurse places a blood pressure* *cuff and pulse oximeter and begins to look for IV access. The little girl begins to have* **rocking chest movements** *and* **no bag movement or mask fogging** *is seen. Despite a chin lift and jaw thrust with a good mask fit, the airway remains obstructed. An oral airway is placed and* **continuous positive airway pressure (CPAP)** *is administered with 8% sevoflurane and 100% oxygen. The child begins to desaturate and the airway is suctioned for a moderate amount of clear mucus.* **High-pitched inspiratory stridor** *is now heard, and her oxygenation begins to stabilize and then improve. After securing an IV and deepening the anesthetic, the patient is intubated without difficulty. Anesthesia is maintained with oxygen/nitrous oxide/desflurane, supplemented with morphine, dexamethasone, and ondansetron.*

After the surgeon confirms that the airway is free of blood, the patient is extubated asleep with spontaneous respirations (deep extubation). As the patient is being transported to the recovery room, **stridor**, *followed by silence and rocking chest movements, is noted. CPAP is applied without benefit and the child becomes slightly cyanotic. Upon arrival to the PACU, propofol 1 mg/kg is administered with good results. As the propofol wears off, the stridor recurs. This time,* **lidocaine (lignocaine)** *1.5 mg/kg is administered through the IV, but before the dose has reached the patient, the IV becomes dislodged. Now the patient begins to desaturate. As a dose of succinylcholine (suxamethonium) is prepared, a jaw thrust is applied, adding pressure against the* **styloid processes** *bilaterally. The succinylcholine is administered via sublingual injection and another IV is placed. As the patient begins to have air exchange, the heart rate drops precipitously. A dose of atropine 0.01 mg/kg is given intravenously with resolution of the* **bradycardia**. *Her airway is suctioned for a small amount of blood and she recovers uneventfully from that point and is discharged home.*

DISCUSSION

1. What are the risk factors for laryngospasm?
Multiple risk factors for perioperative respiratory complications in children have been identified (Flick et al., 2008). Risks factors

that increase the incidence of laryngospasm in particular include exposure to secondhand smoke at home, asthma, atopy, young age, and airway surgery. An upper respiratory infection also increases the risk for laryngospasm, especially if the symptoms have been present within the previous 2 weeks. This child had a **cough** that is present mostly in the **morning**, suggesting postnasal drip etiology rather than a lower respiratory etiology. Other risk factors to consider are seen in Table 14.1.

2. What is the significance of stridor?

Stridor is the **high-pitched inspiratory sound** that results from incomplete closure of the vocal cords, partial closure of the arytenoids, or both. In this case, it can be a sign of **partial laryngospasm** or a sign of resolving laryngospasm, depending on the context. If a patient begins to have stridor on induction, the initial response is to ensure a patent airway with anterior displacement of the mandible, deepen the anesthetic, and apply positive

---

Table 14.1

LARYNGOSPASM RISK FACTORS

Young age

Recent upper respiratory infection

Asthma

Parental smoking history

Airway surgery, operations associated with bleeding in the airway -T+A, nasal surgery, palate surgery

Inhalational induction, deep intubation without use of muscle relaxants, deep extubation

Light plane of anesthesia

Strong family history of asthma and atopy

Gastroesophageal reflux

"Choking" episodes at home when sleeping

Elongated uvula

LMA

---

pressure. The insertion of an oropharyngeal airway should not be performed, as there is potential to irritate the periglottic area and turn a partial laryngospasm into **complete laryngospasm**. Administering positive-pressure ventilation may also be stimulating and force any secretions or blood in the hypopharynx further down onto the glottis. At this point in a laryngospasm episode, it is best not to stimulate or move the patient. Instead of touching the patient, assistants ensure that IV lines and medications are ready and assist as directed. In most cases, the combination of CPAP, oxygen, and higher concentrations of inhaled anesthetic will break the laryngospasm episode. If secretions are heard or suspected in the oropharynx (mucus from an upper respiratory infection, tears from crying, or blood from intraoral/pharyngeal procedures), then gentle suction can relieve the glottic stimulation. Stridor is a sign that the airway is partially compromised and the patient is vulnerable to worsening airway compromise; it indicates a time to be gentle in handling the airway.

If stridor disappears and there is no air movement, complete laryngospasm has occurred. Signs of complete airway obstruction include rocking chest wall motion, retractions, tracheal tug, loss of the capnography trace, and no movement of the anesthesia bag. While breath holding can look like laryngospasm, the absence of respiratory effort in the former differentiates the two.

3. What measures can be taken to prevent laryngospasm?
Prevention is the best treatment for laryngospasm (Table 14.2). High-risk patients must be managed expectantly, especially if they are undergoing airway surgery.

4. What are effective measures to treat laryngospasm?
Immediate recognition and intervention are required to prevent the progression of laryngospasm to complete airway obstruction with the development of hypoxemia, hypercarbia, bradycardia, and cardiac arrest (Table 14.3). Five out of 1,000 patients who

---

Table 14.2

MEASURES TO PREVENT LARYNGOSPASM

- Avoid stimulation of the airway and surgical stimulation while the patient is lightly anesthetized.
- Apply topical lidocaine to the larynx prior to intubation, or give intravenous lidocaine shortly before extubation.
- Suction the airway for secretions and blood.
- Prior to extubation, give 100% oxygen to provide a margin of safety
- Hold the breathing bag at full inspiration with positive pressure of 15 to 20 cmH$_2$O as the trachea is extubated.
- Extubate the patient once fully awake rather than while still asleep.

---

develop laryngospasm have a cardiac arrest (Olsson & Hallen, 1998).

Once an episode begins, a determination needs to be made to whether it is a **partial or complete obstruction**. If stridor is heard (partial laryngospasm), then the following approach should be taken: appropriate monitoring with pulse oximetry and ECG, delivery of 100% oxygen and positive pressure via a tightly fitting face mask, anterior mandible displacement, suctioning the airway to clear blood and secretions, and applying continuous positive airway pressure (CPAP). On inspiration, there is often a brief moment of relaxation of the larynx during which a firm squeeze on the bag in phase with inspiration promotes continued oxygenation and resolution of the laryngospasm. Further, distending the hypopharynx is a basic step in relieving an obstructed airway and can help ensure that there is no soft tissue upper airway obstruction in addition to the laryngospasm. While high levels of CPAP may be necessary, avoid excessive pressure that can cause gastric distention and subsequent compromise of ventilation and possible regurgitation. If the stomach becomes distended, the stomach should be suctioned after the laryngospasm

---

Table 14.3

APPROACH TO LARYNGOSPASM

Signs

Incomplete laryngospasm: Reduced air movement
- Stridor
- Decreased movement of the anesthesia bag
- Retractions, rocking or paradoxical chest wall motion
Complete laryngospasm: No air movement
- No stridor, no breath sounds
- No bag movement
- No $ETCO_2$

Treatment

Incomplete laryngospasm:
- Optimize airway position (head tilt, jaw thrust, good mask seal)
- 100% oxygen, CPAP
- Minimize stimulation
- Deepen anesthetic
- Suction airway if needed
Complete laryngospasm, or partial with decompensation:
- Start as for incomplete spasm
- "Laryngospasm notch pressure," "flutter the bag"
- IV present: Atropine, succinylcholine, or propofol
- No IV: Intramuscular or sublingual succinylcholine and atropine
- Intubate as needed

---

is resolved. Since laryngospasm occurs in a light plane of anesthesia, it can be effectively treated by deepening the anesthetic or awakening the patient, depending on whether the spasm occurs during induction, maintenance, or emergence.

Another useful technique of treating laryngospasm is called "fluttering the bag," in which the anesthesia bag is squeezed and released very rapidly in a staccato rhythm. Larson (1998) describes an interesting technique of very firm pressure on the "laryngospasm notch" located just behind and below both ears, pressing very firmly toward the base of the skull with both fingers while at the same time lifting the mandible forward.

If laryngospasm is complete, the interventions mentioned above should be taken but may not improve the airway obstruction. It is important to call for help early on and to begin aggressive intervention immediately. When the laryngospasm persists, the prompt administration of succinylcholine is indicated. Atropine (10 mcg/kg) should be given prior to succinylcholine to prevent **bradycardia**. Both drugs can be given intravenously, intramuscularly, or sublingually if no venous access is available. Intravenous doses of succinylcholine range from 0.1 to 2 mg/kg. Smaller doses can break the spasm, while larger doses are given if emergency intubation is needed. The dose of intramuscular atropine is 20 mcg/kg and the dose of intramuscular succinylcholine is 4 mg/kg. Do not delay the administration of succinylcholine by looking for venous access. Once bradycardia occurs, the onset of drug effect is prolonged and effective treatment is delayed. If intravenous access is present when laryngospasm occurs, propofol 0.5 to 2 mg/kg can be given instead of succinylcholine.

If after all these measures the airway has not been secured, cricothyrotomy or emergent tracheostomy may be required. Negative-pressure pulmonary edema has been associated with laryngospasm. The large negative intrapleural pressure generated in an attempt to overcome the airway obstruction may lead to pulmonary edema (Lee & Downes, 1983).

5. What could have been done differently to prevent the laryngospasm episodes?

The age of the child and the need for T+A, while important risk factors, are not modifiable ones. Postponing surgery for 2 weeks after upper respiratory infection symptoms resolve could be considered. Parental smoking is unlikely to be altered within an effective time frame. Anesthetic factors are the major, controllable variables for the anesthesiologist. Of the inhalational anesthetics, desflurane and isoflurane are associated more strongly with laryngospasm than sevoflurane. Propofol is less associated with laryngospasm than thiopental (thiopentone) and ketamine. There is conflicting evidence that intravenous lidocaine may be helpful in reducing episodes. Whether this effect is due to direct relaxing effects on the glottis or a more general deepening of anesthesia is not clear. However, spraying lidocaine 2% to 4% onto the glottis can help prevent laryngospasm. Awake extubation ensures that the patient will not have laryngospasm while emerging from anesthesia.

SUMMARY

1. While one may not be able to alter the preoperative risk factors, prudent anesthetic technique and a high level of vigilance may result in earlier recognition and prompt treatment should laryngospasm occur.
2. Stridor and incomplete laryngospasm can progress rapidly to complete laryngospasm.
3. Aggressive airway management and prompt administration of atropine, succinylcholine, or propofol, as indicated, should quickly reestablish a patent airway.

ANNOTATED REFERENCES

- Alalami AA, Ayoub CM, Baraka AS. Laryngospasm: review of different prevention and treatment modalities. *Pediatr Anesth* Apr 2008; 18(4): 281–288.

  This is one of four articles published together in one volume of *Pediatric Anesthesia*. It is a good, basic overview of the risk factors for and recognition and treatment of laryngospasm.
- Flick RP, Wilder RT, Pieper SF, van Koeverden K, Ellison KM, Marienau ME, Hanson AC, Schroeder DR, Sprung J. Risk factors for laryngospasm in children during general anesthesia. *Pediatr Anesth* Apr 2008; 18(4): 289–296.

Another one of the four articles published together. Using information drawn from a quality improvement database, risk factors are identified and incidence rates provided.

- **Hampson-Evans D, Morgan P, Farrar M. Pediatric laryngospasm. *Pediatr Anesth* Apr 2008; 18(4): 303–307.**

One of a cluster of articles on the topic, this one gives an algorithm for treatment of laryngospasm. Unfortunately, it is limited in scope, with reliance on succinylcholine and atropine as pharmacological interventions. It does discuss two mechanical approaches, which are worth reading.

- **Wittkugel EP. Laryngospasm. In JL Atlee, ed. *Complications in Anesthesia*, 2nd ed. Philadelphia: Saunders, 2007: 599–602.**

An excellent overview of laryngospasm in children, with two flowcharts that outline the effective management of incomplete and complete laryngospasm.

Further Reading

Burgoyne LL, Anghelescu DL. Intervention steps for treating laryngospasm in pediatric patients. *Pediatr Anesth* 2008; 18: 297–302.

Larson PC. Laryngospasm: the best treatment. *Anesthesiology* 1998; 89(5): 1293–1294.

Lee KWT, Downes JJ. Pulmonary edema secondary to laryngospasm. *Anesthesiology* 1983; 39: 347–349.

Olsson GL, Hallen B. Laryngospasm during anaesthesia: A computer-aided incidence studying 136,929 patients. *Acta Anaes Scand* 1984; 28: 567–575.

von Ungern-Sternberg BS, Oda K, Chambers NA, Rebmann C, Johnson C, Sly PD, Habre W. Risk assessment for respiratory complications in paediatric anaesthesia: a prospective cohort study. *Lancet* 2010; 376(9743): 773–783.

15

Tonsillar Bleed

ELIZABETH A. HEIN AND
JUDITH O. MARGOLIS

INTRODUCTION

Adenotonsillectomy is one of the most frequently performed surgical procedures of childhood: approximately 250,000 tonsillectomies are performed a year in the United States alone. Postoperative bleeding, although rare, is a potentially serious complication following adenotonsillectomy. Identifying and implementing appropriate care of these patients can be lifesaving.

LEARNING OBJECTIVES

1. Identify risk factors for postoperative bleeding in patients undergoing an adenotonsillectomy.
2. Estimate blood loss using clinical signs and symptoms when patients present with postoperative bleeding.
3. Develop a safe anesthetic plan for a patient undergoing a surgical procedure to stop post-adenotonsillectomy bleeding.
4. Describe common postoperative complications after cauterization of the bleeding tonsil.

CASE PRESENTATION

A 7-year-old boy presents to the operating room from the emergency department (ED) for cauterization of a bleeding tonsil.

*The **adenotonsillectomy was performed 8 days ago** for recurrent adenotonsillitis. His mother states that he has not been eating or drinking well in the past few days and that she noticed some blood-tinged secretions during the previous night. The patient is otherwise healthy with no family history of bleeding disorders. On examination in the ED, the patient appeared dehydrated—lethargic, with **dry lips** and **pale skin**—and he complains of **nausea**. The boy's vital signs are HR 110, RR 28, BP 85/45, with a **capillary refill of 4 seconds**. Bleeding was noted from one of the tonsil beds. His last oral intake was 6 hours previously. An intravenous line was placed in the ED and the patient was fluid resuscitated with lactated Ringer's. A **hemoglobin level** drawn on admission is 8.5 g/dL.*

*After fluid resuscitation, the patient is brought to the operating room and standard monitors are placed. After preoxygenation with 100% oxygen via mask, **a rapid-sequence induction** using etomidate and succinylcholine (suxamethonium) is undertaken. A **cuffed** oral RAE **endotracheal tube,** one half size smaller than previously used, is placed. The surgeon stops the bleeding with electrocautery and packing. The stomach is lavaged and then suctioned with an orogastric tube. Anti-emetic and pain medications are given. The patient is **extubated** when fully **awake** and airway reflexes have returned. He is transferred to the recovery area for observation. The patient develops **wheezing** on the right side and his oxygen saturation falls to 92%. After nebulized albuterol (salbutamol) and 2 L of oxygen by nasal cannula are administered, the oxygen saturation improves to 99%. A **chest radiograph** demonstrates mild opacification in the right lower lobe consistent with atelectasis or aspiration. The child is **admitted overnight for observation**.*

DISCUSSION

1. When does post-adenotonsillectomy bleeding occur?

The postoperative bleeding rate after adenotonsillectomy is estimated to be 0.5% to 2%. The bleeding is predominantly seen from the tonsillar fossa but can be seen from the adenoid bed in the nasopharynx. There are two periods in which postoperative bleeding typically occurs. *Primary bleeding* occurs within the *first 24 hours* of the operation and is usually brisk and easy to identify. Inadequate surgical hemostasis is the predominant cause. When primary bleeding is identified, one must investigate the possibility that the patient has an undiagnosed bleeding disorder. Blood samples should be drawn to look for a coagulation factor deficiency and consultation with a hematologist is warranted. If blood loss is significant, obtaining a **hemoglobin** level after fluid resuscitation will identify the need for a blood transfusion.

Secondary bleeding occurs most commonly between **5 and 10 days postoperatively**, but it can occur up to 28 days postoperatively. Secondary bleeding is traditionally attributed to sloughing of eschar tissue. This type of postoperative tonsillar bleeding can present as oozing over a few days. Hypovolemia from blood loss may be complicated by hypovolemia from poor oral intake due to pain and vomiting. Therefore, two sources of hypovolemia may be present, making the evaluation of blood loss and volume status more difficult.

2. What are the risk factors for post-tonsillectomy bleeding?

While many studies have been undertaken to identify patient attributes that predispose children to post-adenotonsillectomy bleeding, the studies have conflicting conclusions. One study (Collison & Mettler, 2000) found male gender, surgery in the spring and summer when patients are active, and use of vasoconstrictors and steroids as risk factors for postoperative tonsil bleeding. Another more recent article (Fields et al., 2010) cited prior work recognizing age >5 years and preoperative use of NSAIDs or aspirin as other risk factors for post-tonsillectomy bleeding. Gunter et al. (1995) compared ketorolac and morphine in terms of analgesic efficacy and side effects, specifically drowsiness, respiratory depression, and emesis. Although both groups needed the same rescue dose of opioid in the recovery room, the ketorolac group had fewer episodes of emesis in both the recovery room and at home after discharge. While the overall incidence of bleeding was not significantly different, patients in the ketorolac group had significantly more episodes of major bleeding. For this reason, the authors terminated the study prematurely. Ketorolac is therefore contraindicated in the perioperative period for children undergoing tonsillectomy. Dexamethasone is commonly used to control postoperative nausea and vomiting (PONV), and some debate was recently generated when a study (Czarnetzki et al., 2008) examining PONV incidentally found an increase in postoperative bleeding. However, the authors stated that the data are preliminary. Other studies found no compelling evidence that the perioperative administration of dexamethasone increases the risk of bleeding after tonsillectomy (Brigger et al., 2010; Gunter et al., 2006). Dexamethasone administration for the prevention of PONV after tonsillectomy is an evidence-based intervention commonly practiced internationally.

The otolaryngology literature also focuses on surgical technique as a contributing cause to post-tonsillectomy bleeding. The general comparison is made between cold steel technique and techniques employing electrocautery, either monopolar, bipolar, or coblation. The cold steel technique uses nonthermal instruments such as a scalpel or snare to remove tonsillar tissue and uses suture and packing to control bleeding. Electrocautery, either monopolar or bipolar, is used for both dissection and hemostasis. Coblation is a newer technology that is touted as having less postoperative bleeding with the added benefit of less pain for patients. These benefits of coblation have not been universally demonstrated. Electrocautery techniques provide better operative hemostasis and therefore less primary bleeding. However, electrocautery causes more thermal tissue injury and eschar development and thus increases the potential for secondary bleeding.

3. What are the signs and symptoms of hypovolemia due to blood loss?

Hypovolemia in children presents with *tachycardia*, *tachypnea*, and, when severe, *hypotension*. Children will typically maintain their blood pressure despite loss of blood volume for a longer period than adults, but will deteriorate rapidly and severely once they do begin to decompensate. **Mucous membranes** will be **dry**. When blood loss is the primary cause of hypovolemia, the skin is **pale** and **capillary refill** is prolonged. Laboratory testing might show decreased **hemoglobin** levels, but if the patient is **dehydrated** as well, the hemoglobin may be normal or even elevated due to hemoconcentration. If the child has swallowed blood, he or she may present with **nausea** and bloody emesis, but keep in mind that these symptoms may be masked if the patient received ondansetron during or after surgery. There have been reported incidences of patients vomiting large amounts of blood 9 to 22 hours postoperatively after receiving ondansetron as part of their perioperative anesthetic care (Hamid et al., 1998). Evaluation for orthostatic hypotension can help quantify blood loss that is hidden in the gastrointestinal system.

4. What are the anesthetic considerations in this case?
Once the diagnosis of tonsillar bleeding that requires surgical hemostasis is made, appropriate fluid resuscitation should begin immediately, before beginning the operation. While brisk bleeding is more common after early hemorrhage, significant hypovolemia may still occur in all these children. As in the case presentation, the child with signs of hypovolemia should be volume resuscitated before induction of anesthesia.

All patients with post-adenotonsillar bleeding should be considered as having *a full stomach, regardless of NPO status,* and a **rapid-sequence induction** is recommended. At least one large-bore intravenous line is needed to *replace intravascular volume loss* and possibly transfuse blood. Resuscitation should begin with an intravenous bolus of crystalloids. Packed red blood cells may be necessary based on clinical signs and the hematocrit. Two laryngoscopes and two suctions should be available and ready for use. The otolaryngologist should be present for the induction of anesthesia since this can be a hazardous time with a high risk of aspiration, difficult intubation, and loss of the airway. The potential for *hypovolemia* must be evaluated in order to choose a safe anesthetic. Traditional induction choices are etomidate or ketamine. If hypovolemia is not an issue, propofol may be used judiciously. Muscle relaxant choices include succinylcholine or rocuronium. A *difficult intubation* must be anticipated as blood is expected in the airway. If the patient is actively bleeding, an assistant may need to place a Yankauer suction into the oropharynx during intubation to allow visualization of the glottis for intubation. Placement of a **cuffed oral RAE tube** (named after inventors, Ring, Adair, and Elwyn) helps to protect the airway from aspiration and facilitates surgical access. Pain medication is used judiciously. With use of an orogastric tube, the stomach should be lavaged with normal saline and suctioned at the end of the case, but keep in mind that this does not guarantee an empty stomach. Keep suction available because a blood clot can be dislodged from the stomach and become lodged in the airway. **Awake extubation** in the operating room is the safest conclusion of the anesthetic. Pain control, vigilance for rebleeding, and reevaluation of hydration status should continue in the recovery period.

5. How should one proceed with an anesthetic if no IV line is in place?

How to anesthetize a child who has active tonsillar bleeding, has symptoms of hypovolemia, is at risk for aspiration on induction, and has no IV catheter in place presents a true clinical dilemma. The risk of aspiration with an inhaled induction is high, so an IV line should be placed. A skilled hand is needed to successfully place an IV in a dehydrated child who is cooperative, but it is even more difficult in a crying, uncooperative child. The parent can help calm the child and increase cooperation for placement of an IV catheter. If multiple attempts at IV line placement are unsuccessful, and the patient is hemodynamically stable, an inhalational induction, although not ideal, can be undertaken if steps are taken to help limit aspiration risk. These steps include keeping the patient breathing spontaneously, having large-bore suction readily available, and having equipment and personnel ready to gain vascular access and to intubate quickly. If a peripheral IV catheter cannot be placed in a patient who is severely dehydrated and/or displays symptoms of shock, an intraosseous or central line should be placed and resuscitation should be undertaken prior to induction to avoid cardiovascular collapse.

6. What issues should be anticipated in the postoperative period?

Patients with *primary bleeding* continue to be at risk for *rebleeding* in the recovery period. They should be extubated awake in the operating room and brought to the recovery area with airway reflexes intact. Coagulation studies, including PT, PTT, and platelet count, should be drawn to rule out a bleeding disorder. Hemoglobin and hematocrit levels will guide the need for blood transfusion. If a coagulopathy is suggested by history or laboratory studies, consultation with a hematologist is indicated. IV fluid administration is continued and pain is controlled so oral intake can be started. **Wheezing** may indicate aspiration and a **chest radiograph** may be helpful. Since the patient has been intubated twice in a short time span, the risk of *airway edema and obstruction* increases. Post-intubation croup should be treated with racemic epinephrine. IV dexamethasone is given to prevent and treat airway edema. Plan for the patient to be **admitted overnight for observation**.

In the case of secondary bleeding requiring cauterization in the operating room, hydration status and replacing blood loss are the main issues in the recovery room. Fluid resuscitation is continued if needed. Laboratory analysis of the hemoglobin level guides the need for transfusion. Because patients may continue to vomit blood or blood clots, vigilance for aspiration is necessary. Stridor, wheezing, or retractions should be evaluated and treated. Overnight hospital admission for further observation may be indicated.

SUMMARY

1. Post-tonsillectomy hemorrhage, an infrequent but serious complication, occurs most commonly within the first 24 hours and then again at 5 to 10 days postoperatively.
2. Major anesthetic issues include hypovolemia due to blood loss and poor oral intake, the risk of aspiration, and the potential for difficult intubation and loss of the airway due to bleeding.
3. Volume resuscitation, appropriate choice of anesthetic drugs, rapid-sequence induction with the surgeon present, and awake extubation are keys to safe anesthetic management.
4. Evaluation for a coagulopathy may be indicated after post-tonsillectomy hemorrhage.

ANNOTATED REFERENCES

- Collison PJ, Mettler B. Factors associated with post-tonsillectomy hemorrhage. *Ear Nose Throat J* 2000; 79(8): 640–646.

This study identifies patient risk factors that predict post-tonsillectomy bleeding. It also references other studies that both agree and disagree with the findings and provides insight into the complexity involved in identifying preoperative risk factors.

- Schmidt R, Herzog A, Cook S, O'Reilly R, Deutsch E, Reilly J. Complications of tonsillectomy: a comparison of techniques. *Arch Otolaryngol Head Neck Surg* 2007; 133(9): 925–928.

This study compares the postoperative complications such as bleeding, pain, and readmission for dehydration of different surgical techniques.

- Windfuhr JP, Schloendorff G, Baburi D, Kremer B. Serious post-tonsillectomy hemorrhage with and without lethal outcome in children and adolescents. *Int J Pediatr Otorhinolaryngol* 2008; 72(7): 1029–1040.
  This article reviews the history and outcomes of patients with life-threatening post-adenotonsillar bleeding. Morbidity and mortality rates and causes are discussed.

Further Reading

Brigger MT, Cunningham MJ, Hartnick CJ. Dexamethasone administration and postoperative bleeding risk in children undergoing tonsillectomy. *Arch Otolaryngol Head Neck Surg* 2010; 136: 766–772.

Czarnetzki C, Elia N, Lysakowski C, Dumont L, Landis BN, Giger R, Dulguerov P, Desmeules J, Tramèr MR. Dexamethasone and risk of nausea and vomiting and postoperative bleeding after tonsillectomy in children: a randomized trial. *JAMA* 2008; 300(22): 2621–2630.

Fields R, Gencorelli F, Litman R. Anesthetic management of the pediatric bleeding tonsil. *Pediatr Anesth* 2010; 20(11): 982–986.

Gunter JB, McAuliffe JJ, Beckman EC, Wittkugel EP, Spaeth JP, Varughese AM. A factorial study of ondansetron, metoclopramide, and dexamethasone for emesis prophylaxis after adenotonsillectomy in children. *Pediatr Anesth* 2006; 16(11): 1153–65.

Gunter J, Varughese A, Harrington J, Wittkugel E, Patankar S, Matar M, Lowe E, Myer C, Willging P. Recovery and complications after tonsillectomy in children: a comparison of ketorolac and morphine. *Anesth Analg* 1995; 81: 1136–1141.

Hamid S, Selby I, Sikich N, Lerman J. Vomiting after adenotonsillectomy in children: a comparison of ondansetron, dimenhydrinate, and placebo. *Anesth Analg* 1998; 86: 496–500.

16

Difficult Airway

PETER HOWE

INTRODUCTION

Airway management in otherwise healthy children is normally easy in experienced hands and an unexpected difficult intubation should be uncommon. Predictors of difficult intubation include mandibular hypoplasia, limited mouth opening, facial asymmetry, and a history of stridor or obstructive sleep apnea. Many of these features occur in conditions such as Treacher Collins syndrome, Goldenhar's syndrome, and the Pierre Robin sequence.

LEARNING OBJECTIVES

1. Describe important ways in which the airway management of children differs from adults.
2. Recognize aspects of the preoperative assessment in a child that are associated with difficult intubation.
3. Develop a plan for managing an expected difficult intubation in a child, including fiberoptic intubation.

CASE PRESENTATION

A 2-year-old girl with Pierre Robin sequence sustained a dog bite to the face. She has a 3-cm full-thickness lip laceration. She last ate 6 hours ago. She is terrified and will not let any member of staff approach her. Her past history includes cleft palate repair at 9 months of age.

On that occasion, she was intubated by a senior anesthetist. The anesthetic record reads: "Anterior larynx. Grade III laryngoscopy despite laryngeal pressure. Easy fiberoptic intubation."

The approach to the anticipated difficult intubation is discussed with her parents and her surgeon. It is agreed that a general anesthetic with an endotracheal tube and throat pack will enable the best possible surgical result. After she receives midazolam 0.4 mg/kg **premedication, in a monitored area** in the preoperative holding bay she allows anesthetic cream to be applied to her hand. After 20 minutes she comes to the induction area with her father in attendance. She has become less agitated but will not allow anything to be placed near her face. She does allow insertion of an intravenous cannula and placement of ECG leads and pulse oximetry. Titrated ketamine 1 mg/kg, with glycopyrrolate to control secretions, helps her to tolerate a face mask. Inhalation induction is completed with sevoflurane in 100% oxygen. Once she has lost consciousness, her father leaves the room. **2 mL 1% lidocaine (lignocaine) is trickled into the back of her pharynx** in preparation for laryngoscopy.

First laryngoscopy provides a view of the tip of the epiglottis only. External laryngeal pressure brings more of the epiglottis into view, but not the larynx. 4% lidocaine is sprayed directly onto the epiglottis.

Her head position is **changed to give greater neck extension.** With this the view is worse, her breathing becomes obstructed, and her oxygen saturation begins to fall. Her obstruction corrects with a return to the original position. A second anesthetist then performs the third laryngoscopy with a straight blade, using the free hand to apply laryngeal pressure, while the first attempts to intubate with an endotracheal tube (ETT) over an angled stylet. The epiglottis and the posterior aspect of the larynx are visible and the ETT is advanced. On auscultation, breath sounds seem present, but **there is no capnograph trace.** The tube is presumed to be esophageal and is removed.

Further attempts at laryngoscopy seem ill advised and preparations are made for fiberoptic intubation. The anesthetic circuit is connected to a nasopharyngeal airway placed in the left nostril. Intubation with fiberoptic guidance proceeds smoothly through the right nostril. The case proceeds uneventfully. At the end of the case *the patient is extubated awake, and then observed in the hospital overnight, with no evidence for airway injury.*

DISCUSSION

1. How does airway management of children differ from that of adults?

Head positioning is extremely important in neonates and young children. The optimal position for mask ventilation is obtained when the head is in a neutral or slightly extended position, but the relatively large size of the head tends to place the neck in flexion, making airway management more difficult. A small gel pad under the shoulders may improve positioning, especially in neonates. As airway tone decreases during induction of anesthesia, some degree of airway obstruction frequently occurs, especially if the patient has a history of snoring or obstructive sleep apnea. The anesthetist should review the **head position** and ensure that the mouth is open and the tongue is not pressed against the palate. Wide mouth opening in combination with a jaw thrust is often useful.

Gastric air insufflation is common during mask ventilation of small children, especially when ventilation has been difficult. A distended stomach may impair movement of the diaphragm and should be emptied by passing a suction tube.

It is often difficult to visualize the laryngeal inlet in small children by conventional laryngoscopy. The larynx is more cephalad, and the epiglottis is long, narrow, omega-shaped, and angled into the lumen of the airway covering the laryngeal inlet. Fortunately, these difficulties are offset by the relative ease with which the larynx can be manipulated by external pressure, either by the little finger of the laryngoscope hand, or by the operator's free hand; in the latter case, a colleague may pass the tube under direct vision. Remember that extending the neck of an infant can compress the glottis against the cervical spine, making the view worse, which differs from the usual results seen in older children and adults.

The relatively cephalad location of the larynx also means that the "sniffing position" is of little benefit in small children, and a pillow under the large head only makes airway management more difficult by flexing the neck. During the first years of life, the larynx moves distally until the age of 4, when it is located at the adult level of C5–C6, and the sniffing position becomes increasingly useful.

The laryngeal mask airway (LMA) is usually easy to insert in children, but in infants the long epiglottis is frequently caught and down-folded by the tip of the LMA. Therefore, many pediatric anesthetists prefer to insert smaller LMAs in a reverse fashion, with the opening against the palate, and then rotate it into place when fully inserted.

2. Why do small children tend to become hypoxic on induction more quickly than adults?

Preoxygenating an upset child is often difficult and ineffective. The oxygen reserve is also much smaller, due to a lower functional residual lung capacity and higher oxygen consumption. Desaturation therefore occurs much more rapidly.

3. How should fiberoptic devices be used in children?

Awake fiberoptic intubation is impractical in an uncooperative child, and most published methods are designed to accompany spontaneously breathing anesthesia. A common method is to use a nasopharyngeal airway attached to an anesthetic circuit, while intubation is performed through the mouth or opposite nostril. Fiberoptic video laryngoscopes are available in small sizes but require practice in elective situations.

The LMA has been shown to provide a reasonable airway in a large proportion of patients with a difficult airway, and the fiberoptic view obtained through the LMA provides a good view of the larynx in most cases. A well-known method is to load an ETT over the scope and intubate through the LMA. The problem then becomes how to remove the LMA. It is possible to pass an ETT exchanger over the scope, intubate through the LMA under vision, and railroad an ETT over the exchanger once the scope and LMA have been removed, as described in detail by Thomas (Thomas & Barry, 2001). Walker has described a similar method, where a guide wire is passed through the scope's suction port and the catheter is advanced blindly over the wire (Walker & Ellwood, 2009). Although costly, these methods are a practical choice for even the relatively inexperienced bronchoscopist and minimize the incidence of the "can't intubate, can't ventilate" scenario. Ellis et al. have published a useful table showing the uncuffed ETT size that can be passed completely through LMAs of different sizes, enabling the LMA to be removed without an exchanger (Ellis et al., 1999).

4. What is the risk and benefit of applying topical local anesthetic to a child's airway? What is the best way to apply it?

The aim is to provide an anesthetized airway, which allows the passage of an airway device without coughing or laryngeal spasm. To avoid toxicity, care should be taken calculating the dose of the local anesthetic. Preoperative administration is ideal, allowing emergency placement of an LMA in a relatively light plane of anesthesia, but most techniques used in an adult are unacceptable to an anxious child. Nebulized local anesthesia is often successful, especially if the child has had nebulized medication before and is familiar with the nebulization mask. Spraying the larynx directly is the most efficient method but requires a deep plane of anesthesia and an adequate view of the larynx, both of which may be difficult to achieve in a child with airway obstruction. Blind **administration of local anesthesia into the back of the mouth** without laryngoscopy works reasonably well to cover key laryngeal structures (Beringer et al., 2010).

5. Can the ASA Difficult Airway Algorithm be applied to children?

The principles can be directly applied, but many of the advanced techniques are impractical in an uncooperative child. In practice, this usually means that once one has decided to start the case, one proceeds directly to the "Preservation of Spontaneous Ventilation" step. Given that the practical airway management algorithm is truncated, it is important to consider some basic steps in a mental checklist before starting a potentially difficult case, as shown in Table 16.1.

6. How many attempts at laryngoscopy are appropriate?

Repeated attempts at laryngoscopy lead to trauma to the larynx and are associated with a worse outcome. In general, if the first laryngoscopy has been unsuccessful, one should ventilate while changing the position or equipment in preparation for the second laryngoscopy. If the second laryngoscopy is also unsuccessful, it is prudent to ask an experienced colleague to try. Beyond three laryngoscopies, the team should recognize that the patient is now at a significantly increased risk of laryngeal trauma, and a fiberoptic or other alternative approach to intubation is warranted. For expected difficult intubation it is important to have a clear plan and have experienced assistance available.

Table 16.1
OPTIONS TO CONSIDER IN PLANNING AN ANTICIPATED DIFFICULT INTUBATION IN A CHILD
1. Preparation
* Are the right people and equipment available in this facility?
* Is the necessary equipment prepared and on hand?
2. Mode of anesthesia
* Could the procedure be done under local anesthetic only?
3. Awake intubation
* Is awake fiberoptic intubation or awake tracheotomy an option?
4. Intubation under anesthesia
*Maintain spontaneous ventilation. Consider ketamine in addition to, or in place of, inhalational agents.
* Positive-pressure ventilation is a last resort. Be mindful of removing the patient's ability to breathe.

7. Should anxious children with an anticipated difficult airway receive sedative premedication?

Many anesthetists feel that the use of sedative premedication in a child with an obstructed or potentially obstructed airway is contraindicated. Anything that reduces the child's ability to breathe is potentially counterproductive. On the other hand, it is sometimes difficult even to approach a terrified child, let alone attach monitoring, apply a face mask, or insert an intravenous cannula. A crying child produces lots of airway secretions and increases the anxiety of parents and staff alike. The ability to induce anesthesia in a smooth and calm atmosphere with full monitoring applied intuitively adds safety to the process.

8. How should one confirm the position of an ETT tube in a child?

As in adults, placement should be confirmed by **capnography** and by direct visualization if possible. Auscultation of the chest is often unreliable. In many cases of esophageal intubation, auscultation of the chest can lead to the erroneous conclusion that the ETT was correctly located in the trachea.

SUMMARY

1. Unexpected difficult intubation in pediatric practice is rare. Potential identifiers include mandibular hypoplasia, facial asymmetry, limited mouth opening, and a history of stridor or sleep apnea.
2. Before starting the case, ensure that adequate assistance and a fiberoptic device are available. Consider not starting the case at all if proper equipment is not available.
3. Maintain spontaneous ventilation if possible.
4. Apply topical local anesthesia to the patient's airway.
5. Performing more than three laryngoscopies places the patient at increased risk.

ANNOTATED REFERENCES

- Benumof JL. Difficult laryngoscopy: obtaining the best view. *Can J Anaesth* 1994: 41(5): 361–365.
  A master class in how to perform direct laryngoscopy.
- Holm-Knudsen RJ, Rasmussen LS. Pediatric airway management: basic aspects. *Acta Anaesth Scand* 2009; 53(1): 1–9.
  An excellent introduction to airway management in children with normal airways.
- Walker RW, Ellwood J. The management of difficult intubation in children. *Pediatr Anesth* 2009; 19(Suppl. 1): 77–87.
  A well-referenced summary of difficult airway management, which focuses on principles and practical suggestions rather than a rigid protocol.

Further Reading

Beringer R, Skeahan N, Sheppard S, Ragg P, Martin N, McKenzie I, Davidson A. Study to assess the laryngeal and pharyngeal spread of topical local anesthetic administered orally during general anesthesia in children. *Pediatr Anesth* 2010; 20: 757–762.

Caplan RA, Posner KL, Ward RJ, Cheney, FW. Adverse respiratory events in anesthesia: a closed claims analysis. *Anesthesiology* 1990; 72(5): 828–833.

Ellis DS, Potluri PK, O'Flaherty JE, Baum VC. Difficult airway management in the neonate: a simple method of intubating through a laryngeal mask airway. *Pediatr Anesth* 1999; 9(5): 460–462.

Holm-Knudsen RJ, Eriksen K, Rasmussen LS. Using a nasopharyngeal airway during fiberoptic intubation in small children with a difficult airway. *Pediatr Anesth* 2005; 15(10): 839–845.

Holm-Knudsen RJ. The difficult pediatric airway—a review of new devices for indirect laryngoscopy in children younger than two years of age. *Pediatr Anesth* 2010; 21(2): 98–103.

Practice guidelines for the difficult airway: A report by the American Society of Anesthesiologists Task Force on Management of the Difficult Airway. *Anesthesiology* 1993; 78: 597–602.

Thomas LB, Barry MG. The difficult pediatric airway: a new method of intubation using the laryngeal mask airway, Cook airway exchange catheter and tracheal intubation fiberscope. *Pediatr Anesth* 2001; 11(5): 618–621.

Walker RW. The laryngeal mask airway in the difficult pediatric airway: an assessment of positioning and use in fibreoptic intubation. *Pediatr Anesth* 2008; 10(1): 53–58.

Wiess M, Engelhardt T. Proposal for the management of the unexpected difficult pediatric airway. *Pediatr Anesth* 2010; 20(5): 454-464.

Airway Reconstruction

ELIZABETH A. HEIN AND
GRESHAM T. RICHTER

INTRODUCTION

Pediatric airway reconstruction is undertaken to correct airway obstruction, which may be congenital or iatrogenic. Congenital airway obstruction can be located at any level of the respiratory system, from the nares to the bronchi. It can be complete obstruction, such as choanal atresia in a newborn, or incomplete, such as adenotonsillar hypertrophy or tracheomalacia. Iatrogenic obstruction is often the result of prolonged intubation in a premature infant, which results in subglottic stenosis (SGS) after extubation. As these children grow, their airway growth may not keep pace, resulting in restrictive symptoms limiting their activity. Laryngotracheoplasty (LTP) or tracheal resection procedures may be needed to reconstruct and enlarge the airway. If the premature infant has concurrent lung disease, long-term intubation is often followed by tracheostomy placement. The timing of decannulation depends on the patient's airway patency and respiratory reserve. Understanding the process of evaluation and treatment of patients with SGS helps the anesthetist provide safe anesthesia for this challenging group of children.

LEARNING OBJECTIVES

1. List the common causes of subglottic stenosis requiring pediatric airway reconstruction.

2. Describe associated problems of prematurity that might influence the outcome of airway reconstructive surgery.
3. Recognize common complications that occur during airway reconstructive surgery.
4. Understand the difference between a single-stage and double-stage repair of a pediatric airway.

CASE PRESENTATION

A 4-year-old, former 28 week premature infant, who was ventilated for 4 weeks at birth and then successfully extubated, presents for laryngotracheoplasty (LTP) with anterior and posterior costal cartilage grafts. He has **stridor and dyspnea** *with vigorous physical activity, occasionally uses an albuterol nebulizer, and uses supplemental oxygen when he has a respiratory illness. He has been well recently and has not required albuterol for several months. On examination, he weighs 14 kg and has a respiratory rate of 38 breaths per minute, a room air oxygen saturation of 96%, mild suprasternal retractions, and a clear chest.*

The patient undergoes an inhalation induction with oxygen, nitrous oxide, and sevoflurane. Before an intravenous line is placed, the patient shows signs of upper airway obstruction and his oxygen saturation drops to 91%. An oropharyngeal airway is placed, nitrous oxide is discontinued, and slow assisted breaths with an inspiratory hold are initiated. The oxygen saturation returns to 99% and the intravenous line is successfully placed. **Spontaneous respiration** *anesthesia is maintained with oxygen and sevoflurane, and the vocal cords are sprayed with lidocaine. While the patient is breathing spontaneously with insufflation of oxygen and sevoflurane, laryngoscopy and rigid bronchoscopy reveal a grade II subglottic stenosis. An uncuffed 4-mm oral ETT is placed and secured. The initial part of the operation is the harvest of a piece of costal cartilage from the lower* *ribs, which is to be used as a graft to augment the size of the trachea. At the end of the* **harvest of the rib graft**, *the field is flooded with saline and a Valsalva maneuver is undertaken to ensure there is no* **air leak**.

Next, an incision is made over the anterior neck and the trachea is exposed. The trachea is opened and the oral ETT is replaced with a sterile, reinforced **ETT placed directly by the surgeon into the trachea. Intermittent removal of the ETT** *is required during the airway reconstruction to gain access to the trachea. While the ETT is removed, the* **oxygen saturation falls** *to 89%. The ETT is replaced and the saturation climbs to 92% but does not increase further. Higher inspiratory pressure is required to ventilate the patient, and the breath sounds from the precordial stethoscope on the left chest are decreased. The surgeon pulls back the ETT, which has* **slipped into the right main bronchus** *and breath sounds return. Later during the procedure, the* **end-tidal CO_2 curve flattens** *despite the presence of breath sounds. The oxygen saturation falls to 90% and the ETT is found to have slipped out of the trachea. Once the surgeon replaces the ETT into the trachea, the saturation returns to 98%. Bronchospasm occurs later and is treated with endotracheal suction and inhaled albuterol (salbutamol). The* **posterior tracheal wall is opened** *and the* **rib graft is sutured into place**. *At this point, the ETT in the field is removed and an appropriate-size nasal ETT is immediately advanced into the trachea with direct laryngoscopy. Another* **rib graft is secured to the anterior wall** *of the trachea and the incision is closed. The patient* **is taken to the ICU intubated and sedated**. *The patient returns to the operating suite 7 days later for a repeat bronchoscopy to evaluate the airway. A nasal ETT one size smaller is placed. The following day, he is extubated awake in the ICU with a good airway.*

DISCUSSION

1. How is this patient a "typical" LTP patient?

This patient is typical in that he is an ex-premature infant with SGS secondary to prolonged intubation. He has progressive

stridor and dyspnea that are exacerbated by exercise and respiratory illnesses. Other issues associated with prematurity that can have an impact on outcome are bronchopulmonary dysplasia (BPD), reactive airway disease (RAD), severity of subglottic stenosis (grade III and above on the Myer-Cotton SGS scale), gastroesophageal reflux disease (GERD), feeding disorders, growth failure, neurological impairment such as cerebral palsy, and prior tracheostomy placement. Common causes of SGS include congenital SGS, prolonged intubation, traumatic intubation, and placement of an ETT that is too large. Cotton and Myer developed a classification scheme for grading circumferential SGS from I to IV based on the percent of cross-sectional area that is obstructed (Myer et al., 1994); examples are shown in Fig. 17.1.

2. **What complications are associated with airway reconstructive surgery?**
Complications specific to LTP involve compromise of the airway and ventilation. With the airway being the operative site, the

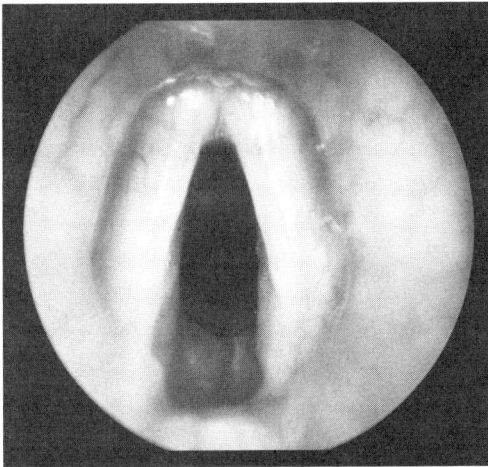

FIGURE 17.1a Grade I SGS (0–50%).

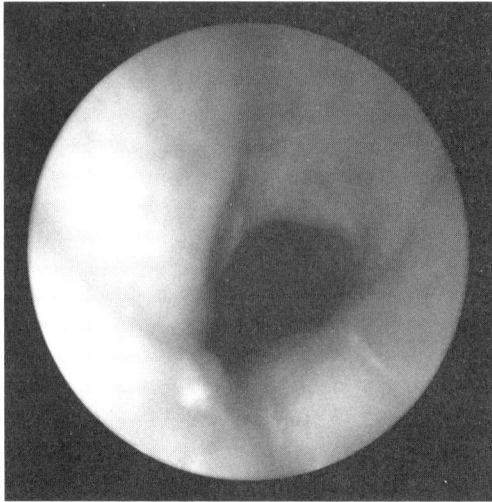

FIGURE 17.1b Grade II SGS (51–70%).

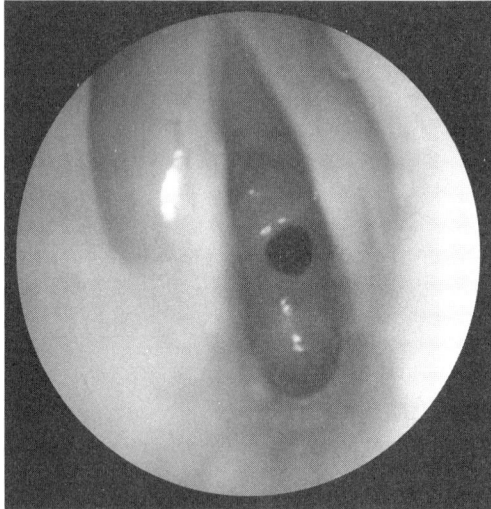

FIGURE 17.1c Grade III SGS (71–99%).

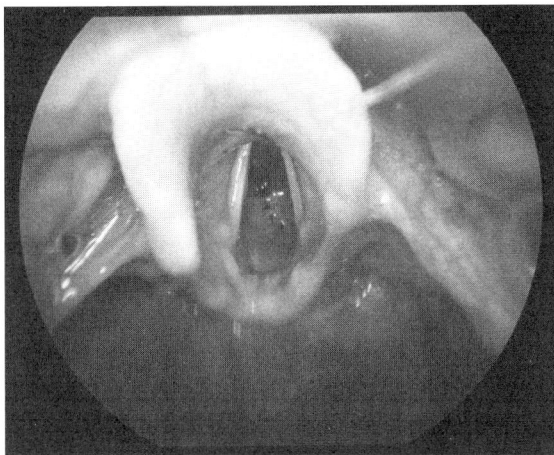

FIGURE 17.1d Grade IV SGS (no lumen).

airway must be safely shared by the surgeon and the anesthesia team. Constant communication with the otolaryngologist and constant observation of the airway are the keys to a safe anesthetic and avoiding a potentially catastrophic loss of the airway.

During the harvest of the costal graft, a pneumothorax can develop. Before wound closure, the surgical field is flooded with saline and a Valsalva maneuver is performed to exclude an **air leak**. Using spontaneous ventilation instead of positive-pressure ventilation decreases the possibility of expanding a small pneumothorax should it develop. *A postoperative chest radiograph should always be obtained.*

The necessity of repeatedly removing the ETT for surgical access requires constant vigilance to make sure it is properly reinserted into the trachea every time. Increased peak airway pressures and oxygen desaturation may indicate unintended **bronchial intubation**. The risk of creating a *false passage* exists each time the ETT or tracheostomy is returned to the airway. If the patient has a history of reactive airway disease, airway instrumentation and blood in the airway might trigger **bronchospasm**, requiring suctioning and inhaled bronchodilators.

Postoperatively, the child must be appropriately sedated and the ETT must be securely maintained because it acts as a stent that supports the newly placed rib graft. If **unintended extubation** occurs, the graft may become dislodged and the airway can be critically compromised with catastrophic results.

3. **What are the advantages and disadvantages of spontaneous and controlled ventilation during airway reconstruction?**

Intraoperative **spontaneous ventilation** has two advantages. First, it helps with visualization as blood and tissue are not "blown" into the operative field. Second, it helps entrain anesthesia and oxygen into the lungs compared to positive-pressure ventilation, which may result in much of the inspired volume escaping through the surgically created opening in the trachea. It is important to remember that with spontaneous ventilation, breath sounds via a precordial stethoscope can be present even with a dislodged ETT. As illustrated in the case, the **capnography trace flattened** and the **oxygen saturation decreased**. One disadvantage of using spontaneous ventilation is the development of intraoperative atelectasis, which may require treatment with positive-pressure ventilation and PEEP. The use of neuromuscular blockade and positive-pressure ventilation is another acceptable technique that prevents intraoperative atelectasis, ensures immobility, and facilitates a smooth anesthetic.

4. **What is the significance of this patient needing both an anterior and a posterior graft?**

SGS is not always a concentric reduction in airway diameter. An anterior graft and a posterior graft are required when there is significant airway stenosis. When the SGS is not concentric, a single anterior or posterior graft is placed to make the airway "round" again. If the segment of stenosis is concentric and short in length, a cricotracheal resection can be performed in which the entire section of stenosis is removed and the two ends of the trachea are reanastamosed. If the section of stenosis is too long for repair by grafting, a slide tracheoplasty performed while on cardiopulmonary bypass may be necessary.

5. **What is the difference between a single-stage and a double-stage LTP repair?**

LTP is a group of surgical procedures undertaken to correct stenosis or to stabilize the larynx or trachea. The patient may or may not have a tracheostomy in place. Some patients may have had prior LTP surgery. The choice of single- or double-stage repair depends on the individual airway anatomy and comorbidities. In a single-stage repair, a stent (usually a nasal ETT) is placed through the glottis into the trachea under direct observation of the operative field to brace the airway and help secure the surgically placed grafts. At the end of the procedure, the patient is transported to the intensive care unit, where he or she remains intubated and sedated. After 2 to 7 days, the child returns to the operating room for evaluation of the airway under general anesthesia. The ETT is removed and the airway is examined with a rigid or flexible bronchoscope. Spontaneous respiration is maintained throughout to evaluate airway dynamics. If the repair is healing well, an uncuffed ETT, usually one size smaller, is placed and secured. The patient returns to the ICU, sedation is discontinued, and the patient is extubated once fully awake. If the graft is dislodged or the repair is not healing as anticipated, any further repair is undertaken, the ETT is replaced, and the postoperative process is repeated.

In a double-stage repair, the airway reconstruction takes place as a two-part procedure. At the end of the initial airway reconstruction, a tracheostomy or a T-tube is placed. A T-tube is an intraluminal stent with an arm (shaped like a T) that protrudes through a tracheostomy to the anterior neck. It functions as a tracheostomy while simultaneously acting as an airway stent. Patients do not need postoperative intubation and ventilation in the ICU. They can recover from anesthesia in the PACU and then transfer to a specialized airway unit. The child undergoes repeat bronchoscopy in the future to assess the effectiveness of the repair and to ensure that restenosis has not occurred prior to decannulation. A trial of capping the tracheostomy may also be performed to be sure the patient will do well without the tracheostomy. The child then returns for the second stage when the T-tube or tracheostomy is removed.

SUMMARY

1. Subglottic stenosis, either congenital or iatrogenic in nature, is repaired with a laryngotracheoplasty.
2. Patients with SGS are often ex-premature infants with other associated medical problems such as bronchopulmonary dysplasia, reactive airway disease, GERD, feeding problems, growth failure, and developmental delay.
3. Spontaneous ventilation and controlled ventilation can both be used effectively during a LTP. Each has advantages and disadvantages.
4. Potential complications related to LTP are bronchospasm, atelectasis, pneumonia, pneumothorax, unintended extubation, bronchial intubation, loss of the airway, airway disruption, and creation of a false passage.
5. Communication and teamwork with the otolaryngologist are the keys to a safe anesthetic.

ANNOTATED REFERENCES

• deAlarcon A, Rutter MJ. Revision pediatric laryngotracheal reconstruction. *Otolaryngol Clinics North Am* 2008; 41(5): 959–980.

This review offers insight into the decision-making process involved with preparing a child for LTP. It discusses preoperative workup, specific surgical options, and common causes for failure in airway reconstruction. The intraoperative photographs and diagrams are very helpful.

- **Rutter MJ. Evaluation and management of upper airway disorders in children.** *Semin Pediatr Surg* **2006; 15(2): 116–123.**

This is an excellent overview of upper airway disorders that might present for surgical repair in the pediatric population.

- **Hein E, Rutter MJ. New perspective in pediatric airway reconstruction.** *Int Anesthesiol Clin* **2006; 44(1): 51–64.**

An excellent overview of airway reconstruction, including anterior cricoid split, LTP, cricotracheal resection (CTR), and slide tracheoplasty. It includes many diagrams, photos, and schematics that clearly explain the procedures. Anesthetic management is discussed in detail.

Further Reading

Myer CM, O'Connor DM, Cotton RT. Proposed grading system for subglottic stenosis based on endotracheal tube sizes. *Ann Otol Rhinol Laryngol* 1994; 103: 319–323.

Nguyen CV, Bent JP, Shah MB, Parikh SR. Pediatric primary anterior laryngotracheoplasty: thyroid ala vs. costal cartilage graft. *Arch Otolaryngol Head Neck Surg* 2010; 136(2): 171–174.

Santos D, Mitchell R. The history of pediatric airway reconstruction. *Laryngoscope* 2010; 120(4): 815–820.

Wooten CT, Rutter MJ, Dickson JM, Samuels PJ. Anesthetic management of patients with tracheal T tubes. *Pediatr Anesth* 2009; 19(4): 349–357.

18

Laryngeal Papillomatosis

ELIZABETH PRENTICE

INTRODUCTION

The incidence of recurrent juvenile laryngeal papilloma caused by human papilloma virus has been rising (Dalmeida et al., 1996). A child with this potentially life-threatening condition requires surgical resection to avoid respiratory obstruction; this surgery may need to be repeated regularly for many years. Laser therapy to the airway provides specific challenges to the anesthesiologist. In particular, the risks of a shared compromised airway as well as the hazards of the laser itself must be appreciated by all medical personnel. The key to success is thorough preoperative assessment, good continuous communication with surgical and nursing staff, preparation for the management of critical incidents, and familiarity with the surgical and anesthetic equipment.

LEARNING OBJECTIVES

1. Review the assessment of severity of upper airway compromise.
2. Develop a plan to deliver a safe general anesthetic in the presence of airway compromise and shared airway surgery.
3. Summarize the airway management and ventilation options for laryngeal surgery.
4. Review laser safety in the context of CO_2 laser microlaryngoscopy.

CASE PRESENTATION

*A 15-kg, 3-year-old girl with a history of progressive **stridor** presents to the emergency department. The parents have noticed a progressively **hoarse voice** and **swallowing difficulty** over the past 14 days. She now becomes **short of breath** when she becomes upset or tries to run for a few seconds. There is no history of choking, trauma, or recent cough or cold. After walking down the corridor into the examination room, she develops stridor with intercostal and substernal retractions with a respiratory rate of 45 breaths per minute. Auscultation is difficult due to transmitted sounds from the upper airway. There is no urticaria, drooling, or facial/neck swelling. She is afebrile. Oxygen saturation is 91% to 94% on room air. A lateral neck x-ray and AP chest x-ray show **no signs of foreign body**. An awake flexible direct laryngoscopy performed by the surgeon reveals extensive papilloma covering two thirds of the glottic opening (Fig. 18.1). She is booked for urgent rigid bronchoscopy, suspension laryngoscopy, and surgical or laser papilloma resection.*

*Induction proceeds for the unpremedicated, fasted child in the OR with sevoflurane in 100% O$_2$. She develops worsening signs of obstruction. A **second anesthesiologist** inserts an intravenous cannula, and 0.5 mg/kg **dexamethasone** is given for postoperative airway edema. Hand ventilation is not successful. The airway is maintained with a mask while the patient breathes spontaneously. Laryngoscopy confirms the papilloma obstructing more than two thirds of the glottic opening. The larynx and upper trachea is sprayed with lidocaine (lignocaine) 4 mg/kg. After topical phenylephrine, a 4.5-mm ETT is passed into the left nostril with the tip in the upper nasopharynx; it is connected to an oxygen supply carrying 2% sevoflurane. Propofol infusion is started at 200 mcg/kg/minute (13 mg/kg/hour) and a bolus of 0.2 mcg/kg of fentanyl is given. The rigid bronchoscope is inserted and airway obstruction worsens; saturations drop to 86%. A **long 3.5-mm ETT** is inserted through the cords to allow ventilation while the surgeon performs an initial **blunt dissection** of the papilloma. Hand ventilation is unsuccessful; saturations continue fall to 75%. A suction catheter cannot be passed through the tube, so the*

ETT is removed and replaced. Ventilation is now easy. The first ETT is **blocked with fragmented papilloma**. *After blunt dissection and hemostasis, spontaneous breathing resumes and the patient is extubated to allow laser surgery to the remaining papilloma. Sevoflurane 2% is reconnected to the nasopharyngeal tube. During periods of active laser work, the FiO$_2$ is reduced to 21%. The patient emerges and is taken to recovery with mild stridor.*

DISCUSSION

1. How does one interpret the examination findings?

Stridor and intercostal and **substernal retractions** with **reduced SpO$_2$** indicate a significant degree of obstruction. A child with **obstruction of up to two thirds of the glottic opening** will often only have symptoms of hoarse voice, nocturnal breathing changes, and a moderate degree of reduction in physical activity (can walk around but not run). SpO$_2$ is often normal; healthy children compensate very well until the airway is critically narrow. A pedunculated growth that can flip into the airway, causing sudden profound airway obstruction, can also be present with minimal symptoms (Fig. 18.1). Please note: If the child had been drowsy this would indicate a highest-priority emergency.

2. What special investigations should be performed?

Specific preoperative evaluation will depend on the certainty of diagnosis. Chest and lateral neck x-rays are reasonable if a foreign body or other intrathoracic diagnosis is considered (and if clinical urgency permits). An awake flexible direct laryngoscopy using local anesthesia to the nose is usually the next step if laryngeal papilloma is suspected. Arterial blood gas sampling will likely cause worsening of symptoms and not add to the diagnostic and treatment pathway. Venous blood may be drawn to support or exclude a diagnosis of bacterial infection. CT imaging does not add information if a diagnosis has been made.

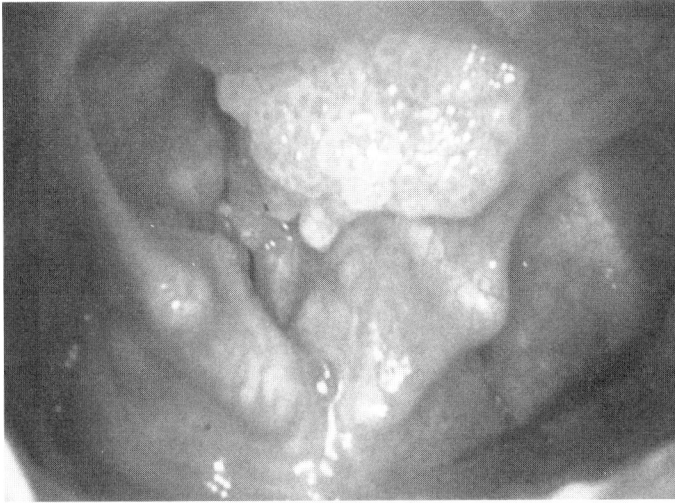

FIGURE 18.1 Laryngeal papillomas obstructing the glottis

3. What are the general options for airway management during laryngeal surgery? How suitable are they for use in a 3-year-old child?

A plan for providing oxygen during the laser surgery will depend on surgical preference, available equipment, and severity of obstruction. Apart from cardiopulmonary bypass, there are four main options for oxygenation:

a) Jet ventilation

This could either involve **subglottic** jet ventilation or **supraglottic** high/low-frequency jet ventilation. Subglottic ventilation may not allow adequate exhalation in small pediatric airways; it therefore has limited usefulness. Barotrauma, air trapping, CO_2 accumulation, pneumothorax, pneumomediastinum, or subcutaneous emphysema may occur. Even small cannulas can impair the surgical field and obstruct air outflow. If used, it is essential to have tightly controlled insufflation pressures. Supraglottic high/low-frequency jet ventilation is usually provided via a jet ventilator cannula within the lumen of the laryngoscope; this technique with deep anesthesia and paralysis has been described in the pediatric literature (Mausser et al., 2007). It carries a theoretical (but not described) risk that the jet may force papilloma fragments or the laser plume deeper into the airway (Best, 2009).

b) Tubeless field and spontaneous ventilation

An ETT or suction catheter (or similar) is placed via the nose to the nasopharynx (ensuring the tip is high and well away from the laser beam), through which gases and volatile agents can be delivered. This technique has the advantages of an unobstructed surgical field, less airway manipulation by the anesthesiologist, less CO_2 accumulation than other techniques, and minimal risk of pneumothorax or barotrauma. The disadvantages are that there is no definitive airway and it is not possible to monitor $EtCO_2$; the anesthesiologist is reliant on visual "clues" such as a hand on the upper abdomen to assess depth of anesthesia and adequacy of airway. There will be some CO_2 accumulation, and the technique requires more skill and experience with drug titration. Smaller patients or patients with marked obstruction may tolerate this for a short surgical time, but if the case is lengthy, progressive atelectasis may cause hypoxia; this may necessitate intermittent orotracheal intubation and supported ventilation in between laser attempts. Practically, if a large papilloma is obstructing most of airway at induction, it may be necessary to insert an ETT for initial surgical blunt dissection before using the laser.

c) Apneic ventilation with intermittent endotracheal intubation

This has limited applicability in young children, as hypoxia ensues rapidly due to higher oxygen consumption and loss of up to 45% of functional residual capacity during general anesthesia. This limits the surgical time to very short episodes. Intermittent intubation with an ETT carries the theoretical risk of seeding papilloma fragments distally in the airway. A standard ETT carries the potential risk of airway fire.

d) Laser ETT

Laser ETTs are available in size 3.0 and 4.0 internal diameter, but the external diameters are larger than a regular ETT. In a child even these small sizes impair the surgical view, making it difficult to perform laser surgery.

4. What preparations need to be made before induction of anesthesia?

Communication with the surgical team is essential; the plan for critical incidents, including complete airway obstruction, needs to be discussed and equipment checked.

Although unlikely, it may also be difficult to pass a standard ETT through the papilloma. There should be **two anesthesia providers** present who are familiar with pediatric airway surgery. A skilled anesthetic assistant with prepared anesthetic equipment is essential, as is the immediate availability of laryngoscopes and a variety of sizes of ETTs (as well as extra-long tubes for intubating through the surgical laryngoscope). The ENT surgeons need to be available at induction with a rigid bronchoscope and equipment to perform an emergency cricothyrotomy.

5. What is a suitable anesthetic induction technique?

The ideal situation is to induce while maintaining spontaneous ventilation. A volatile induction with sevoflurane is the safest as it is easiest to reverse and is unlikely to produce significantly prolonged apnea. It would be ideal to have IV access with the use of topical local anesthetic cream before induction. Practically, however, the second anesthesiologist can insert the IV line after induction. IV access should be on the limb closest to the anesthesiologist to allow direct vision of IV anesthetic agent delivery. Topical local anesthetic (lidocaine) is administered via an atomizer when the patient is deep enough to tolerate laryngoscopy. The volume and concentration depend on the size of the child, using a dose not exceeding 5 mg/kg.

6. What hypnotic agents can be used to maintain anesthetic depth?

Sevoflurane can be used for maintenance but is not ideal as the sole anesthetic agent because the end-tidal sevoflurane concentration cannot be measured and intermittent airway obstruction may occur during the procedure. The inability to scavenge not only causes environmental pollution, but also can affect the surgeon, who spends 45 to 90 minutes inhaling the volatile "spill." Sevoflurane is useful for intermittent supplementation to anesthesia when vocal cord movement is not controlled by propofol and opioid alone. The dose of propofol will depend on the opioid and volatile agent used; however, 166 to 250 mcg/kg/min (10–15 mg/kg/hour) is often used in combination with an opioid. Propofol boluses should be small to preserve ventilation.

7. What opioid agents can be used to supplement anesthesia?

To decrease coughing and airway irritability, low-dose opioid is recommended to supplement the hypnotic agent(s). Bolus doses should be fairly conservative to maintain spontaneous ventilation. In this example, if 2 mcg/kg fentanyl were made up to 10 mL with 0.9% saline, it allows an intermittent bolus dose of 1 mL (= 0.2 mcg/kg). Alternatively, remifentanil or alfentanil infusions can be used as effective adjuncts.

8. How can the depth of anesthesia and adequate ventilation be ensured?

During the surgery, the view of the patient is obscured with drapes and a table to support the suspension laryngoscopy equipment (Fig. 18.2). There is no end-tidal anesthetic agent or end-tidal CO_2 monitoring. Appropriate depth is important; too deep will predispose to apnea and too light is associated with coughing, splinting, and desaturation. The anesthesiologist has to rely on other monitoring and clinical signs to assess anesthetic depth and effectiveness of ventilation, such as:

- Direct visualization of vocal cord movement on video screen

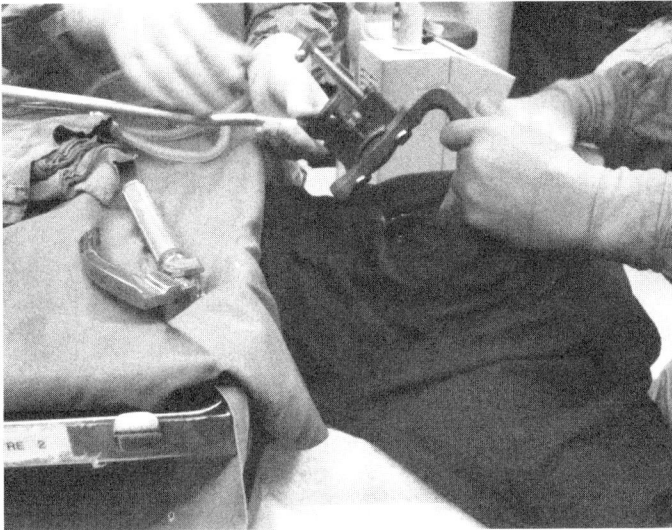

FIGURE 18.2 Suspension laryngoscopy for papilloma excision

- Maintaining a hand on the upper abdomen can gauge depth and rate of ventilation and give a feel of early airway obstruction.
- Pulse oximetry and heart rate
- BIS/entropy; the value of this is questionable in smaller children (<3 years)

9. What are the risks associated with laser airway surgery?

Risks of laser airway surgery include airway fire, damage to healthy tissue, and injury to OR staff. All staff must communicate clearly and be familiar with laser surgery and safety protocols. Laser-safe eye goggles need to be worn and the patient's face and eyes need to be protected with swabs soaked in warm saline. Fire can occur only if flammable materials are present within the airway. Both nitrous oxide and oxygen support combustion. Inspired oxygen concentrations need to be as low as possible (ideally 21%). It should be remembered that there is potential for cross-infection from papillomas. Specifically designed masks are required due to protect against inhalation of virus-laden particles.

10. What is the emergency management of an airway fire?
In the event of a fire, the "four Es" mnemonic is helpful (Werkhaven, 2004):

- **Extract**: Combustible material (ETT, pledgets)
- **Eliminate**: Oxygen
- **Extinguish**: A large prefilled syringe of 0.9% saline should be available.
- **Evaluate**: Operative field and tracheobronchial tree

SUMMARY

1. Juvenile laryngeal papillomas present with potentially life-threatening airway obstruction, which can be precipitated during general anesthesia.
2. Safe management of these patients requires good planning and communication between skilled anesthetic, surgical, and nursing staff.
3. Balancing adequate depth of anesthesia for surgery against the maintenance of spontaneous ventilation can be difficult.
4. All members of the staff need to be familiar with laser safety protocols.

ANNOTATED REFERENCES

- Best C. Anesthesia for laser surgery of the airway in children. *Pediatr Anesth* 2009; 19(s1): 155–165.

An excellent recent review on both the physics and use of laser and airway management for laser surgery in children.

- **Theroux MC, Grodecki V, Reilly JS, Kettrick RG. Juvenile laryngeal papillomatosis: scary anaesthetic!** *Paediatr Anaesth* **1998; 8(4): 357–361.**

This article reviews the clinical presentation and course of papillomatosis as well as citing an interesting case report.

- **Werkhaven JA. Microlaryngoscopy-airway management with anaesthetic techniques for CO$_2$ laser.** *Paediatr Anaesth* **2004; 14(1): 90–94.**

Another good summary of airway management for laser surgery.

Further Reading

Dalmeida RE, Mayhew JF, Driscoll B, McLaughlin R. Total airway obstruction by papillomas during induction of general anesthesia. *Anesth Analg* 1996; 83(6): 1332–1334.

English J, Norris A, Bedforth N. Anaesthesia for airway surgery. *Contin Educ Anaesth Crit Care Pain* 2006; 6(1): 28–31.

Kailey J, Cranston A, Moriarty A. Intravenous anaesthesia for laser surgery of the airway in children with recurrent laryngeal papillomatosis. *Paediatr Anaesth* 2002; 12(9): 819–820.

Malherbe S, Whyte S, Singh P, Amari E, King A, Ansermino M. Total intravenous anesthesia and spontaneous respiration for airway endoscopy in children: a prospective evaluation. *Pediatr Anesth* 2010; 20(5): 434–438.

Mausser G, Friedrich G, Schwarz G. Airway management and anesthesia in neonates, infants and children during endolaryngotracheal surgery. *Paediatr Anaesth* 2007; 17(10): 942–947.

19

Bacterial Tracheitis Versus Epiglottitis

JUNZHENG WU AND C. DEAN KURTH

INTRODUCTION

Both acute epiglottitis and bacterial tracheitis can cause severe airway obstruction, respiratory distress, and sudden respiratory arrest in young children. The early and prompt differential diagnosis between the two is crucial to select the type of airway intervention to ensure a safe outcome.

LEARNING OBJECTIVES

1. List the differential diagnoses of these two diseases.
2. Describe the key differences in airway intervention between the diseases.
3. Identify the criteria for extubation.

CASE PRESENTATION

*A 3-year-old boy presents at 2 a.m. to the emergency department (ED). The child has a high fever and signs of upper airway obstruction. His mother states that he was put to bed in good health but woke up 4 hours later crying, with **difficulty breathing**, complaining of **a sore*** *throat* and **refusing to eat or drink**, and had a **soft voice**. *Physical exam shows the child to be flushed, **drooling, sitting upright and leaning forward,** with significant **inspiratory stridor** and marked suprasternal retractions. An intraoral exam is unsuccessful due to increased patient agitation and dyspnea. A flexible nasolaryngoscopy is also unsuccessful. The vital signs are heart rate 148/min, respiratory rate 30/min, the temperature 39.5°C, SpO_2 92% with 5 L/min blow-by O_2. Although emergently intubating the child is considered in the ED to control the airway and improve the oxygen saturation, the medical, anesthesia, and otorhinolaryngology (ENT) surgical team decide to bring the child to the operating room (OR) to manage the airway. The patient is **transported to the OR** by the anesthesiologist, ENT surgeon, and nurse **in the company of the parents.***

*In the OR, the patient undergoes an **inhalation induction** with sevoflurane and 100% O_2, monitored by pulse oximetry and capnography, while leaning on the mother's shoulder. Once asleep, the patient is laid supine on the operating table. Ventilation is manually assisted with continuous positive airway pressure (CPAP) while the patient breathes spontaneously. After intravenous cannulation, atropine 20 mcg/kg is administered. The patient is intubated with a styletted 3.0 cuffed endotracheal tube (ETT) under direct laryngoscopy after adequate anesthesia depth is ensured. The periglottic region is beefy red, and the epiglottis and arytenoids are notably edematous. The cuff is not inflated after an air leak at 28 cmH_2O is confirmed. Once the airway is secured, the patient is paralyzed, a throat culture is obtained, and the airway is converted to nasal intubation. He is then transported to the pediatric intensive care unit (PICU) under continuous sedation.*

*In PICU, the patient receives **antibiotics** and dexamethasone. The child is kept mechanically ventilated with pressure-support while sedated with an IV infusion of dexmedetomidine and midazolam, and intravenous boluses of fentanyl PRN. The patient defervesces and is extubated after swelling of the airway is significantly reduced as evidenced by an **air leak** of less than 15 cmH_2O around the ETT, confirmed with flexible laryngoscopy.*

DISCUSSION

1. What is the diagnosis in this patient? What are the major common and differential features between epiglottitis and bacterial tracheitis?

The diagnosis is acute epiglottitis and is made from history, physical appearance, and radiography. Due to of the risk of sudden and complete occlusion of the airway, epiglottitis is a truly life-threatening disease in children that demands immediate intervention once the diagnosis is strongly suspected.

The common features for epiglottitis and bacterial tracheitis include occurrence in a similar age group (2–8 years), presence of high fever (>38.5°C), and toxic appearance with marked restlessness, irritability, dyspnea, and extreme anxiety. Both could cause severe **stridor** and sudden upper airway obstruction. There are some major differences between them to differentiate the diagnosis (Table 19.1). Epiglottitis is characterized by abrupt onset without a prodrome and rapid progression to respiratory obstruction, shock, and death in a matter of hours. By contrast, bacterial tracheitis has a gradual onset starting with a viral respiratory tract infection, usually reaching a peak within days. The patient with epiglottitis commonly has a severe **sore throat and pain with swallowing or eating** (dysphagia) and a **muffled voice**; cough is rare. The child with tracheitis usually has a barking, croup-like cough and hoarseness. Copious **drooling**, caused by dysphagia, frequently presents in the patient with epiglottitis but is usually absent in bacterial tracheitis. In the ED, patients with epiglottitis typically are **sitting** with their chin hyperextended and body **leaning forward** (tripod or sniffing position) to maximize air entry and improve diaphragmatic excursion. The mouth may be open wide and the tongue may protrude. An erythematous and swollen epiglottis may be seen in the oropharynx by physical exam or flexible laryngoscopy. However, a throat exam should not be performed in an uncooperative child because the exam and restraint of the child may precipitate complete airway obstruction. Complete blood count may show an elevated white blood cell count, and the lateral airway radiograph may

Table 19.1

COMPARISON OF ACUTE EPIGLOTTITIS VERSUS BACTERIAL TRACHEITIS

	Acute Epiglottitis	*Bacterial Tracheitis*
General		
Age (years)	2–8	2–8
Onset/Progress	Abrupt, in hours	Insidious, in days
Prodrome	No	Often follows a viral URI
Pathogen(s)	β-hemolytic streptococcus *N. meningitides* *H. influenzae* type b	*Staphylococcus aureus* β-hemolytic streptococcus
Pathology	Inflammation/ swelling of epiglottis and supraglottic structures	Swelling/narrowing at glottis and subglottis, mucopurulent and necrotizing membrane
Symptoms		
Cough	No or minimal	Deep, barking, croup-like
Dyspnea	Yes	Yes
Dysphonia	Yes, muffled voice	Normal or hoarse
Dysphagia	Yes, severe sore throat	No
Drooling	Continuous, copious	No
Signs		
Fever/ appearance	>38°C, toxic	>38°C, toxic
Stridor	Inspiratory	Inspiratory
Respiratory pattern	Slow, usually quiet	Rapid, struggling
Retraction	Suprasternal, intercostal	Suprasternal, intercostal
Position	Sitting, leaning forward, mouth open, neck extended	Any position except supine

(continued)

Table 19.1 (*continued*)

	Acute Epiglottitis	Bacterial Tracheitis
X-ray finding	Thick epiglottis "thumb sign"	Subglottic narrowing, "steeple sign," tracheal membranes
Treatment Plan		
Humidified O_2	Yes	Yes
Hospitalization	Immediate	Depends on severity
Patient's position	Keep sitting	As is comfortable
Airway exam	Avoid prior to intubation	Performed prior to intubation
Induction of choice	Inhalation with sevoflurane	Inhalation or intravenous
Intubation urgency	Emergently in all patients	Decided after airway exam
Where to intubate	In the OR under GA	In the OR or ED
Ventilation in ICU	Mechanical, PS	Mechanical, PS
Antibiotics	Empirically first, then by culture sensitivity	Empirically first, then by culture sensitivity
Steroids	May be beneficial	Not beneficial
Extubation	Swelling receded, air leak	Air leak, after airway exam

show enlargement and thickness of the epiglottis ("thickened thumb" sign). As with the throat exam, laboratory tests should be deferred until the airway is secured if there is any doubt as to the child's ability to cooperate.

2. What are the pathophysiologic characteristics of epiglottitis and bacterial tracheitis?

Epiglottitis, more appropriately called supraglottitis, consists of inflammation and swelling of structures above the glottis, including the lingular surface of the epiglottis, aryepiglottic folds and arytenoids, and occasionally the uvula, with little to no involvement of subglottic structures or the laryngeal surface of the epiglottis. The condition is almost always caused by a bacterial infection. Since the widespread vaccination against *Haemophilus influenzae* type b (Hib), which was the most common pathogen causing epiglottitis, the overall incidence of the disease among children has dropped dramatically. The primary pathogens now are *Neisseria meningitides*, group A streptococcus, and *Candida albicans*. Blood or throat culture will usually reveal the pathogen. Acute epiglottitis carries significant morbidity and mortality because of the high risk of sudden airway occlusion leading to respiratory arrest.

Bacterial tracheitis (also called bacterial croup) consists of a diffuse inflammation of the larynx, trachea, and bronchi with mucopurulent membranes within the trachea. The major site of disease occurs at the level of the cricoid cartilage, the narrowest part of the trachea. Severe airway obstruction develops secondary to subglottic edema and sloughing of epithelial lining or accumulation of a mucopurulent membrane within the trachea. Because of the narrow, funnel shape of the pediatric subglottic airway, relatively little inflammation is required to significantly reduce the diameter of the airway and dramatically increase the resistance to airflow and **work of breathing**. Although the pathogenesis of bacterial tracheitis remains unclear, mucosal damage and immune impairment arising from a preceding viral infection, recent intubation, or airway trauma predisposes the mucosa to invasive infection with common pyogenic organisms such as *Staphylococcus aureus* or streptococcus species. The patient can present with toxic shock syndrome if the pathogen is staphylococcus or toxic shock-like syndrome if the pathogen is streptococcus. Direct laryngobronchoscopy and the lateral neck soft tissue x-ray consistently reveal a normal epiglottis and aryepiglottic folds, along with marked subglottic mucosal edema. Intratracheal irregularities and membranes may also be seen on the lateral airway radiograph.

3. What are the key differences in airway management?

The anesthesiologist needs to decide quickly which entity he or she is seeing. Acute epiglottitis represents a medical emergency and mandates immediate action. Due to the risk of sudden, complete airway occlusion, endotracheal intubation should be emergently performed in all patients who manifest symptoms and signs of airway obstruction. In the absence of imminent airway occlusion, the child should **remain sitting up**, monitored, but otherwise **not disturbed during transport** to the location for intubation. Any maneuvers that would agitate the child might precipitate acute airway obstruction. Thus, attempts at intraoral exam with tongue depressor and flexible laryngoscopy, blood draws, and insertion of intravenous catheters should be deferred or approached with great caution. The diagnosis should be made by lateral neck soft tissue x-ray and confirmed by direct inspection of the airway in the OR under general anesthesia immediately before intubation to secure the airway. It may be of comfort (therefore safety) for the **parents to accompany the child to the OR** to help the child remain calm. An ENT or pediatric surgeon skilled in performing tracheostomy should be present in the OR during the intubation. **Inhalation induction** with sevoflurane is the method of choice with the patient in sitting position, breathing spontaneously, assisted with CPAP. After the IV is established, atropine is administered before laryngoscopy to limit oral secretions, maintain heart rate (hence, cardiac output) with deep anesthesia, and prevent vagally mediated bradycardia. Muscle relaxants are contraindicated because they may precipitate complete airway collapse. It is important to ensure a deep plane of anesthesia before laryngoscopy and oral intubation is attempted. Due to the severe supraglottic edema, styletted ETTs a few sizes smaller than usually expected should be prepared. Visualization of the glottis may be very difficult due to profound supraglottic edema. After securing the airway, the oral tracheal tube is replaced with a nasotracheal tube as long as the laryngoscopy and oral intubation are straightforward. If the laryngeal inlet cannot be observed during laryngoscopy because of swelling and secretions, an assistant can compress the chest and the anesthesiologist can often find the laryngeal inlet by bubbles from the trachea. Oral intubation should not be converted to nasal intubation in this scenario. If intubation can not be achieved, then the surgeon performs a tracheostomy while the patient is ventilated by mask.

Compared to epiglottitis, the development of airway obstruction in bacterial tracheitis occurs slowly and insidiously. As a result, there is time to evaluate the airway and an IV may be established to start **antibiotics** sooner. Once the diagnosis is suspected, the case is scheduled in the OR under general anesthesia for flexible bronchoscopy and rigid micro-laryngoscopy and bronchoscopy (MLB) to assess the airway. The key decision regarding intubation is made following an MLB airway exam.

MLB is not only important to confirm the diagnosis and evaluate the tracheal ulceration and extent of edema, but it also has a therapeutic purpose by allowing the surgeon to perform tracheal toilet and remove thick, mucopurulent secretions and sloughed mucosal membranes. Tracheal intubation is required only in patients with severe airway obstruction and respiratory distress. To minimize trauma in the inflamed subglottic area, ETTs 0.5 to 1.0 size smaller than ordinarily used are recommended for intubation. A tracheostomy kit should be handy prior to proceeding with the airway exam and intubation. Both IV and inhalation inductions can work well; muscle relaxants may be avoided but are not contraindicated.

4. What are the criteria for extubation in PICU?

For epiglottitis and bacterial tracheitis, the patient initially remains sedated and mechanically ventilated. As the patient's condition improves, the patient can be switched to spontaneous ventilation with pressure support. While intubated, sedation may be maintained with intravenous infusions, per local practice. Broad-spectrum antibiotics are administered empirically until the cultures direct a specific antibiotic. In epiglottitis, the majority of patients are ready for extubation in 24 to 48 hours. The criteria for extubation include symptomatic improvement (**reduction of fever** and toxic appearance), an **audible air leak** of less than 20 cmH$_2$O around the ETT, and minimal swelling of the epiglottis and supraglottic tissues as confirmed by laryngoscopy. In bacterial tracheitis, frequent suctioning and high inspired gas humidity are required to maintain the ETT patency. MLB may be performed to reevaluate the airway to ensure that the patient is ready for extubation. Tracheostomy is rarely necessary unless there is a failed attempt at emergent intubation and failed extubations leading to prolonged intubation despite appropriate medical management.

SUMMARY

1. Epiglottitis is a medical emergency that requires immediate intubation; bacterial tracheitis is an urgent condition that allows a wider range of response.
2. Due to airway swelling and secretions, the ETT size will be much smaller than expected for both conditions.
3. A team approach (anesthesiology, ENT/surgery, nursing, parents) is crucial for both conditions so that a safe airway can be established without further complications.

ANNOTATED REFERENCES

- Hannallah RS, Brown KA, Verghese ST. Otorhinolaryngologic procedures. In CJ Cote, J Lerman, eds. *A Practice of Anesthesia for Infants and Children*. Philadelphia: Saunders, 2009: 657–683.

  A focused discussion on the clinical course and airway intervention.
- Metha R, Hariprakash SP, Cox PN, Wheeler DS. Diseases of the upper respiratory tract. In DS Wheeler, HR Wong, eds.

Pediatric Critical Care Medicine: Basic Science and Clinical Evidence. London: Springer, 2007: 480–505.

Detailed description with a well-illustrated table to compare acute epiglottitis and bacterial tracheitis.

Further Reading

Graf J, Stein F. Tracheitis in pediatric patient. *Semin Pediatr Infect Dis* 2006; 17: 11–13.

Katori H, Tsukuda M. Acute epiglottitis: analysis of factors associated with airway intervention. *J Laryngol Otol* 2005; 119: 967–972.

Narkeviciute I, Mudeniene V, Petraitiene S. Acute epiglottitis in children: experience in diagnosis and treatment in Luthuania. *Acta Medica Lituanica* 2007; 14: 54–58.

Tebruegge M, Pantazidou A, Yau C. Bacterial tracheitis—tremendously rare, but truly important: A systematic review. *J Pediatr Infect Dis* 2009; 4(3): 199–209.

PART 4

CHALLENGES IN PATIENTS

WITH PULMONARY DISEASE

Intraoperative Wheezing

LINDY CASS

INTRODUCTION

Wheezing is an important sign for anesthesiologists. At the preoperative consult it usually indicates bronchospasm from poorly controlled asthma, though many other causes are possible. Intraoperative wheezing also has many potential causes, including bronchospasm, airway obstruction, anaphylaxis, or aspiration. Intraoperative wheezing is an anesthetic emergency that can lead to life-threatening respiratory and cardiac complications. Prompt action to maintain oxygenation, removal of any trigger factors, and, if indicated, bronchodilator administration will usually result in a safe outcome.

LEARNING OBJECTIVES

1. Know the causes of wheezing.
2. Recognize the risk factors for perioperative bronchospasm.
3. Know how to manage the child with intraoperative wheezing.

CASE PRESENTATION

An 18-month-old boy is scheduled for a cochlear implant. He was full-term and healthy at birth. At 9 months he had meningitis with consequent deafness. *He previously had two episodes of wheezing with respiratory tract infections that were treated symptomatically with an albuterol (salbutamol) inhaler with spacer; neither required hospitalization. He has been well for the previous 2 weeks. He previously had an uneventful general anesthetic for CT and MRI scanning.*

*On examination, he is happy, appears well, and weighs 10 kg. He is afebrile, his oxygen saturation on air is 99%, and chest examination is clear. Anesthesia is induced using sevoflurane, oxygen, and nitrous oxide. He is given morphine 0.5 mg and propofol 20 mg to deepen anesthesia for intubation. No muscle relaxation is used because VIIth nerve monitoring is to be used intraoperatively. A 4.5-mm internal diameter endotracheal tube (ETT) is placed to a depth of 4.5 cm at the cords and 12 cm at the lips. Hand ventilation demonstrates a normal $ETCO_2$ trace on the capnograph and auscultation reveals equal air entry bilaterally. Anesthesia is maintained using **desflurane** with an end-tidal concentration of 7.5% in air and oxygen. He is ventilated using pressure control with an inspiratory pressure of 15 cmH_2O. Prophylactic antibiotics (cefazolin 50 mg/kg) are given intravenously.*

*Five minutes later, before the start of surgery, the oxygen saturation drops from 99% to 94% on a FiO_2 of 0.4. The expired tidal volume decreases from 80 mL (7.6 mL/kg) to 45 mL (4 mL/kg). The $ETCO_2$ is now 52 mmHg and the **capnograph** trace changes from a square wave to an **upsloping ramp**. Auscultation reveals a bilateral high-pitched wheeze and the ventilating bag feels tight on manual ventilation.*

*The inspired oxygen is increased to 100% and the ETT is inspected. It is **not kinked** and remains secure at 12 cm at the lip. A suction catheter is passed down the ETT with **no** evidence of **obstruction**. His blood pressure and pulse are unchanged at 70/40 and 110 and his skin color is normal. **Anaphylaxis** is therefore thought to be unlikely. The volatile agent is changed to sevoflurane. Oxygen saturation improves to 96% and the tidal volumes rise to 60 mL (5.7 mL/kg). Two puffs of **albuterol** are administered into the breathing circuit. Within 5 minutes the wheezing has resolved, $ETCO_2$ trace returns to a normal square wave, and oxygen saturation improves to 99%. The FiO_2 is reduced back to 0.4 and the oxygen saturations are maintained.*

A decision is made to proceed and surgery is completed without recurrence of wheezing. Recovery is uneventful.

DISCUSSION

1. What is wheezing?

Wheezing is a high-pitched, musical whistle heard in expiration. In the healthy child, the velocity of airflow is too low to produce sound and breathing is inaudible without a stethoscope. Wheezing occurs from increased speed of airflow and turbulence in narrowed airways. In asthma, bronchospasm, and bronchiolitis, the small airways are affected, but in fact the wheezing comes from the trachea and major bronchi, which are narrowed from secondary compression during expiration. Small airway obstruction leads to forced expiration with positive (rather than the usual negative) intrapleural pressure. This positive intrapleural pressure exceeds the intraluminal pressure in the trachea and major bronchi and results in compression and dynamic expiratory narrowing of these airways.

While obstruction of the small airways is the most common reason for wheezing, obstructive lesions in the trachea or main bronchi may also generate an increase in velocity of airflow causing wheezing. Foreign bodies in the large airways or compression from lymph nodes may also manifest as wheezing.

Extrathoracic obstructive causes of wheezing usually have an inspiratory noise. This distinguishes them from bronchospasm, which usually just has the expiratory wheeze. "Stridor" is the term used to describe the inspiratory noises.

2. What causes wheezing?

There are many potential causes. A useful classification of possible causes is based on age (Table 20.1). Wheezing is common, and 40% to 50% of children less than 6 years of age will wheeze at some time. The majority of these have a condition known as transient infant wheeze; as did the child in this scenario. This is a

Table 20.1

ETIOLOGY OF WHEEZING BY AGE GROUP

Causes of preoperative wheezing in infants, toddlers, and preschoolers

Obstruction of small airways

> Acute viral bronchiolitis (RSV)
> Aspiration
> Asthma/bronchospasm
> Bronchiectasis
> Chronic lung disease of prematurity
> Transient infant wheeze

Obstruction of large airways

> Airway and vascular malformations
> Inhaled foreign body
> Mediastinal cysts/masses

Causes of preoperative wheezing in school-age children/ adolescents (5–15 years)

Obstruction of small airways

> Asthma
> *Mycoplasma pneumoniae* infection
> Bronchiectasis

Obstruction of large airways

> Bronchial adenoma
> Alpha 1-antitrypsin deficiency
> Inhaled/ingested foreign body
> Mediastinal tumors/masses
> Hysterical wheezing

benign condition that appears to be related to the relatively small caliber and floppiness of the airways. Most children outgrow the condition by age 6 years, but 5% to 7% of all children (30–40% of those who wheeze) continue to wheeze and are diagnosed with persistent wheezing or asthma (Henry, 2007).

3. What is the management of the child who is wheezing at the preoperative consult?

First, the cause of wheeze should be determined. The age of the child, a history of prematurity, respiratory tract infection, or reactive airways disease will give clues as to the likely cause. In a child with transient wheeze or asthma, further history is required to determine how well controlled the symptoms are. A history of chronic cough and diurnal or nocturnal symptoms are typical of poorly controlled asthma. Factors that trigger bronchospasm should be recorded. A history of recent viral infection or an exacerbation of asthma requiring hospitalization is associated with an increased risk of perioperative bronchospasm refractory to simple measures and is of particular concern.

Poor weight gain suggests other causes for wheezing, such as gastroesophageal reflux disease, cystic fibrosis, or immunodeficiency.

The child with chronic pulmonary disease, such as bronchopulmonary dysplasia, needs to be assessed with regard to optimization. Parental assessment of the child's current status and a history of recent respiratory infection or productive cough are important. The requirement for home oxygen therapy in the past or currently should be noted as an indicator of significant disease. An objective measure, such as pulse oximetry breathing air, is useful and may be compared with previous readings. The question that must be asked is, "Is this child in the best possible condition?" If so, it is appropriate to proceed with caution.

On physical examination, the anesthesiologist should decide if the child looks unwell. The temperature should be checked and the work of breathing should be assessed. Transient wheezers generally do not have significant respiratory distress and hypoxia.

Tachypnea and the use of intercostal and supraclavicular muscles are indicative of more severe asthma. Unilateral wheezing suggests aspiration of a foreign body or bronchomalacia. Wheezing together with crackles suggests an interstitial lung disease such as infection, bronchopulmonary dysplasia, or pulmonary edema (e.g., in a child with congenital heart disease). Wheezing together with stridor and noises transmitted from upper airway narrowing would suggest an upper and lower airway process such as croup, tracheomalacia, or bronchomalacia.

4. How is intraoperative wheezing managed?

A rapid diagnosis of the cause of intraoperative wheezing must be made. Wheezing usually occurs under light anesthesia as a result of bronchial or carinal stimulation. It may also result from bronchospasm subsequent to aspiration or **anaphylaxis** or might be drug-related via a variety of other mechanisms. The clinical context will help ascertain the cause. Mechanical causes of **airway obstruction** (e.g., kinking or mucous plugging of the ETT) need to be recognized by inspecting the circuit and inserting a suction catheter to the tip of the ETT. Other mechanical causes are rare but may include incidental inhaled foreign body (this may not have been witnessed or suspected), obstructive mass, vascular ring, and vocal cord dysfunction.

Anaphylaxis is likely when all of the following three criteria are met:

- Sudden onset and rapid progression of symptoms
- Life-threatening airway and/or circulation problems
- Skin and/or mucosal changes (flushing, urticaria, angioedema)

In the child in this scenario, a mechanical cause was excluded and anaphylaxis was thought to be unlikely. The child had *persistent wheezing*. This is best managed by deepening the anesthesia with a bolus of propofol (1–2 mg/kg) or by increasing the inspired sevoflurane concentration. **Desflurane** causes a marked increase in airway resistance, particularly in children with airway irritability, and should have been avoided (Von Ungern-Sternberg et al., 2008). In this scenario a beta-2 agonist was also given to treat acute bronchospasm via the inhalational route. Short-acting agents such as **albuterol** (salbutamol) may be given through the breathing circuit. One puff is equivalent to 100 mcg. Alternatively, a 0.5% solution (5 mg/mL) may be nebulized, either diluted (0.5 mL in 4 mL) or undiluted. Other beta-2 agonists include terbutaline and metoproterenol. In life-threatening bronchospasm, a bolus of epinephrine (adrenaline) 1 to 2 mcg/kg IV (one-tenth the resuscitation dose) or an intravenous infusion of a beta-2 agonist is indicated.

Systemic corticosteroids are used in more severe attacks than seen in this scenario. They are slower in onset than the beta-2 agonists. Methylprednisolone 0.5 to 1 mg/kg or hydrocortisone 2 to 4 mg/kg may be given intravenously. Corticosteroids enhance and prolong the response to beta-adrenergic agents within one hour, while 4 to 6 hours are required for the anti-inflammatory effects. Lidocaine (lignocaine) (1.5 mg/kg IV) may reduce the airway response to instrumentation and drug-induced bronchospasm. However, paradoxically, lidocaine can itself also cause a significant increase in airway tone and narrowing when given by inhalation or intravenously (Chang et al., 2007). Magnesium may also be used in severe asthma attacks (Cheuk et al., 2005). Aminophylline is not recommended as a therapy under anesthesia because it may cause cardiac dysrhythmias (Streetman et al., 2002).

The wheezing child should be observed closely in the postanesthesia care unit for increasing work of breathing, respiratory distress, and changing oxygen requirement. Children with a past history of reactive airways disease may develop wheezing as they emerge from anesthesia. Volatile agents are good bronchodilators; an effect that wanes on emergence. The possibility of NSAIDs triggering asthma should be remembered, although this phenomenon is more common in adults.

Persistent oxygen dependence may indicate a need for arterial blood gas measurement. A chest radiograph may be normal in reactive airways disease; however, typical findings include peribronchial thickening, subsegmental atelectasis, and hyperinflation. Unusual causes of wheeze such as congenital lung malformations or vascular malformations may be detected. A pulmonologist (respiratory pediatrician) may be consulted if symptoms do not resolve.

5. How can intraoperative wheezing be avoided?

Elective surgery should be postponed in children at high risk (i.e., those with concurrent respiratory infection or poorly controlled asthma and those with preoperative wheezing). A careful anesthetic plan is required for the child considered to be at risk if surgery is to go ahead. All asthma medications should be continued until surgery. *Premedication with a beta-2 agonist* (e.g., albuterol) decreases the incidence of perioperative bronchospasm and should be considered in high-risk children. A course of preoperative *corticosteroids* might also be considered in high-risk children.

Inhalational induction with sevoflurane may be preferred, as volatile agents generally are bronchodilators and the mask is often familiar and well tolerated. Intravenous induction may be safely performed, bearing in mind the effects of the different agents on bronchomotor tone. Propofol causes significant upper airway relaxation, while ketamine has weak sympathomimetic actions and causes bronchodilation; however, the disadvantage is that it increases secretions.

For maintenance of anesthesia desflurane should be avoided, and sevoflurane may be superior to isoflurane (Rooke et al., 1997). Adequate depth of anesthesia is critical before airway instrumentation is attempted. Endotracheal intubation is associated with a lower incidence of respiratory events but is more likely to provoke bronchospasm than placement of a laryngeal mask airway (Kim & Bishop, 1999; Mamie et al., 2004). Extubation of the trachea under deep anesthesia is often recommended. Emergence in patients with irritable airways is associated with laryngospasm and bronchospasm.

A number of drugs routinely used in anesthesia can induce bronchospasm through histamine release or muscarinic activity or by provoking allergic reactions. Atracurium has histamine-releasing effects, while cisatracurium does not. Rocuronium may be used for rapid-sequence intubation, although succinylcholine is not contraindicated in those at risk of bronchospasm. As for all cases, care must be taken that nondepolarizing neuromuscular block is fully reversed. The use of morphine in asthmatics has been controversial, although there is little objective evidence to validate these concerns (Eschenbacher et al., 1984).

SUMMARY

1. Wheezing is common and has many potential causes.
2. Risk factors for developing intraoperative wheezing include intercurrent respiratory infection and poorly controlled asthma. In these cases, consider postponing surgery.
3. A careful anesthetic plan will decrease the risk of intraoperative wheezing. Premedication with albuterol, avoidance of desflurane, and maintenance of a deep plane of anesthesia minimize the likelihood of wheezing.
4. In cases of intraoperative wheezing due to bronchospasm, cease triggering agents, deepen anesthesia, and administer inhaled beta-2 agonists. Exclude anaphylaxis, aspiration, and mechanical obstruction of the ETT.

ANNOTATED REFERENCES

- Von Ungern-Sternberg BS, Saudan S, Petak F, Hantos Z, Habre W. Desflurane but not sevoflurane impairs respiratory tissue mechanics in children with susceptible airways. *Anesthesiology* 2008; 108: 216–224.

This excellent article demonstrates the adverse effect that desflurane has on the respiratory mechanics of children with recent respiratory infection or asthma.

• **Von Ungern-Sternberg BS, Boda K, Chambers NA, Rebmann C, Johnson C, Sly PD, Habre W. Risk assessment for respiratory complications in paediatric anaesthesia: a prospective cohort study.** *Lancet* **2010; 376: 773–783.**

This paper outlines the risk factors for perioperative respiratory complications in children, including asthma.

• **Woods BD, Sladen RN. Perioperative considerations for the patient with asthma and bronchospasm.** *Br J Anaesth* **2009;103 Suppl 1: i57–65.**

This comprehensive review of asthma and anesthesia is essential reading.

Further Reading

Chang HY, Togias A, Brown RH. The effects of systemic lidocaine on airway tone and pulmonary function in asthmatic subjects. *Anesth Analg* 2007; 104: 1109–1115.

Cheuk DKL, Chau TCH, Lee SL. A meta-analysis on intravenous magnesium sulphate for treating acute asthma. *Arch Dis Child* 2005; 90: 74–77.

Eschenbacher WL, Bethel RA, Boushey HA, Sheppard D. Morphine sulfate inhibits bronchoconstriction in subjects with mild asthma whose responses are inhibited by atropine. *Am Rev Respir Dis* 1984; 130(3): 363–367.

Henery, R. "Wheezing disorders other than asthma" in Roberton DM, South M, eds. *Practical Paediatrics*. 6th edition. Edinburgh: Churchill Livingstone; 2007. 459–463.

Kim ES, Bishop MJ. Endotracheal intubation, but not laryngeal mask airway insertion, produces reversible bronchoconstriction. *Anesthesiology* 1999; 90: 391–394.

Mamie C, Habre W, Delhumeau C, Argiroffo CB, Morabia A. Incidence and risk factors of perioperative respiratory adverse events in children undergoing elective surgery. *Paediatr Anaesth* 2004; 14: 218–224.

Rooke GA, Choi JH, Bishop MJ. The effect of isoflurane, halothane, sevoflurane, and thiopental/nitrous oxide on respiratory system resistance after tracheal intubation. *Anesthesiology* 1997; 86: 1294–1299.

Streetman DD, Bhatt-Mehta V, Johnson CE. Management of acute, severe asthma in children. *Ann Pharmacother* 2002; 36: 1249–1260.

Von Ungern-Sternberg BS, Saudan S, Petak F, Hantos Z, Habre W. Desflurane but not sevoflurane impairs respiratory tissue mechanics in children with susceptible airways. *Anesthesiology* 2008; 108: 216–224.

21

Cystic Fibrosis

DAVID MARTIN AND JUNZHENG WU

INTRODUCTION

Cystic fibrosis (CF) is an inherited chronic disease that affects about 30,000 children and adults in the United States and 70,000 worldwide. CF is the most common fatal inherited disorder affecting Caucasians in the United States. While its presentation can vary in severity, the most common clinical manifestations are progressive lung damage and chronic digestive problems due to exocrine gland dysfunction and the production of thick viscous mucus. Careful perioperative management is important to avoid respiratory complications.

LEARNING OBJECTIVES

1. Understand the pathophysiology of CF and its clinical implications.
2. Know how to evaluate and optimize the patient with CF preoperatively.
3. Explain the key principles of intraoperative management.
4. Develop a plan to avoid postoperative respiratory complications.

CASE PRESENTATION

*An 11-year-old girl with CF is scheduled for flexible bronchoscopy and bronchopulmonary lavage due to a worsening **productive cough**,* *low-grade fever, and* **increased breathing effort** *in the past few weeks. Her history is significant for* **meconium ileus** *requiring bowel resection in infancy. Her chest x-ray shows* **hyperinflation** *and diffuse interstitial disease with* **bronchiectasis** *and nodular densities of mucoid impaction. She is on oral supplementation of pancreatic enzymes and fat-soluble vitamins and uses inhaled tobramycin.*

In the OR, propofol and fentanyl are used to induce anesthesia after thorough preoxygenation. Vigorous gagging and breath holding are noticed during the process of intubation. The SpO_2 quickly drops from 97% to 65% and moderate **bilateral wheezing** *is heard over the chest after the endotracheal tube (ETT) is pulled back 2 cm from carina. The anesthetic plane is deepened and two rounds of nebulized albuterol (salbutamol) are given via the inspiratory limb of the anesthesia circuit. She is given positive-pressure ventilation with a FiO_2 of 1.0. The SpO_2 returns to 96% over a few minutes and the wheezing dramatically improves. The pulmonologist proceeds with flexible bronchoscopy. A thick, yellow layer of mucus is seen throughout the bronchial tree. After lavage and* **extensive** *suction of visible* **secretions,** *the procedure is completed. The patient returns to spontaneous breathing with SpO_2 97% at FiO_2 = 1.0 and is extubated fully awake and transported to the post-anesthetic care unit (PACU).*

In the PACU, the first set of vital signs is within the normal limits, but over the next 30 minutes the patient develops an increased frequency of her productive cough. The PACU nurse initiates manual **chest physiotherapy** *with postural drainage. The patient expectorates copious thick mucus from the respiratory tract and maintains SpO_2 at 96% on room air. The patient is sent to the ward for overnight observation.*

DISCUSSION

1. What are the genetic and molecular abnormalities in CF?

CF is an autosomal recessive genetic disorder. The CF transmembrane conductance regulator (CFTR), which is widely localized on the surface of epithelia lining the respiratory tract, pancreas, intestine, sweat and salivary glands, and reproductive tract, is responsible for the pathophysiologic process of this disease. Up to 300 mutations on a gene that directs the synthesis of CFTR have been identified on the long arm of chromosome 7 in CF patients. CFTR loses its chloride-regulating mechanism, resulting in the impermeability of epithelial cells to chloride ions. Diagnostic tests for CF include DNA sequencing to identify mutations and sweat testing, which demonstrates an excessive amount of sodium and chloride in the sweat.

2. **What are the pathophysiologic features and the clinical manifestations of CF in the respiratory and GI system?**
Respiratory system: Pulmonary involvement accounts for more than 90% of the morbidity and mortality in CF patients. In the normal airway epithelium, chloride ions are actively transported into the airway lumen with sodium and water to hydrate the airway secretions. In CF, the abnormal CFTR protein causes an inability to actively secrete Cl⁻ ions. As a result, sodium and water are attracted into the epithelial cells from the airway lumen, leading to the viscid, thick, and dehydrated airway secretions that are the hallmark of the disease. This thick mucus leads to airway inflammation and mucociliary dysfunction. The resulting inability to clear secretions causes mucus plugging and increased bacterial colonization. The upper airway involvement includes an increased volume of thick mucus, hyperactive mucus-secreting glands, edema and hypertrophy of the mucous membranes, chronic nasal congestion, sinusitis, and nasal polyps. The involvement of the lower respiratory tract in CF usually dominates the clinical picture. Small airway obstruction by thick secretions causes progressive **bronchiectasis** and **hyperinflation** of the lungs due to air trapping, **atelectasis**, and frequent pulmonary infection with a wide variety of pathogens (most commonly *Staphylococcus aureus* and *Pseudomonas aeruginosa*). Wheezing is the result of airway hyperreactivity, especially accompanying pulmonary infection. Over time, pulmonary function deteriorates as measured by decreases in FEV_1 and exercise tolerance. Hypoxia and respiratory

failure result from acute exacerbation, pulmonary infections, or progressive loss of lung function due to chronic lung disease. With advanced disease, hypoxemia leads to pulmonary hypertension, cor pulmonale, and right ventricular failure. Pneumothorax and hemoptysis may occur in advanced stages.

GI system: GI complications of CF have several implications for the anesthesiologist. **Meconium ileus** in neonates results in intestinal obstruction; the babies can present to the OR with volvulus, atresia, and/or peritonitis from perforation. Pancreatic duct blockage by thick exocrine secretions results in two major consequences. First, the enzymes are prevented from reaching the intestine, leading to malabsorption of protein, fat, and the fat-soluble vitamins A, D, E, and K. Vitamin K deficiency is closely associated with coagulopathy and bone disease, frequently seen in CF patients. Delayed puberty and vitamin D and calcium deficiencies also contribute to osteoporosis. Second, duct plugging causes progressive pancreatic fibrosis. This eventually leads to pancreatic endocrine dysfunction and insulin-dependent diabetes in a small portion of patients. Biliary cirrhosis, portal hypertension, and cholelithiasis can develop in the late stages of this disease.

3. How should one assess and optimize the patient for elective surgery?

CF is a lifelong chronic and progressive disease. CF patients coming to the OR may therefore have different issues depending on when and why they present. Pre-anesthetic assessment of the CF patient should account for the dynamics of the disease and focus on the most commonly affected organs and systems. The severity of pulmonary disease is assessed by *exercise tolerance,* symptoms of *cough,* the *quality and quantity of mucus* production, *baseline oxygen saturation, the need for supplemental oxygen,* and the presence of active and persistent *wheezing.* About 40% of patients are responsive to bronchodilators, but in some "paradoxical responders," the FEV_1 may in fact deteriorate. The most likely explanation is that albuterol reduces smooth airway tone;

CF patients who have damaged, bronchiectatic airways require this tone to prevent airway collapse. One should inquire about recent fever and pulmonary infection. Pulmonary function tests and chest x-rays should be reviewed. ECG and echocardiogram should be obtained when cor pulmonale, pulmonary hypertension, or other cardiac abnormality is suspected. Arterial blood gas analysis should be considered to analyze the baseline of pO_2 and pCO_2 prior to any major and prolonged surgery. Clinical measures that can be taken (in consultation with the respiratory physician) to optimize the patient for surgery include (a) *a full course of antibiotics* for ongoing active pulmonary infection prior to elective surgery; (b) *oral and inhaled corticosteroids* to treat coexistent allergic pulmonary aspergillosis and reactive airway disease; (c) *daily bronchodilators* and/or steroid for active wheezing if a good response to the drug is observed; (d) *intensive pulmonary therapy* including incentive spirometry, daily regimens of postural drainage, and manual and mechanical chest physiotherapy (percussion, clapping, and vibration) to facilitate bronchial airway drainage; and (e) *aerosol therapy* with inhaled mucolytic agents (N-acetylcysteine) or inhaled DNAase. *Mucolytic agents* decrease sputum viscosity and improve mucus clearance; inhaled tobramycin has the benefit of reaching distal sites of lung infection in high concentrations. Inhalation of hypertonic saline (7% NaCl) accelerates mucus clearance and improves lung function and is now part of the routine management of CF patients. It should be continued throughout the perioperative period. When possible, surgery should be scheduled later in the day to allow enough time for ambulation and chest physiotherapy in the morning to facilitate expectoration of secretions retained overnight.

Review of the GI system should focus on nutritional status and gastroesophageal acid reflux (GER), which can be seen in nearly 50% of pediatric patients. Insulin-dependent diabetes and coagulopathy should be suspected and evaluated with preoperative testing if indicated. Clinical optimization of the CF patient includes acid suppression to control GERD, blood sugar management regimens if indicated (see Chapter 46), preoperative administration of oral or intramuscular vitamin K to reduce the risk of coagulopathy, nutritional therapy such as pancreatic enzymes, and vitamin replacement to increase immune function.

Numerous metabolic disturbances are seen in patients with CF, including *decreased plasma albumin levels* (which may affect drug binding and wound healing), *intravascular volume depletion* (due to chronic diarrhea, poor oral intake, and diuretic therapy), and *electrolyte imbalances*, which may be caused by excessive chloride and sodium loss from sweat.

4. What are key points of intraoperative management?

The anesthetic plan for the CF patient depends upon the nature of the operation and the condition of the patient. The goal is to provide minimal long-term ventilatory depression and to enhance clearance of secretions.

Premedication: Daily medications, particularly bronchodilators, corticosteroids, and cardiotonic drugs, should be continued into the perioperative period. Preoperative oral benzodiazepines have been used successfully to treat the anxiety that may be seen in children with chronic diseases such as CF. Prophylactic treatment with bronchodilators should be considered before induction if reactive airways and bronchospasm are significant components of the disease. Premedication with anticholinergic agents such as atropine and glycopyrrolate has historically been used to reduce bronchial secretions and suppress vagal tone. Anticholinergics offer little advantage and their use should be avoided. The use of H_2 receptor antagonists and antacid premedication is recommended in patients with poorly controlled GERD. Provided that coagulation is normal, regional anesthesia can be considered when appropriate as a method of reducing the systemic side effects of anesthetic drugs, especially opioids.

Induction/intubation: If general anesthesia is selected, preoxygenation to maximize hemoglobin saturation before induction is especially important. CF patients with moderate to severe lung disease may have an altered hypoxic respiratory drive, so close attention should be paid to the adequacy of respiration during preoxygenation. Inhalation induction may be used in young CF patients as it would be for any other appropriate patient. Pronounced V/Q mismatch and large FRC and small tidal volumes may significantly prolong inhalation induction. In patients with poorly controlled GERD, rapid-sequence induction and intubation should be considered to reduce the risk of aspiration. Propofol is favored for intravenous induction due to its bronchodilating effect and minimal airway irritation. Ketamine, despite its bronchodilating properties, is less desirable as it tends to increase bronchial secretions and may promote laryngospasm. Intubation should be performed at a deep plane of anesthesia to avoid coughing, breath holding, and bronchospasm. Cuffed ETTs offer the advantage over uncuffed tubes for permitting higher ventilation pressure, if required. Humidification of inspired gases is important to reduce dessication and inspissation of already thick secretions. One should be prepared to suction thick secretions from the ETT, which can become plugged or narrowed by mucus. Intravenous fentanyl and the application of lidocaine spray to the upper airway may smooth the intubation process. Nasal polyps causing nasal obstruction may complicate mask ventilation and present a relative contraindication to nasotracheal intubation. Muscle relaxation is preferred in CF patients with severe respiratory involvement; note that concurrent use of aminoglycoside antibiotics (tobramycin) may prolong the duration of action of a nondepolarizing muscle relaxant. Short-acting muscle relaxants are preferred so that recovery of strength is not delayed postoperatively. Stress-dose steroids and parenteral vitamin K can be administered if indicated.

Maintenance of general anesthesia: Inhalation agents, particularly sevoflurane, are advantageous in producing bronchodilation with minimal airway irritation. Higher concentrations of oxygen should be delivered because of increased oxygen consumption in the CF patient. Even though nitrous oxide has been safely used by some anesthesiologists, it should be used cautiously because of the potential risk of sudden rupture of emphysematous bullae, resulting in pneumothorax. To reduce the risk of pneumothorax, adequate ventilation should be achieved with minimal peak ventilatory pressures. Adequate intravenous hydration and humidified and warmed inspired gases are important in preventing intraoperative inspissation of secretions. Frequent suctioning through the ETT or by bronchoscopy reduces the risk of mucous plugging and helps to maintain adequate oxygenation and ventilation. Although the LMA is an option for short cases, disadvantages include the inability to suction, obstruction of the LMA by thick secretions, and the risk of laryngospasm and aspiration. Attention to maintaining euthermia is important since CF patients have less subcutaneous fat and tend to develop hypothermia during and after surgery. Blood sugar should be monitored in patients with diabetes. Lastly, due to sweat chloride losses, patients can dehydrate easily. Careful attention must be paid to the patient's volume status, starting preoperatively.

Extubation: Avoidance of prolonged intubation and mechanical ventilation reduces the risk of postoperative pulmonary infection. The ETT should be thoroughly suctioned and lung recruitment maneuvers should be performed prior to extubation. Complete reversal of neuromuscular blockade should be confirmed and the patient should be extubated fully awake, meeting standard extubation criteria.

5. What post-anesthetic interventions facilitate patient recovery?

Post-anesthetic care must be directed toward continued *aggressive respiratory therapy*, *oxygen supplementation*, and *clearance of respiratory secretions*. Good pain management is important in reducing the effect of splinting on pulmonary function and sputum clearance. Patient-controlled analgesia may be particularly useful to allow patients to time administration of analgesia along with their need to cough. Either opioid- or regional anesthesia-based techniques can be used. Care must be used when considering NSAIDs in patients with a history of hemoptysis. Opioids must be administered very carefully and titrated to effect to minimize respiratory depression. The effect of opiates on bowel motility should also be monitored. **Chest physiotherapy** should be included in the perioperative care of the CF patient. Treatment with bronchodilators and prolonged oxygen supplementation are expected in the recovery room for many postoperative CF patients. Patients should be restarted on their maintenance pulmonary regimen as soon as possible. Admission to the hospital for overnight observation or even an intensive care unit stay may be required, depending on baseline pulmonary status and perioperative changes.

SUMMARY

1. CF manifests from birth with a number of medical problems that require surgery or complicate anesthesia. Optimal preoperative preparation of the patient is important and differs at varying stages of the disease.
2. Adequate depth of anesthesia for intubation is important to reduce coughing, bronchospasm, and desaturation. Volatile agents promote bronchodilation and frequent suctioning is helpful in removing copious thick secretions.
3. Postoperative care emphasizes chest physiotherapy and pain control to optimize pulmonary function.

ANNOTATED REFERENCES

· Boucher R, Knowles M and Yankaskas J. Chapter 41, Cystic fibrosis. In Mason R, Broaddus VC, Martin T, King T, Schraufnagel D, Murray J, Nadel J, eds. *Murray and Nadel's Textbook of Respiratory Medicine*, 5th ed. Philadelphia: Saunders, 2010.

Comprehensive evaluation and treatment from a medicine perspective.

- **Huffmyer JL. Perioperative management of the adult with cystic fibrosis.** *Anesth Analg* **2009; 109: 1949–1961.**

An updated review focusing on perioperative anesthetic management.

- **Karlet M. An update on cystic fibrosis and implications for anesthesia.** *AANA J* **2000; 68: 141–146.**

A thorough review with a detailed description of pathophysiology and perioperative anesthetic management and good tables.

Further Reading

Baum VC, O'Flaherty JE. Cystic fibrosis. In Anesthesia for Genetic, Metabolic, and Dysmorphic Syndromes of Childhood, 2nd ed. Philadelphia: Lippincott Williams and Wilkins, 2007: 94–96.

Cowl CT, Prakash UB, Kruger BR. The role of anticholinergics in bronchoscopy. A randomized clinical trial. *Chest* 2000; 118: 188–192.

Sanchez I, Holbrow J, Chernick V. Acute bronchodilator response to a combination of beta-adrenergic and anticholinergic agents in patients with cystic fibrosis. *J Pediatr* 1992; 120: 486–488.

22

Pectus Excavatum Repair

DAVID L. MOORE AND
KENNETH R. GOLDSCHNEIDER

INTRODUCTION

Pectus excavatum is a defect in the proper growth of the sternum and adjacent costal cartilages, causing posterior depression of the chest. Pectus deformities account for more than 90% of congenital chest wall deformities. Evidence supports surgical repair, as many patients experience progressive cardiopulmonary symptoms over time. The most common symptoms include dyspnea with exercise and loss of endurance. An increasingly common method of repair is the Nuss minimally invasive technique, in which rigid bars are placed under the sternum and the costal cartilages with thoracoscopic guidance for a period of time until permanent remodeling of the chest is achieved.

LEARNING OBJECTIVES

1. Understand the risks of repair of pectus excavatum as they apply to anesthetic technique.
2. Review techniques involved with thoracic epidural catheters.
3. Learn how to manage postoperative pain following pectus repair.

CASE PRESENTATION

A 14-year-old otherwise healthy boy with a severe pectus excavatum deformity presents for surgical repair using the Nuss minimally invasive technique. The patient originally came to the surgeon after his parents inquired about correcting his pectus deformity a year before. The defect, while noticeable at an earlier age, has progressed as the patient has grown over the past 2 years. He had no symptoms initially but has since noted **dyspnea** *on exertion, as well as difficulty keeping up with his friends. The preoperative CT scan reveals the pectus deformity with leftward shift of the heart and an* **epidural space depth** *of 4 cm. The* **Haller index** *is noted to be 8 (Fig. 22.1). His workup is otherwise unremarkable.*

After securing intravenous access, the patient is **lightly sedated** *and assisted to the sitting position. His back is cleansed with povidone–iodine and draped with sterile barriers. After subcutaneous lidocaine (lignocaine) local anesthetic is injected, an 18g Touhy needle is inserted between the spinous processes of T6 and T7 and the epidural space is entered with a continuous-pressure, loss-of-resistance technique using preservative-free saline. The catheter is advanced 4 cm into the epidural space, the needle is removed, and the site is dressed in sterile fashion. Test dosing is unremarkable.*

The patient is returned to the supine position, general endotracheal anesthesia is induced, and two large-bore IV catheters are placed. The patient's arms are extended to just less than 90 degrees to allow surgical access to the lateral thorax. Through a small incision in each side of the chest, an introducer and then the pectus bar is passed under the sternum anterior to the heart and lungs. A thoracoscope is used to help guide the bar. During the placement of the bar, brief ventricular ectopy occurs, which needs no treatment. The bar is then flipped and the sternum pops out. Stabilizer bars and sutures affix the pectus bar to the ribcage. At the end of the case, a small **pneumothorax** *is noted on the left side.*

Following the case, the patient is **extubated deep** *to prevent coughing on the ETT. The patient is then taken to the recovery room and maintained on face mask oxygen. As the patient emerges,*

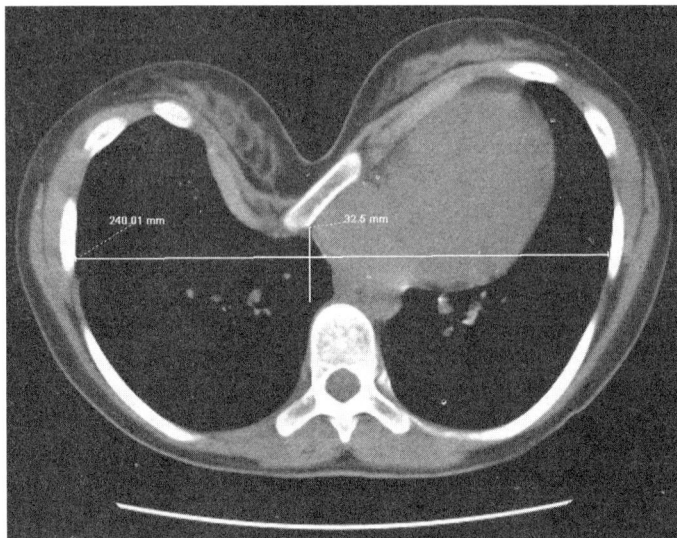

FIGURE 22.1 Preoperative computed tomography scan. Haller index = 8 (severe).

intravenous methocarbamol is given for **muscle spasms**. *The epidural is effective, though some mild pain on coughing is reported and the patient says his* **breathing feels "tight"** *and "strange." A 3-day course of epidural analgesia is planned.*

DISCUSSION

1. On what should the preoperative evaluation focus?

A thorough preoperative history and physical examination is important to determine the clinical severity of the pectus excavatum and to assess for associated medical problems. Pectus excavatum can be seen in patients with inherited connective tissue disorders such as Marfan syndrome, homocystinuria, and Ehler-Danlos syndrome. Patients with pectus excavatum may have scoliosis and mitral valve prolapse. Although severe pectus deformities can cause a leftward shift of the heart with some compression, most patients with this deformity are healthy. They may present to the surgeon initially with concerns over the cosmetic appearance of their chest, but eventually proceed to surgery because of dyspnea with exercise and loss of endurance. **CT scans** are performed to determine the severity of the pectus deformity using the **Haller index**, which is defined as the ratio of the transverse diameter of the thorax to the anterior–posterior diameter of the thorax. In the original description of the Haller index, patients with indices of 3.25 and greater all had operative correction of their pectus deformities (Haller et al., 1987). While the CT scans are of primary benefit to the surgeon, the anesthesiologist may find them useful preoperatively in **determining the approximate depth from the skin to the epidural space**. In the case of a patient with scoliosis, the scans can be invaluable in enabling the anesthetist to anticipate the angle of approach to the epidural space. Depending on the severity of the deformity and the presence of associated medical problems, preoperative evaluation with an electrocardiogram, echocardiogram, and pulmonary function testing may be indicated.

2. What complications may occur with endoscopic pectus repair?

Endoscopic pectus excavatum repair is a minimally invasive approach to treating the cosmetic and progressive, functional cardiopulmonary compromise of the defect. Although the patients are often healthy, the surgical procedure can be associated with serious complications. Bilateral pneumothoraces and injury to the heart and other mediastinal structures have been described with this procedure; they can occur at the time of placement of the retrosternal bar or later when the bar is removed. The most common risks include bar displacement, **pneumothorax**, and infection, but complications may also include cardiac injury, sternal erosion, arterial pseudo-aneurysm, and persistent cardiac arrhythmias (Hebra et al., 2000). Death from exsanguination due to cardiac or vascular injury has been described, and although rare, vigilance, good venous access, and availability of packed red cells are essential. While an arterial line is not required, two large-bore peripheral IVs are necessary. Compared with the open procedure, endoscopic repair is performed with minimal blood loss and no resection of bony or cartilaginous structures and allows a quicker return to normal activity. While highly successful and less invasive than open pectus repair, "minimally invasive" endoscopic repair still causes significant postoperative pain.

A smooth emergence without coughing is important to prevent complications. If the patient coughs on the endotracheal tube, the increased intrathoracic pressure may force air in the pleural cavity from a residual pneumothorax and cause subcutaneous emphysema, which may be extensive. Short-acting opioids, lidocaine, a small dose of propofol prior to extubation, or **deep extubation** (as done in this case) may be performed to avoid coughing against the endotracheal tube.

3. How can pain control be provided?

Pain control is achieved using a multimodal approach. A well-functioning epidural can avoid issues with opioid usage, which include poor dynamic pain relief, sedation, nausea and emesis, pruritus, hallucinations, ileus, urinary retention, and respiratory depression. However, evidence for one modality being superior to the other is modest. The technical aspects for epidural catheter insertion in adolescents do not differ from those for adult patients. Since many younger patients may not be able to cooperate with having the catheter placed while they are awake, placement of catheters in anesthetized patients is standard practice in pediatric anesthesia. On the other hand, many adolescents will tolerate placement quite well with modest sedation, if they are brought to understand that the procedure is not particularly painful or scary. Epidural analgesia is maintained until the third postoperative day for single-bar pectus repairs and until the fourth postoperative day for repairs with more than one bar. Beyond incisional and bony pain, the conformational change of the thoracic cavity can cause considerable **spasmodic pain**. This is relieved by a combination of methocarbamol around the clock and diazepam as needed. The anti-inflammatory drug ketorolac can be started immediately postoperatively, assuming intraoperative bleeding is absent. If there is no functional epidural, then opioids provided via a patient-controlled analgesia pump can be used effectively. The adjunct medications are used as with the epidurals.

The transition to an oral regimen requires some forethought, as no oral regimen will be able to match the comfort of an effective epidural. One technique is to begin long-acting opioids roughly 6 hours before the catheter is to be discontinued so that therapeutic blood levels of the opioid are established before the onset of significant pain. The adjunct medications are then transitioned to oral equivalents at the time the epidural is removed. Informing the patient and family that the transition can be a little rocky will set expectations appropriately and maintain satisfaction with care, even though the analgesic regimen may need adjustment to achieve optimal comfort.

4. What are the advantages and limits of epidural analgesia for pectus repairs?

Patients undergoing thoracic surgery have been shown to have better pain control and improved postsurgical ventilation with epidural analgesia than patients using opioid-based analgesia (Weber et al., 2007). This is true in the pectus population, particularly as they get older and the thoracic cage becomes particularly rigid. Thoracic epidurals typically are inserted at the T5–T7 level. It is important to recognize that pain from endoscopic pectus repairs is felt as superiorly as T1, and the most common mistake in placing epidural catheters is to insert them too low. Patients need to be educated that their respirations will feel different postoperatively. A **"tight" sensation** is often described and can be distressing even though it is not painful. No mode of analgesia will completely relieve that feeling. Preoperative education will help patients have realistic expectations for their

Table 22.1

POSTOPERATIVE ANALGESIA PROTOCOL FOR PECTUS EXCAVATUM REPAIR

Education

Pain is significant despite "minimally invasive" approach.
The chest will feel tight and breathing will feel different from preoperatively. Patients need to know this is normal.
Transition from epidural to oral regimen may be challenging.

Epidural/PCA

Epidural:
- T5–T6 entry
- Optimal mixture of local anesthetic and opioid is unclear; consider a hydrophilic opioid as multiple dermatomes are involved

PCA:
- Consider basal infusion.
- Opioid choice as per local preference

Intravenous Regimen

Methocarbamol scheduled, for continuous relief of spasmodic pain
Ketorolac scheduled, for general musculoskeletal pain
Diazepam: for acute muscle spasm

Oral Regimen

Start prior to discontinuing the epidural to smooth the transition:
- Ibuprofen
- Methocarbamol scheduled
- Diazepam as needed for muscle spasm
- Oxycodone: scheduled long-acting form with immediate release as needed for breakthrough pain

Duration of Treatment

Epidural/PCA regimen:
- Run until POD #3 for single bar
- Run until POD #3–4 for double bar
- Older patients may need longer

PO regimen:
- Up to 2–4 weeks
- Older patients may need longer

postoperative course, reduce their anxiety, and prevent unneeded adjustments to the epidural analgesia. A change in the location or type of pain may indicate that the pectus bar has shifted, which can be confirmed radiographically. Some surgeons prefer that the patient sits straight up rather than rolling to the side when sitting to avoid dislodging the pectus bar. Keep this in mind when examining the epidural insertion site. The postoperative timing of the transition from epidural to oral analgesia varies but generally will be a day or so longer for patients having two bars placed than for those receiving one. Table 22.1 presents an overall approach to analgesia in pectus repair patients.

SUMMARY

1. While rare, complications of the endoscopic pectus repair can be catastrophic.
2. Comfort can be maintained with either epidural or PCA-based analgesia. Special attention needs to be paid to the transition to the oral regimen.
3. Educate the patient regarding the limits of analgesia and the likelihood of a prolonged analgesic requirement postoperatively.

ANNOTATED REFERENCES

- Hebra A, Swoveland B, Egbert M, Tagge E, Georgeson K, Otherson HB, Nuss D. Outcome analysis of minimally invasive repair of pectus excavatum: review of 251 cases. *J Pediatr Surg* 2000; 35(2): 252–258.

  This is the first analysis of outcomes for the Nuss procedure. It discusses the unique complications and the learning curve of the procedure.

- Nuss D, Kelly R, Croitoru D, Katz M. A 10-year review of a minimally invasive technique for correction of pectus excavatum. *J Pediatr Surg* 1998; 33(4): 545–552.

  This landmark article began the change from the open Ravitch procedure to the Nuss procedure.

- Weber T, Matzl J, Rokitansky A, Klimscha W, Neumann K, Deusch E. Superior postoperative pain relief with thoracic epidural analgesia versus intravenous patient-controlled analgesia after minimally invasive pectus excavatum repair. *J Thor Cardiovasc Surg* 2007; 134(4): 865–870.

  In this prospective randomized trial, thoracic epidural analgesia had statistically significant better results in pain scores, usage of supplemental oxygen, and need for additional pain medications in the 72 hours following surgery.

Further Reading

Conti ME. Anesthetic management of acute subcutaneous emphysema and pneumothorax following a Nuss procedure: a case report. *AANA J* 2009; 77(3): 208–211.

Haller JA Jr, Kramer SS, Lietman SA. Use of CT scans in selection of patients for pectus excavatum surgery: a preliminary report. *J Pediatr Surg* 1987; 22(10): 904–906.

Hosie S, Sitkiewicz T, Petersen C, et al. Minimally invasive repair of pectus excavatum—the Nuss procedure. A European multicentre experience. *Eur J Pediatr Surg* 2002; 12(4): 235–238.

Jaroszewski D, Notrica D, McMahon L, Steidley DE, Deschamps C. Current management of pectus excavatum: a review and update of therapy and treatment recommendations. *J Am Board Fam Med* 2010; 23(2): 230–239.

Liu S, Carpenter R, Neal J. Epidural anesthesia and analgesia: their role in postoperative outcome. *Anesthesiology* 1995; 82(6): 1474–1506.

Soliman IE, Apuya JS, Fertal KM, Simpson PM, Tobias JD. Intravenous versus epidural analgesia after surgical repair of pectus excavatum. *Am J Ther* 2009; 16(5): 398–403.

23

Difficult Ventilation During Laparoscopic Fundoplication

MATTHIAS W. KÖNIG AND
JOHN J. McAULIFFE, III

INTRODUCTION

An ever-increasing number of surgical procedures are now performed via the laparoscopic approach, and it is estimated that about 60% of abdominal surgeries in children can be performed laparoscopically today. The creation of a pneumoperitoneum has significant effects on the respiratory system, particularly in small children. Further, laparoscopic procedures have the potential for unique complications not typically seen with conventional "open" surgical techniques.

LEARNING OBJECTIVES

1. Know the respiratory complications specifically related to laparoscopy.
2. Understand how to manage the respiratory changes that can occur after creation of a pneumoperitoneum.
3. Identify the advantages and disadvantages of volume- versus pressure-controlled ventilation strategies in relation to laparoscopic surgery.

CASE PRESENTATION

A 16-month-old girl presents for elective laparoscopic Nissen fundoplication. Her past medical history is significant for premature birth at 28 weeks gestational age, developmental delay, gastroesophageal reflux not responsive to medical therapy, recurrent aspiration, and failure to thrive. Her weight is 9.8 kg; vital signs are within normal limits with the exception of a saturation of 95% on room air. On the day of surgery, she appears to be at her baseline state of health, but copious secretions and "noisy" breathing are noted. After an uneventful anesthesia induction and intubation, the patient is ventilated in **volume control** *mode and the surgical team commences with the insertion of ports and* **insufflation of CO_2** *to create a* **pneumoperitoneum***. After approximately 1 minute, pulse oximetry saturation decreases from 97% to 89%. At the same time,* **peak airway pressure increases** *from 18 to 26 cmH_2O.*

DISCUSSION

1. **What respiratory effects are expected as a consequence of a pneumoperitoneum in children?**

Creation of a **pneumoperitoneum** "pushes" the diaphragm cephalad, leading to a reduction in functional residual capacity (FRC). If FRC falls below closing capacity, oxygen saturation will fall as a consequence of ventilation–perfusion mismatching due to atelectasis. The upward displacement of the diaphragm causes a restriction of lung excursion during the respiratory cycle, thereby lowering lung compliance. In neonates and infants, these effects are exacerbated by the large size of the liver and the fact that their closing capacity is relatively high compared to FRC.

Typical changes in respiratory parameters during pediatric laparoscopy (CO_2 pneumoperitoneum and Trendelenburg position) are:

• Reduced pulmonary compliance by ~30%

- Reduced FRC by ~30%
- Altered gradient between end-tidal and arterial pCO_2 (the end-tidal pCO_2 exceeds arterial pCO_2)
- Increased pulmonary vascular resistance due to changes in lung volumes and effects of CO_2

It is important to remember that these respiratory system changes have associated changes in the cardiovascular system (Table 23.1). Transperitoneal CO_2 absorption is rapid, but prolonged CO_2 pneumoperitoneum (>1 hour) increases the likelihood of hypercarbia. This effect seems to be more pronounced in children than in adults due to the thinner peritoneal lining.

Most of the respiratory changes caused by a pneumoperitoneum will resolve spontaneously after the intra-abdominal gas is released at the end of surgery, and respiratory parameters will return to normal. However, some children will require supplemental oxygen postoperatively to maintain saturation, a phenomenon

---

Table 23.1

PATHOPHYSIOLOGIC CHANGES DUE TO INCREASED ABDOMINAL PRESSURE WITH PNEUMOPERITONEUM

Cardiovascular	*Respiratory*	*Neurologic*
IAP <15 mmHg: cardiac output ⇔ or ⇧ due to venous return from splanchnic vessels IAP >15 mmHg: progressive ⇧ of IAP leads to ⇩ cardiac output and ⇩ blood flow to kidneys, liver, and intestines	Compliance ⇩ FRC ⇩ Gradient end-tidal to arterial pCO_2 ⇧ PVR ⇧	IAP >25 mmHg: ICP ⇧ and CPP ⇩

IAP, intra-abdominal pressure; FRC, functional residual capacity; ICP, intracranial pressure; CPP: cerebral perfusion pressure; PVR: pulmonary vascular resistance
Reprinted from Pennant JH. Anesthesia for laparoscopy in the pediatric patient. *Anesth Clin North Am* 2001; 19: 69–88. Copyright 2001, with permission from Elsevier.

that has been attributed to temporarily altered diaphragmatic function due to surgery.

2. What are other causes of increased peak pressures and desaturation in laparoscopic cases?

In particular, the following three complications need to be considered since they are uniquely related to the laparoscopic approach:

Secondary endobronchial intubation: This is not uncommon in younger children since the upward displacement of the diaphragm also causes upward movement of the relatively short trachea. Head-down positioning will further increase this risk. In very small children, endobronchial intubation may not be easily diagnosed by auscultation, and a high index of suspicion is needed. Changes in end-tidal CO_2 after one-sided intubation in children do not necessarily follow a predictable, diagnostic pattern, and increased, decreased, and unchanged readings have been described. In a study by Rolf and Coté (1992), a *decrease in oxygen saturation was the most consistent vital sign change associated with an unintended endobronchial intubation*.

Pneumothorax or pneumomediastinum is possible at any time during laparoscopic surgeries, more so if the surgery is close to the diaphragm. Insufflated gas can reach the pleural/mediastinal space along surgically created passages or via congenital defects or the esophageal aperture. Hallmark signs of pneumothorax include diminished breath sounds on the affected side, hyperresonance on percussion, increased end-tidal CO_2 and—potentially—hemodynamic instability secondary to a mediastinal shift.

Unintended intravascular insufflation of CO_2 with subsequent *gas embolism* has been described as a potentially fatal complication related to laparoscopic surgery. The estimated incidence is around 0.6% in adults, with most cases manifesting shortly after the initial gas **insufflation** via a misplaced Veress needle (Magrina, 2002). Symptoms of a massive gas embolism include a sudden drop in end-tidal CO_2, desaturation, normal airway pressures, hemodynamic instability (hypotension, dysrhythmias), and pulseless electrical activity (PEA). Slow continuous entry of gas into the venous system may produce a "mill wheel" murmur on auscultation.

3. How should ventilatory management be adjusted during laparoscopic surgery?

Depending on the ventilation mode, the following changes can be seen:

Volume-controlled ventilation (VCV): Unless compliance is very significantly reduced, tidal volume and minute ventilation will remain unchanged but **peak airway pressures** will increase.

Pressure-controlled ventilation (PCV): tidal volume will decrease in proportion to the decrease in compliance; **peak airway pressures** will remain unchanged.

At first glance, volume-controlled ventilation would appear to be the obvious choice since, at least in theory, it should maintain minute ventilation better and thus avoid hypoxia and hypercarbia in the face of altered lung compliance. However, two other factors should be recognized in the setting of laparoscopic surgery:

Endotracheal tube leak: According to traditional teaching, an uncuffed endotracheal tube should be used in preschool-age children. This will frequently lead to a significant leak and make effective ventilation and accurate end-tidal CO_2 monitoring difficult, particularly in VCV. PCV is less affected by a small leak around the endotracheal tube and will still achieve adequate tidal volumes. Recent data suggest that cuffed endotracheal tubes may be safely used in young children (Weiss et al., 2009).

PCV does have advantages in the setting of decreased lung compliance. At least in the adult critical care experience, PCV is advantageous in patients with decreased lung compliance (e.g., adult respiratory distress syndrome) with regards to oxygenation, lung recruitment, and risk of barotrauma. When using PCV during laparoscopic cases, minute ventilation needs to be monitored since tidal volumes will vary with changes in intra-abdominal pressure.

Increases in minute ventilation are often necessary to achieve normocapnia during laparoscopy. This can be realized by either increasing tidal volume (higher preset volume in VCV; higher inflation pressure and/or increasing I:E ratio in PCV) and/or by increasing respiratory rate. Increasing tidal volume is the more "efficient" way to increase minute ventilation since the relative contribution of dead space ventilation will then decrease. Peak inspiratory pressures need to be monitored closely when using VCV to avoid barotrauma. Increasing the I:E ratio will help to reduce peak inspiratory pressures in VCV. Excessive increases in respiratory rate (>30/min) may be taxing for some anesthesia ventilators and they may be unable to still deliver the desired tidal volumes.

The end-tidal pCO_2 may exceed arterial pCO_2 during prolonged laparoscopic cases. Attempting to "normalize" the end-tidal pCO_2 may result in undesirable hyperventilation. In otherwise healthy children, mild permissive hypercapnia may increase cardiac output and improve splanchnic oxygen delivery. In many cases, it is possible to allow end-tidal pCO_2 to remain in the range of 45 to 50 mmHg unless there are mitigating conditions. If precise control of arterial pCO_2 is indicated, an arterial catheter should be placed for blood gas determination.

4. How can respiratory effects of the pneumoperitoneum be minimized?

Limit intra-abdominal pressure (IAP): Modest evidence is available regarding the relationship between IAP from the CO_2 pneumoperitoneum and the degree of respiratory and cardiovascular changes (e.g., DeWaal & Kalkman, 2003). In children, IAP should be limited to *no more than 10 to 15 mmHg*. However, the literature does not provide much information on the ideal IAP in neonates and infants, and there have been cases of poor physiologic tolerance of IAPs of less than 10 mmHg. Close communication with the surgical team about any observed respiratory changes in response to abdominal CO_2 **insufflation** is vital. When in doubt, the IAP should be temporarily released to stabilize the patient.

Positive end expiratory pressure (PEEP): The protective effects of PEEP to prevent small airway collapse have not been studied in children during laparoscopic surgery but are described in the adult literature. With the exception of the smallest patients, the application of a moderate amount of PEEP (3–5 cmH_2O) is probably safe and beneficial in children. However, it must be recognized that PEEP may add to the detrimental effects of IAP on venous return and cardiac preload, particularly in neonates and infants, in whom it should be used only with caution.

5. What are the risks of hypercarbia, and who is at particular risk?

Most healthy children will not suffer any adverse consequences from transient, moderate hypercarbia during laparoscopic surgery. In the following settings, however, hypercarbia may not be tolerated, even transiently:

Intracranial pressure (ICP): Both cerebral blood flow and ICP increase in children undergoing laparoscopic surgery even without evidence of intracranial pathology, as well as in adult and pediatric patients with a ventriculoperitoneal shunt (VPS). Clinically, children with a functioning VPS have been reported to tolerate laparoscopic procedures well, and the presence of a VPS should therefore not constitute a contraindication *per se*. Avoidance of hypercarbia is recommended in at-risk patients who may have *reduced cerebral compliance* (e.g., in a trauma victim with closed head injury, consideration should be given to open technique rather than laparoscopic abdominal exploration).

Pulmonary hypertension: Hypercarbia can increase pulmonary vascular resistance. This may be poorly tolerated in patients with preexisting moderate to severe pulmonary hypertension or in those with congenital cardiovascular abnormalities, where it may produce an imbalance between pulmonary and systemic blood flow. Nevertheless, cardiac anomalies do not automatically preclude laparoscopic techniques. A small review of neonates with hypoplastic left heart syndrome found no adverse effects (Slater et al., 2007), but the anesthesia provider needs to be aware of the potential consequences of hypercarbia-induced increases in pulmonary vascular pressure.

Finally, end-tidal CO_2 monitoring may not always accurately reflect arterial pCO_2 during laparoscopic surgery. A small case series showed an age-dependent discrepancy between the two values that increases at younger ages, particularly in infants. In cases where hypercarbia is a concern, arterial cannulation may be beneficial to measure $PaCO_2$ directly.

SUMMARY

1. CO_2 pneumoperitoneum reduces lung compliance and may lead to atelectasis, hypoventilation, and direct CO_2 absorption, causing hypoxia and hypercarbia.
2. Migration of the endotracheal tube into a mainstem bronchus is not uncommon in laparoscopic surgery in small children. Oxygen desaturation is the most consistent sign.
3. Pneumothorax, pneumomediastinum, and gas embolism are rare complications related to laparoscopic technique.
4. Patients with increased intracranial pressure, those with moderate to severe pulmonary hypertension, and those with certain congenital cardiac abnormalities may not tolerate hypercarbia.
5. Pressure-controlled ventilation and PEEP can be advantageous to prevent hypoxia and hypercarbia.

ANNOTATED REFERENCES

- Durkin ET, Shaaban AF. Recent advances and controversies in pediatric laparoscopic surgery. *Surg Clin North Am* 2008; 88: 1101–1119.

This review presents the surgical perspective and an outlook on future applications of laparoscopic techniques.

- **Pennant JH. Anesthesia for laparoscopy in the pediatric patient.** *Anesth Clin North Am* **2001; 19: 69–88.**
  Succinct and complete overview of pertinent physiologic changes during laparoscopic surgery in children.
- **Weiss M, Dullenkopf A, Fischer JE, Keller C, Gerber AC. Prospective randomized controlled multi-centre trial of cuffed or uncuffed endotracheal tubes in small children.** *Br J Anaesth* **2009; 103: 967–873.**
  Recent landmark study showing no added risk when using cuffed endotracheal tubes in young children.

Further Reading

De Waal EE, Kalkman CJ. Haemodynamic changes during low-pressure carbon dioxide pneumoperitoneum in young children. *Paediatr Anaesth* 2003; 13(1): 18–25.

Magrina, JF. Complications of laparoscopic surgery. *Clin Obs Gyn* 2002; 45:469-480.

Rolf N, Coté CJ. Diagnosis of clinically unrecognized endobronchial intubation in paediatric anaesthesia: which is more sensitive, pulse oximetry or capnography? *Pediatr Anesth* 1992; 2: 31–34.

Sanders JC, Gerstein N. Arterial to end-tidal carbon dioxide gradient during pediatric laparoscopic fundoplication. *Pediatr Anesth* 2008; 18: 1096–1101.

Stayer S, Olutuye O. Anesthesia ventilators: better options for children. *Anesth Clin North Am* 2005; 23: 677–691.

Slater B, Rangel S, Ramamoorthy C, Abrajano C, Albanese CT. Outcomes after laparoscopic surgery in neonates with hypoplastic heart left heart syndrome. *J Pediatr Surg.* 2007; 42(6):1118-21.

PART 5

CHALLENGES IN BLOOD AND

FLUID MANAGEMENT

24

Massive Transfusion in a Child

STEFAN SABATO

INTRODUCTION

The traditional early management of hemorrhagic shock is currently being challenged, and many centers around the world have already changed their practice. Damage-control resuscitation, in conjunction with damage-control surgery, has been shown to improve major morbidity and mortality outcomes in adults. In children there is little direct evidence for these new approaches, but supporting evidence is accumulating. This chapter will introduce these concepts while also reinforcing the core principles of managing acute hemorrhage in the trauma setting.

LEARNING OBJECTIVES

1. Appreciate the principles of preparation for and early assessment and management of a major pediatric trauma involving major hemorrhage.
2. Understand the concepts of damage-control resuscitation and damage-control surgery.
3. Know how to avoid the complications of a massive transfusion.
4. Understand the basics of the acute coagulopathy of trauma shock.

CASE PRESENTATION

*The **trauma team** arrives to the emergency bay to receive a 4-year-old who has been in a motor vehicle accident. The paramedics have failed to obtain intravenous access. The initial assessment reveals hypovolemic shock due to intra-abdominal hemorrhage. An 18-gauge intravenous cannula is sited in the right antecubital fossa, blood is sent to the laboratory, and an O-negative packed red blood cell (pRBC) transfusion commences. The hospital's **massive transfusion protocol (MTP)** is activated, and a focused secondary survey and trauma series of radiographs are performed. The abdomen continues to become more distended, the patient remains hypotensive, and transfusion continues with a unit of thawed fresh frozen plasma (FFP). The aim is for a palpable pulse, improved conscious state, and **systolic blood pressure within the lower limit of the normal range**. The decision is made to take the child to the operating room (OR) without further investigation, and transfusion of a unit of platelets commences en route (Table 24.1).*

In preparation, the OR has been warmed to 24°C, a rapid infuser has been primed, and the cell salvage machine is available. Blood products have been placed in the OR refrigerator as per the MTP.

Table 24.1

PATIENT'S APPEARANCE IN THE EMERGENCY DEPARTMENT

Primary & Secondary Survey

Patent airway and spontaneous respiration
HR 190
BP 50/-
Child's Glasgow Coma Scale (GCS) score 10
Distended abdomen
Evidence of abrasion to right upper quadrant
No external bleeding
No apparent head injury
No other obvious evidence of trauma

An arterial line is inserted, but it is difficult to obtain further large-bore venous access. After induction with manual in-line stabilization of the cervical spine, the surgeon performs a cutdown to gain large-bore venous access in the left antecubital fossa.

While preparing for surgery, ventilation becomes more difficult due to increasing abdominal distention. The surgeon incises the abdomen and blood immediately pours from the wound. Worsening hypotension ensues. The child is transfused with sequential units of pRBCs/salvaged blood, FFP, and platelets. The surgeon identifies a laceration in the inferior vena cava and clamps the vessel to control the hemorrhage. Further exploration reveals a lacerated liver and perforated transverse colon. The surgeon then places **packs** in the abdominal cavity to allow the patient to be stabilized.

The initial coagulation tests taken earlier demonstrate that the patient was **coagulopathic upon arrival** to the hospital. Approximately 2 blood volumes have been transfused prior to clamping, and further transfusion is now guided by laboratory assessment and **thromboelastography (TEG)**. A **tranexamic acid** infusion is started, 0.5 mL/kg calcium gluconate is given to **correct hypocalcemia,** and 5 mL/kg cryoprecipitate is transfused to treat **hypofibrinogenemia**. To avoid **hypothermia** and **acidosis** the patient is actively warmed, and sodium bicarbonate is slowly titrated to achieve a pH of >7.2. Ongoing microvascular bleeding is observed; therefore, 100 IU/kg of activated **recombinant factor VIIa** (rFVIIa) is administered. The surgery is completed with a defunctioning colostomy, placing packs around the lacerated liver and in the abdominal cavity, and forming a temporary laparostomy.

DISCUSSION

1. **What are the key aspects of the assessment and management of a major pediatric trauma where major hemorrhage is suspected or possible?**

Advance notice prior to a major trauma patient arriving in the hospital is crucial. This allows mobilization of the trauma team and time to ensure that the appropriate locations, such as the CT scanner and an OR, are vacant. The **trauma team** consists of the emergency physician, the general/trauma surgeon, the anesthesiologist, the intensivist, nursing staff, radiographers, and support staff. It is important that the role of the team leader and each individual is clearly defined. The anesthesiologist warms the OR, calculates the estimated body weight and blood volume of the patient, and prepares the correct drugs, rapid infusion device, and cell saver. Continued communication with the paramedics also facilitates preparation.

Most trauma patients will not require a massive transfusion, and existing ATLS guidelines of crystalloid transfusion followed by pRBCs will suffice. However, in major trauma, if death from hemorrhage does occur it is usually within 6 hours of the injury. Therefore it is important to identify which patients are likely to require massive transfusion early, and in these cases facilitate the delivery of blood products. Tachycardia is the first sign of hypovolemia in children, and up to 40% of blood volume can be lost before hypotension ensues. Other early signs of hypovolemia are postural hypotension and a narrow pulse pressure (Barcelona et al., 2005). Institution of a **massive transfusion protocol** (MTP) has been shown to improve survival and reduce total blood product consumption (Riskin et al., 2009). It allows the treating team to focus on the patient's physiology instead of ordering blood products based on laboratory values that may no longer be relevant by the time the result is available (Dressler et al., 2010). The MTP streamlines communication with the blood bank, expedites the delivery of blood products, and engages the support of a hematologist. Inadequate communication between treating physicians and the blood bank is a consistent cause of transfusion-related adverse outcomes (Stainsby et al., 2008).

In this case, the initial assessment revealed hemodynamic instability from intra-abdominal bleeding. Therefore, supradiaphragmatic intravenous access was obtained. The decision on whether to CT scan the child will depend on the stability of the patient and the location of the scanner. If the CT is within the emergency room, then the scan may be performed efficiently while resuscitation continues. In this scenario the child went straight to the OR due to ongoing instability. A focused abdominal ultrasound scan can be performed, but these studies have a high false-negative rate in children. As a rule, the decision to operate is based on hemodynamics rather than imaging.

2. What are the components of damage-control resuscitation?

Damage-control resuscitation includes rapid control of surgical bleeding, avoiding crystalloid/colloid hemodilution, prevention of acidosis/hypothermia/hypocalcemia, and hemostatic resuscitation (Spinella & Holcomb, 2009). Hemostatic resuscitation involves aggressive *volume resuscitation with a 1:1:1 unit ratio of pRBCs:FFP:platelets*. The aim is to deliver "reconstituted whole blood" in a simple manner that is easy in a crisis. This combination avoids exacerbating coagulopathy with excessive crystalloid and pRBC transfusions and helps address consumptive coagulopathy.

While not an exact science, reconstituted whole blood is the best "resuscitation fluid" until hemostasis has been achieved. Subsequent transfusion should be guided by the hematocrit, coagulation profile, platelet count, **TEG**, and the clinical scenario. Laboratory-based coagulation assessment with prothrombin and activated partial thromboplastin times often takes 40 minutes to provide a result and thus is not always helpful in guiding transfusion practice in the actively bleeding patient. **TEG** can provide point-of-care assessment of coagulation and platelet function within 15 minutes and will provide information on the degree of fibrinolysis. After hemostasis is achieved, it is best to then aim to minimize total transfusion volume and donor exposures. Data from the United Kingdom have shown that children have higher rates of adverse outcomes from transfusion than adults, and infants have almost triple the adult rate (Stainsby et al., 2008). Complications relate to both the volume administered and the number of units to which the child is exposed. Thus, each new unit exposure introduces an incremental increase in risk.

Transfusion-related complications may also be reduced by using donor-matched blood products and using pRBCs that are less than 14 days old (Spinella & Holcomb, 2009).

It is important to avoid the "lethal triad" of **hypothermia, acidosis**, and **coagulopathy**. This triad results in further bleeding and hence transfusion, which in turn worsens the hypothermia, acidosis, and coagulopathy, resulting in a "vicious cycle" that may eventually lead to death from hyperkalemia- and hypocalcemia-induced cardiac arrhythmia. Acidosis prolongs clotting time by impairing enzyme activity and depleting fibrinogen levels and platelet counts (Fries & Martini, 2010). It is more important to fix the cause of the acidosis (i.e., hypoperfusion) rather than treating the acidosis itself (Ganter & Pittet, 2010) but if acidosis becomes severe (<7.2), consider administering bicarbonate or tromethamine (Rossaint et al., 2010). Hypothermia affects coagulation protease function below 33°C and worsens coagulopathy, especially in acidosis (Ganter & Pittet, 2010). Hypothermia below 34°C is associated with increased mortality in trauma patients (Fries & Martini, 2010).

Some authors also include permissive hypotension as part of damage control; however, this has been demonstrated to improve morbidity and mortality outcomes only in penetrating torso trauma in adults. Some guidelines recommend moderate hypotension in adult trauma in the absence of central nervous system injury, but in children normotension should be the goal.

3. What does a 1:1:1 transfusion ratio mean in pediatrics?

Although there is an increasing body of evidence in adult military and civilian settings supporting a 1:1:1 ratio of FFP:platelets:pRBC, some recent published guidelines do vary in their recommendations (Duchesne et al., 2008; Holcomb et al., 2008; Rossaint et al., 2010). The exact ratio of products to be used may not be as important as early and aggressive administration of a "high" ratio of FFP and platelets to pRBCs (Riskin et al., 2009). While most guidelines are designed for adults, the modern approach to resuscitation is now being translated into pediatric practice, and there are already published protocols of the use of a 1:1:1 transfusion ratio in hemorrhagic shock in children (Dressler et al., 2010).

In the setting of massive transfusion, it is easier to keep track of what should be given if the team thinks in terms of the number of units transfused rather than volume or mL/kg. Although the volume of each unit will vary slightly between blood banks depending on institutional practice and the method of preservation, the mass of blood product in each unit should be relatively consistent. When considering the use of reconstituted whole blood transfusion in children, it is important to be aware that the literature describes a ratio of 1 adult unit of pRBCs to 1 adult unit of FFP to 1 buffy coat-derived single-random-donor platelet unit. Some centers offer both adult- and neonatal-sized units of pRBCs and FFP, and some blood banks pool platelets into a single bag of 5 units (~300 mL) from three or four donors to reduce the total donor exposure to the recipient. Also, platelets may be collected from the buffy coat of spun donated whole blood, or obtained by apheresis. One unit of apheresis-derived platelets (~180 mL) is equivalent to a pooled bag of buffy coat-derived platelets.

4. What are the adjuncts to reconstituted whole blood?

A large multicenter prospective randomized controlled trial has recently demonstrated improved survival with the use of **tranexamic acid** in adult trauma with significant hemorrhage. The improved survival was seen without an increase in thrombotic complications (CRASH-2, 2010). Although the number needed to treat in this study was large, it still seems reasonable to use tranexamic acid in trauma. In the case presentation, the initial focus was on damage-control resuscitation and surgery as soon as possible. A tranexamic infusion was started when time permitted.

During resuscitation, **fibrinogen** levels may fall as a result of dilution, hypothermia, and acidosis (Fries & Martini, 2010). Some authors believe it is the first factor to reach critically low levels. Published guidelines recommend cryoprecipitate if bleeding occurs with TEG signs of functional fibrinogen deficit, or a plasma fibrinogen level of less than 1.5 to 2 g/L (Rossaint et al., 2010). In the case presentation, the child received fibrinogen early in the FFP in small amounts, and later with cryoprecipitate after laboratory confirmation of hypofibrinogenemia.

Massive transfusion can lead to **hypocalcemia** because blood products are preserved with a citrate-containing solution that chelates calcium. FFP and platelets have the highest citrate concentrations. Citrate is rapidly metabolized by the liver, and therefore citrate-induced hypocalcemia is generally transient, but it can affect hemostasis during resuscitation. Current recommendations are to maintain an ionized calcium level of above 0.9 mmol/L (Rossaint et al., 2010).

Guidelines recommend the use of **recombinant activated factor VII** (rFVIIa) in blunt abdominal trauma in adults as it may be useful in areas of diffuse small vessel bleeding. This is despite the lack of strong supporting evidence. To be effective rFVIIa requires adequate platelets and fibrinogen, normothermia, and a normal pH.In trauma, there are reduced levels of *anti*coagulant factors along with increased *pro*coagulant factors, and thus there may be a risk of thrombosis with rFVIIa. rFVIIa has a short half-life, with an average of 2.7 hours for adults and 1.3 hours for children. The clearance is faster for pediatric patients (67 mL/kg/hr) compared to adults (33 mL/kg/hr). Varying doses have been described in children, but it seems that 80 to 100 IU/kg is sufficient as an initial dose, with a second dose 1 hour later. TEG may guide therapy administration as rFVIIa normalizes the *in vitro* PT and INR.

5. Acute coagulopathy of trauma-shock

The child in the case presentation was already **coagulopathic on arrival** prior to the administration of any intravenous fluid. 25% of major trauma patients are coagulopathic upon arrival to the emergency department prior to any aggressive intravenous crystalloid or colloid resuscitation, or the onset of any hypothermia and acidosis. Extensive tissue damage and tissue hypoperfusion secondary to hemorrhage directly affects coagulation (Ganter &

Pittet, 2010); systemic hypoperfusion has a dose-dependent association with coagulopathy as measured by prothrombin time and partial thromboplastin time. With shock, there is increased plasma-soluble thrombomodulin expressed by the endothelium. Thrombomodulin binds with thrombin, resulting in less available thrombin to cleave fibrinogen into fibrin. Also, the thrombin–thrombomodulin complex activates protein C, which in turn irreversibly inactivates factors Va and VIIIa and deactivates plasminogen activator inhibitor (PAI-1). Inhibition of these coagulation factors further impairs the ability to cleave fibrinogen to fibrin, and deactivation of PAI-1 promotes fibrinolysis (Ganter & Pittet, 2010). This phenomenon may be a protective mechanism to prevent thrombosis in isolated tissues with hypoperfusion, but it is counterproductive in the bleeding patient. Raised tissue plasminogen activator levels from injured vessel walls and reduced thrombin activatable fibrinolysis inhibitor also contribute to fibrinolysis (Ganter & Pittet, 2010). Lastly tissue injury also activates the complement cascade, which in turn affects coagulation.

The acute coagulopathy of trauma-shock (ACoTS, also known as endogenous acute coagulopathy and acute traumatic coagulopathy) is distinct from the more familiar systemic acquired coagulopathy resulting from hemodilution, hypothermia, acidosis, and consumption of coagulation factors. The possible presence of ACoTS is one reason why coagulation factors should be given early, and the possibility of developing ACoTS highlights the importance of correcting tissue hypoperfusion as early as possible.

6. Damage-control surgery

Communication between the surgeon and the anesthesiologist is important in any emergency operation. The case presentation illustrates how good teamwork improves patient outcome. The surgeon assisted in obtaining large-bore intravenous access prior to incising the abdomen and releasing the tamponade. Damage-control surgery is an abbreviated resuscitative laparotomy for control of bleeding, restitution of blood flow where necessary, and control of contamination (Rossaint et al., 2010). Once the inferior vena cava was clamped controlling the hemorrhage, **packing the abdomen** allowed the anesthesiologist to stabilize the patient. The packs will remain *in situ* for 24 to 48 hours, allowing normalization of the coagulation profile, intravascular volume, and electrolytes in the intensive care unit. Then the patient will have definitive surgical repair of the viscera if necessary, and closure of the abdomen.

SUMMARY

1. Establishing appropriate trauma procedures and protocols such as massive transfusion protocols streamlines the institution's management of trauma patients and can improve patient outcomes.

2. In cases of trauma with major hemorrhage, blood products should be given early in a ratio of 1:1:1 for FFP:platelets:pRBC.

3. Massive transfusion may cause coagulopathy, hypothermia, and acidosis. These can result in further bleeding and should be treated aggressively. Hyperkalemia and hypocalcemia should also be treated early.

4. Coagulopathy may develop early after trauma. Along with FFP and platelets, tranexamic acid, fibrinogen, and recombinant factor VII should be considered as ways to reverse coagulopathy.

ANNOTATED REFERENCES

- Holcomb JB, Wade CE, Michalek JE, et al. Increased plasma and platelet to red blood cell ratios improves outcome in 466 massively transfused civilian trauma patients. *Ann Surg* 2008; 248: 447–458.

The best evidence in a civilian population for a 1:1:1 ratio of blood products.

- **Riskin DJ, et al. Massive transfusion protocols: the role of aggressive resuscitation versus product ratio in mortality reduction. *J Am Coll Surg* 2009; 209: 198–205.**

  An excellent illustration of the beneficial impact of an MTP.

- **Spinella PC, Holcomb JB. Resuscitation and transfusion principles for traumatic hemorrhagic shock. *Blood Rev* 2009; 23: 231–240.**

  An excellent recent summary of both ACoTS and damage-control resuscitation.

Further Reading

Barcelona SL, Thompson AA, Cote CJ. Intraoperative pediatric blood transfusion therapy: a review of common issues. Part II: transfusion therapy, special consideration, and reduction of allogenic blood transfusions. *Pediatr Anesth* 2005; 15: 814–830.

CRASH-2 trial collaborators. Effects of tranexamic acid on death, vascular occlusive events, and blood transfusion in trauma patients with significant hemorrhage (CRASH-2): a randomised, placebo-controlled trial. *Lancet* 2010; 376: 23–32.

Dressler AM, Finck CM, Carroll CL, Bonanni CC, Spinella PC. Use of a massive transfusion protocol with hemostatic resuscitation for severe intraoperative bleeding in a child. *J Pediatr Surg* 2010; 45: 1530–1533.

Duchesne JC, Hunt JP, Wahl G, Marr AB, Wang YZ, Weintraub SE, Wright MJ, McSwain NE Jr. Review of current blood transfusion strategies in a mature level 1 trauma center: were we wrong for the last 60 years? *J Trauma* 2008; 65: 272–276.

Fries D, Martini WZ. Role of fibrinogen in trauma-induced coagulopathy. *Br J Anaesth* 2010; 105: 116–121.

Ganter MT, Pittet J-F. New insights into acute coagulopathy in trauma patients. *Best Practice & Research Clinical Anaesthesiology* 2010; 24: 15–25.

Rossaint R, Bouillon B, Cerny V. Management of bleeding following major trauma: an updated European guideline. *Crit Care* 2010; 14: R52.

Stainsby D, Jones H, Wells AW, Gibson B, Cohen H; SHOT Steering Group. Adverse outcome of blood transfusion in children: analysis of UK reports to the serious hazards of transfusion scheme 1996–2005. *Br J Haematol* 2008; 141: 73–79.

25

Management of Acutely Burned Children

ROBERT McDOUGALL

INTRODUCTION

The resuscitation of the child with burns poses a number of challenges to the anesthesiologist. It is vital that there is a systematic approach to managing the airway, breathing, and circulation. This requires an understanding of the pathophysiology of burn injury. Particular attention must be paid to the timing and technique of securing the airway. Appropriate vascular access and pain management are also of high priority in the burned child.

LEARNING OBJECTIVES

1. Understand the approach to resuscitation of the acutely burned child.
2. Know the key issues in developing a plan to secure the airway.
3. Know how to provide effective pain management in the setting of an acute burn.

CASE PRESENTATION

*A 3-year-old, 15-kg boy is brought to the emergency department with face, neck, and trunk burns sustained when he pulled a pot of boiling soup from the stove. The incident occurred 2 hours ago. The ambulance service has placed **an intraosseous line** and has administered 300 mL 0.9% saline and morphine 1.5 mg. He appears to be in severe distress and has obvious facial burns and swelling.*

*Oxygen is administered via a non-rebreathing mask and his airway is assessed. There is no evidence of stridor and his cry sounds normal. His **lips and anterior tongue** are **swollen**. On auscultation, his chest is clear. His **respiratory rate is 40**, SpO$_2$ 100%, **heart rate 200**. It is impossible to get a blood pressure reading but he has strong peripheral pulses. **Capillary refill time is 3 seconds**. An intravenous cannula is placed in the saphenous vein at the ankle and a further dose of morphine 1.5 mg is administered. A fluid bolus of 300 mL 0.9% saline is given and preparations are made for intubation. Five minutes later he is still distressed and a further dose of morphine 1.5 mg is given. His mother is now present and she confirms the history of the injury and states that he is otherwise well. The heart rate has now settled to 130/minute and respiratory rate to 25/minute.*

*A **secondary survey** confirms that he has no other injuries. It is estimated that the size of the burn is 20% to 25% of **body surface area (BSA)**. The burn on the right upper arm appears to be circumferential. A radial pulse is still present. A urinary catheter is inserted and it is elected to take him to the operating room for intubation as his facial swelling has continued to worsen and for possible escharotomy of his right arm.*

*There is some debate between the senior anesthesiologist and the trainee as to the type of induction, particularly the merits of inhalational versus intravenous techniques. Anesthesia is induced with sevoflurane and oxygen and the trachea is intubated with a size 4.0 **cuffed endotracheal tube** (ETT). At laryngoscopy, the tongue is swollen but the larynx appears normal. The cuff is gently inflated to a pressure of 20 cmH$_2$O. He is given ketamine 30 mg and the burn surgeon* *performs an escharotomy to the right upper arm. The burns are dressed and the patient is transferred to the intensive care unit.*

DISCUSSION

1. How should the young child with burns be assessed?

The general approach for the burned child, as for any injured child, should be assessment and management of airway, breathing, and circulation (ABC). A burned child may need immediate intubation due to respiratory distress, or more commonly a child may be intubated early if it is thought likely that intubation may become urgent at a later stage. This is because a delayed intubation may become very difficult due to increased swelling of the face and airway.

Flame burns may involve a significant intraoral and laryngeal burn leading directly to increasing swelling and obstruction. In patients with scalds it is rare for the larynx and pharynx to be swollen directly from the burn, or for the laryngeal anatomy to become significantly distorted. However, scalds may still result in significant facial, **lip, and tongue swelling**, making intubation and airway management difficult.

This child had significant **facial burns** and in the hours following the burn it would be expected that the **face, lips, and tongue** would **swell,** possibly leading to upper airway obstruction. Early intubation was indicated in this patient primarily because of this risk. Later intubation may also have become necessary due to decreased pulmonary function secondary to the systemic inflammatory response to the burn resulting in pulmonary edema and pulmonary hypertension. Lastly, in this child intubation would likely be needed for anesthesia for escharotomy, and early intubation would allow liberal use of opioid analgesia without fear of respiratory depression.

Assessment of the circulation is challenging in the distressed child. **Heart rate** and **respiratory rate** will be elevated due to pain and anxiety as well as due to any hypovolemia. There is a wide range of normal for blood pressure for a 3-year-old child. **Capillary refill time** is highly variable between patients and therefore on its own is an *unreliable sign* to diagnose hypovolemia. *It is unusual for a burn patient to be profoundly hypovolemic secondary to dehydration in the first 2 hours after a burn. Significant hypovolemia immediately post-injury is more likely due to another injury.* In this child the presence of strong peripheral pulses indicates that circulatory compromise was not severe at this stage.

It is important that other injuries are identified during the assessment. Burns often occur in the setting of other injuries. A careful **secondary survey**, looking at each organ system, should be undertaken once ABC has been stabilized. The size of the burn can be assessed at this point.

2. What is the correct approach to securing the airway in a burn patient?

Burn patients with facial, neck, and airway injury should be treated as for any patient with a potentially difficult airway. If airway obstruction is impending, then preparations for intubation should be expedited. In this case, both intravenous and inhalational induction would be possible. An intravenous induction may be quicker and less distressing for the child but may lead to apnea and hypoventilation. This may lead to hypoxia if bag-and-mask ventilation is not possible. Succinylcholine (suxamethonium) may be used as part of a rapid-sequence induction within 48 hours of a burn injury. After this time, proliferation of extrajunctional nicotinic receptors can lead to significant hyperkalemia when succinylcholine is administered. In this case an inhalational induction was chosen because it allowed greater control over a potentially difficult airway. Awake, fiberoptic bronchoscopy is often used in adults with burns to assist with intubation. This technique has limited use in the awake child.

This child may develop lung compliance problems secondary to the inflammatory response to the burn. The use of an uncuffed ETT may lead to increasing air leak, which may make ventilation difficult. It is possible to change ETTs, but increasing facial edema will make this difficult. A **cuffed ETT** was used to avoid these problems.

Securing an ETT in a patient with facial burns is challenging. Conventional adhesive tapes do not stick and may cause further damage to burned tissue. Tracheostomy tapes may be useful but can put pressure on the facial area. A novel way of securing a tube is the use of orthodontic brackets, which are bonded to the maxillary incisors (Sakata et al., 2009). The oral ETT can then be secured to the brackets with wire. This avoids the use of tapes and allows oral and facial hygiene to be maintained

3. What are the options for intravenous access in the child with burns?

Intravenous access in the child with burns may present a challenge to the anesthesiologist; particularly if there have been numerous previous unsuccessful attempts. If possible, intravenous lines should not be placed through burned tissue. An intravenous cannula placed in the burned area may increase the risk of infection and may be difficult to secure. The dorsum of the hand, cubital fossae, and the long saphenous veins at the medial ankle are the most reliable sites. In this case, an **intraosseous needle** was placed. This is an excellent emergency option if peripheral veins cannot be accessed. The usual site is at the anteromedial aspect of the proximal tibia, taking care to avoid the growth plate. Resuscitation fluids and drugs can be given safely and rapidly through the intraosseous needle. Complications such as osteomyelitis are rare, but compartment syndrome can occur if the needle becomes displaced. It can be difficult to secure intraosseous needles, so after initial resuscitation, peripheral access should be attempted again. Central venous access may be attempted after attempts at peripheral access have failed or other indications for central access exist (e.g., inotropic support).

4. How should resuscitation fluids be managed in the child with burns?

As part of the ABC approach, most children with burns of more than 10% **BSA** require intravenous fluid resuscitation.

In estimating the amount of fluid required, the size of the burn is more important than the depth. The fluid loss from burns is predominantly from the extracellular compartment; therefore, an isotonic fluid should be chosen for resuscitation. The following formula is a useful guide to calculating total fluid resuscitation for the first 24 hours: 4 × % burn area × weight (kg). 50% of this amount should be given in the first 8 hours (from the time of burn) and the remainder over the next 16 hours. This formula is a guide only and may lead to over-resuscitation in smaller burns. This calculation *does not include maintenance requirements*. In this patient, part of the calculated resuscitation volume was given a fluid bolus of 20 mL/kg because there was clinical evidence of hypovolemia (**tachycardia**, **tachypnea**, **prolonged capillary refill**).

Most burn patients retain gut activity and oral intake is to be encouraged. Urine output should be closely monitored, aiming for an hourly output of more than 0.75 mL/hr. In large burns blood electrolytes should be checked regularly (q6–12h) as Na^+ and K^+ abnormalities are not uncommon.

5. What are the options for analgesia in the acutely burned patient?

Pain from thermal injury is particularly severe. Strong pain relief should be administered as soon as the primary survey has been completed. In this case morphine was administered and titrated to effect. The correct total dose is the dose that leads to adequate pain relief. Other opioids (e.g., fentanyl) may be used with equal effect. This child is likely to need a continuous opioid infusion for some days. *Multimodal analgesia* is also useful during the acute phase of pain management, and agents such as ketamine, tramadol, acetaminophen (paracetamol), and nonsteroidal anti-inflammatory drugs may be used as adjuncts to opioids.

This patient required escharotomy for a circumferential burn to his arm. Traditional teaching has been that escharotomy requires minimal analgesia or anesthesia because it has been thought that most of the burns causing limb constriction are full thickness and therefore have little sensation. In practice, most scald burns have a significant component of partial-thickness burn, and escharotomy will be a painful procedure as sensory nerves in the burned area will be intact. Escharotomy for children is generally performed under general anesthesia. In this case ketamine was used as it provides anesthesia as well as post-procedure analgesia.

Over the medium term of care, multimodal analgesia will help minimize some of the side effects of opioid administration such as tolerance.

SUMMARY

1. In resuscitation of the acutely burned child, airway, breathing, and circulation are priorities. Perform a careful secondary survey to exclude other injuries and assess the size of the burn. Fluid management depends on the size of the burn and the time of injury.
2. The airway should be secured early if there is a risk of airway obstruction. Inhalational or intravenous induction techniques may be appropriate. Securing the ETT can be challenging.
3. Burn pain is severe and requires strong analgesics. Multimodal analgesia may reduce the side effects from opioids.

ANNOTATED REFERENCES

• Fabia R, Groner JI. Advances in the care of children with burns. *Advances Pediatr* 2009; 56: 219–248.

This summary of current surgical management of children with burns is useful for understanding the overall management of these children.

- Fuzaylov G, Fidkowski CW. Anesthetic considerations for major burn injury in pediatric patients. *Pediatr Anesth* 2009; 19(3): 202–211.

This paper gives a good summary of the pathophysiology of thermal injury and outlines the major complications that must be managed by the anesthesiologist.

- Sakata S, Hallett B, Brandon MS, McBride CA. Easy come, easy go: A simple and effective orthodontic enamel anchor for endotracheal tube stabilization in a child with extensive facial burns. *Burns* 2009; 35: 983–986.

This gives instructions on securing an ETT with an orthodontic bracket.

Further Reading

Light TD, Latenser BA, Heinle JA, et al. Demographics of pediatric burns in Vellore, India. *J Burn Care Res* 2009; 30(1): 50–54.

Quinlan KP, O'Connor A, Robinson M, Gottlieb LJ. Protecting children from fires and burns. *Pediatr Ann* 2010; 39(11): 709–713.

Rogers AD, Karpelowsky J, Millar AJ, Argent A, Rode H. Fluid creep in major pediatric burns. *Eur J Pediatr Surg* 2010; 20(2): 133–138.

26

Management of Burn Patients for Grafting and Excision

ROBERT McDOUGALL

INTRODUCTION

Anesthesia management for excision and grafting of burns in a child can be extremely challenging. Early excision of burned tissue significantly decreases morbidity and mortality but often involves procedures that lead to significant blood loss. Burn patients also have a markedly increased metabolic rate secondary to the inflammatory response to the burn. Burn patients may be difficult to monitor, are at risk of hypothermia, and present complex pain-management problems.

LEARNING OBJECTIVES

1. Understand the factors that determine the timing of burn surgery.
2. Know how to manage the major complications of burn excision and grafting.
3. Know how to provide effective pain management for the burn patient.

CASE PRESENTATION

*A 24-kg, 6-year-old girl sustained burns to approximately **40% of her body**, including trunk (anterior and posterior) and arms, in a **house fire** in the early hours of the morning. There are no burns to the face or neck. In the emergency department, she was intubated, given 20 mL/ kg 0.9% saline and morphine and ketamine for analgesia and transferred to the ICU. She is booked on the afternoon emergency operating list for **early excision and grafting** of her burns. She is on pressure-support ventilation and is requiring an inspired oxygen concentration of 30% to maintain adequate oxygen saturations. Chest x-ray shows her lung fields to be clear. Her heart rate is 110 beats/minute, blood pressure is 110/65, **temperature 38.1°C**, and she has a right radial arterial line, a left femoral central venous catheter, and an 18-g intravenous catheter in her right foot. She has had 1,700 mL of fluid and her urine output has been at least 30 mL/hr since admission. Sedation and analgesia are being provided with infusions of morphine and ketamine. Her hemoglobin (Hb) is 10.5 g/dL. All other blood results are unremarkable. **Three units of packed cells** are requested from the blood bank.*

*The patient is transferred to the operating room, which has been **prewarmed** to 32°C (90°F), and is placed on the operating table, which has a warming mattress. The lower body is covered with a **plastic sheet** and a **forced-air warming blanket**. Anesthesia is induced with propofol and ketamine and maintained with sevoflurane, air, and oxygen. **Morphine and ketamine** infusions are continued and boluses of morphine 5 mg and ketamine 25 mg are given. Bilateral **fascia iliaca blocks** with 0.25% levo-bupivacaine are administered prior to harvesting of donor skin from the thigh (Fig. 26.1). Dressings are removed and the surgeons infiltrate the burned tissue with a solution of 1:200,000 epinephrine (adrenaline) to reduce blood loss (Fig. 26.2). As excision commences, a fluid bolus of 500 mL Ringer's lactate solution is given. There is no hemodynamic response to harvesting of skin but there is some blood loss. A further 500 mL Ringer's lactate is given and Hb is checked and found to be 6.3 g/dL. A unit of packed red blood cells is given over half an hour. Over the*

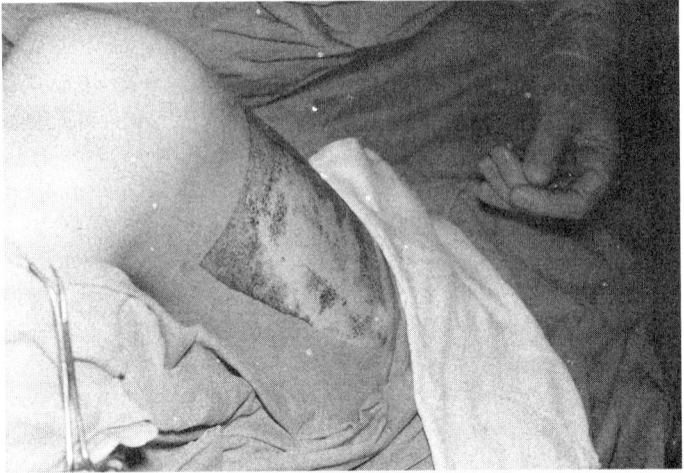

FIGURE 26.1 Donor harvest site, left thigh.

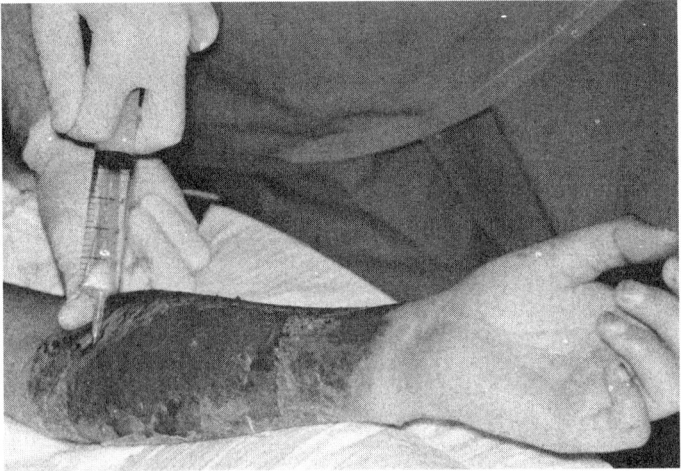

FIGURE 26.2 Injecting epinephrine under eschar to reduce blood loss.

*next 90 minutes, the surgeons excise the burned tissue and attain hemostasis. The patient remains hemodynamically stable and urine output is 38 mL for the last hour. There is enough skin to cover 60% of the burned area, and the remaining area is covered with a temporary skin substitute. At the end of surgery, hemoglobin is 7.5 g/dL. Another unit of packed red blood cells is administered over 2 hours. Over the 2 hours in the operating room, her **temperature has fallen to 35.4°C**. A second forced-air warmer is placed over her now-dressed upper body and she is rewarmed to 36.5°C prior to transfer back to the ICU. In the ICU, **ketamine and morphine infusions are continued**.*

*The patient is booked for **change of dressings and further grafting in 7 days**.*

DISCUSSION

1. What factors determine the timing of burn excision and grafting?

The type of burn, the extent of the injury, and the stability of the patient help determine the timing of the grafting. Excision of burned tissue and covering with skin or skin substitutes within 7 days of injury significantly decreases morbidity and mortality. There is a large systemic inflammatory response in major burns (>25% of body surface area), and this can lead to *significant catabolism*, which is associated with increased morbidity. Early excision and coverage of a major full-thickness burn decreases the risk of sepsis and decreases the inflammatory response. This results in decreased mortality and decreased length of hospital stay (Ong et al., 2006). A flame burn is more likely to cause a full-thickness burn, whereas a hot-water scald is more likely to be superficial or partial thickness due to the lower temperature of boiling water. Therefore, there may be advantages in delaying excision of scald burns (especially if <25% body surface area) as it may not be immediately apparent which areas are deep and need grafting.

Extensive excision and grafting causes *significant blood loss* and the potential for **hypothermia**. Patients with significant comorbidities or who are systemically unwell from their burn injury (e.g., respiratory failure, hypovolemia, sepsis, and coagulopathy) should be stabilized prior to surgery as significant blood loss and hypothermia have the potential to worsen such problems. This child had a significant area of deep burn and was clinically stable and was able to undergo early excision and grafting of her burns.

Patients requiring multiple visits to the operating room for grafting and dressing changes must be carefully scheduled to avoid prolonged fasting. The nutritional requirements of burn patients are greatly increased in the hypermetabolic phase post-injury, and inadequate nutrition will lead to excessive catabolism, which can significantly delay recovery. Continuous feeding via the nasojejunal route, through the perioperative period, may be considered in patients with large burns.

2. What respiratory problems may be encountered in the post-burn period?

Direct thermal injury to the upper airway may cause supraglottic airway swelling and lead to respiratory distress. Facial and neck burns can also lead to supraglottic edema. Patients with such injuries should be intubated early (as discussed in the previous chapter).

Most patients with significant burns will develop some lung dysfunction, either due to inhalational injury or as part of the post-burn inflammatory response. Mechanical ventilation may be required and oxygen should be given to maintain normal oxygen saturations. In this patient, there was no evidence of airway burns, but the history of a house fire suggests that inhalational injury is likely. Her oxygen requirement of 30% is not high, but it is decided to leave her intubated postoperatively as lung dysfunction may still develop. This will also allow adequate doses of opioid analgesics to be given without risk of depression of respiratory drive.

3. How can hypothermia be avoided during burn surgery?

Burn patients are at great risk for hypothermia because of the loss of normal skin which usually acts as a barrier to heat loss. The body's usual homeostatic mechanisms may also be upset by the burn patient's hypermetabolic state, the malfunction of the dermal circulation, and the effects of general anesthesia. Hypothermia may impair wound healing, contribute to rejection of skin grafts, increase wound infection, and lead to coagulopathy. Post-anesthesia, the hypothermic patient will respond by shivering, which increases oxygen consumption by the body and can lead to hypoxia. Heat loss was minimized in this patient by **prewarming the operating room** to 32°C, covering the patient with a **plastic sheet**, and using a warming mattress and a **forced-air warmer**. Prewarming the operating room reduces the temperature gradient between the patient and environment. It is important that enough time for warming up the whole room is allowed, particularly the walls, which contribute significantly to radiant heat loss. The maximum allowable temperature is that which is tolerated by the operating room staff, particularly those in surgical gowns. It is important to cover as much of the patient as possible to reduce evaporative, radiant, and convective heat losses. A warming mattress and forced-air warmers minimize conductive heat loss and can contribute to active warming. Other strategies are the use of overhead radiant heat lamps and the use of warm intravenous fluid and blood warmers. It is important to note the patient's temperature prior to anesthesia and surgery. Most burn patients become relatively hyperthermic in the days after injury as their metabolic rate increases, often with temperatures over 39°C. Normothermia for these patients may be 38° to 39°C rather than 37°C. Therefore, a perioperative temperature drop of 2°C may have significant consequences in terms of postoperative shivering.

4. What strategies are available for blood conservation during surgery?

Minimizing exposure to blood products reduces the risk for blood-borne disease and other complications of transfusion.

Minimizing bleeding will also allow greater surgical time and may lead to fewer visits to the operating room. Strategies for reducing bleeding include using injected or topical vasoconstrictors, tourniquets, electrocautery, and compressive dressings, preventing coagulopathy, and avoiding hypothermia. In this patient, epinephrine 1:200,000 was injected under the eschar prior to excision (Fig. 26.2). The epinephrine causes vasoconstriction in the subcutaneous tissues. During injection, the patient must be monitored carefully for signs of systemic absorption of epinephrine (tachycardia, hypertension). Epinephrine doses of up to 180 mcg/kg given over 15 minutes have been administered in this way without systemic side effects (Robertson et al., 2001). Dressings soaked with dilute epinephrine solutions can also be applied to donor sites. Avoiding tachycardia and hypercarbia may decrease blood loss. Hypothermia, which can lead to coagulopathy, should also be avoided.

5. What factors determine the extent of excision and grafting?

The extent of the surgery is often determined by the blood loss and availability of blood products, the availability of appropriate postoperative care, and the development of intraoperative coagulopathy or hypothermia. Blood loss can be rapid during burn surgery and significant coagulopathy can develop quickly. Hemoglobin and coagulation should be monitored intraoperatively. Adequate supplies of blood products must be promptly available.

6. How can analgesia be optimized in the patient with a major burn?

Burns are particularly painful. Full-thickness burns may not be as painful as superficial and partial-thickness burns, but most thermal injuries are mixed in their depth. A multimodal approach is important in minimizing the side effects from long-term opioid use. The analgesics used in this case, morphine and ketamine, are both strong analgesics and are suitable for use in infusions, which may be titrated to effect. Pain from harvesting skin is particularly severe and may require bolus rescue dosing. The **fascia iliaca block**, used in this case, is a particularly effective block for burn surgery as it provides analgesia to the anterior, lateral, and medial surfaces of the thigh, which are common sites for skin harvesting. This block may provide effective analgesia for 12 to 24 hours. Use of local anesthesia for neural blockade may reduce the need for strong analgesics and their side effects. Patients with significant burns may require weeks of opioid infusions, and this can lead to increasing dose requirements as tolerance to opioids develops. If patients require opioids for more than a few days, rotation of different opioids may reduce opioid tolerance. Use of non-opioids, such as clonidine or ketamine, will help reduce opioid requirements. Acetaminophen (paracetamol), nonsteroidal anti-inflammatory agents, and oral opioids are also very useful adjuncts to intravenous agents in burn patients. These patients often require multiple dressing changes and other procedures during their treatment, which can often be managed without general anesthesia. It is important that nonpharmacological techniques of pain management are considered for these procedures as well as the usual pharmacological agents. These techniques may include hypnosis, distraction, guided imagery, and relaxation techniques. Children should be given some control over parts of the procedure and parents should be present whenever possible. Procedures should be performed in a relaxed environment and consideration given to the type of lighting, music, and temperature of the procedure room.

7. How are the pharmacodynamics and pharmacokinetics of common anesthesia drugs affected by burns?

The volume of distribution and clearance of most commonly used drugs are influenced by burn pathophysiology. In general, anesthesia drugs should be titrated to effect.

The behavior of muscle relaxants is significantly changed by burn injury, particularly after the first 24 hours. In particular, succinylcholine can lead to profound hyperkalemia, which may cause cardiac arrest. This is presumably due to the proliferation of extrajunctional nicotinic receptors on the muscle membrane that occurs after a burn. Succinylcholine is contraindicated in burn patients fter the first 48 hours and should be avoided until the burn has healed and normal activity has resumed. Patients with significant burns, such as this patient, are relatively resistant to nondepolarizing relaxants, and increased loading doses and more frequent dosing may be required to maintain muscle relaxation.

The effect on the pharmacokinetics of opioids is variable following burn injury and depends upon the opioid used and the stage after burn injury. Opioids should be titrated to effect; as mentioned previously, tolerance to opioids will develop, and this will require increased dosing. The development of multisystem organ disease, particularly renal failure, in large burns will also affect clearance, especially of morphine and its metabolites.

SUMMARY

1. The timing of surgery depends on the type of burn, the extent of the injury, and the stability of the patient.
2. Major complications of burn excision and grafting include blood loss, coagulopathy, and hypothermia.
3. Keys to effective pain management for the burn patient include a multimodal approach using pharmacological and nonpharmacological approaches. Regional analgesic techniques may be useful in the perioperative period; opioid rotation may reduce the problem of opioid tolerance.

ANNOTATED REFERENCES

- Fabia R, Groner JI. Advances in the care of children with burns. *Advan Pediatr* 2009; 56: 219–248.

This summary of current surgical management of children with burns is useful for understanding the overall management of these children.

- **Fuzaylov G, Fidkowski CW. Anesthetic considerations for major burn injury in pediatric patients.** *Pediatr Anesth* **2009; 9(3): 202–211.**

This paper gives a good summary of the pathophysiology of thermal injury and outlines the major complications that must be managed by the anesthesiologist.

Further Reading

Ong YS, Samuel M, Song C. Meta-analysis of early excision of burns. *Burns* 2006; 32: 145–150.

Robertson RD, Bond P, Wallace B, Shewmake K, Cone J. The tumescent technique to significantly reduce blood loss during burn surgery. *Burns* 2001; 27: 835–838.

Liver Transplant

XIMENA SOLER, LORI A. ARONSON, AND
GILLIAN DERRICK

INTRODUCTION

Liver transplantation is an established therapy in pediatric end-stage liver failure. Blood loss during orthotopic liver transplantation (OLT) is highly variable. Massive hemorrhage and transfusion of blood products, with its related consequences, is a well-known complication of this operation.

LEARNING OBJECTIVES

1. Understand the risk of bleeding associated with OLT in children.
2. Identify risk factors and discuss current trends in the diagnosis and management of hemorrhage and coagulopathy in the course of pediatric liver transplantation.
3. Review the advantages and disadvantages of antifibrinolytics in pediatric OLT.

CASE PRESENTATION

*A 10-month-old, 7.3-kg boy with **liver failure** secondary to total parenteral nutrition (TPN) cholestasis is admitted for OLT. He was born prematurely at 24 weeks' gestation; perinatal complications included* necrotizing enterocolitis (NEC) that required distal small bowel resection and total abdominal colectomy. This resulted in **short gut syndrome** and dependence on **TPN**. Other perinatal complications included a right grade IV intraventricular hemorrhage, bronchopulmonary dysplasia, and developmental delay. The patient recently had upper gastrointestinal bleeding. His severe portal hypertension has required treatment with octreotide.

Baseline laboratory data show anemia and **thrombocytopenia** (hemoglobin 8.9 g/dL and platelet count 30,000/microliter), elevated liver enzymes, hypoalbuminemia, and **abnormal coagulation (PT 22.3, PTT 51.7, INR 1.84)**. His electrolyte panel is normal. Though considered for a multivisceral transplant, he has been tolerating 75% of caloric intake enterally, so he is scheduled for OLT only. He was granted a split organ, receiving the left lateral segment of a reduced liver graft.

A rapid-sequence induction with propofol and succinylcholine is uneventful. Endotracheal intubation is achieved with a 3.5 cuffed ETT with a leak pressure at 20 cmH$_2$O. A 5.5Fr 8-cm triple-lumen right internal jugular vein **central line** is inserted under ultrasound guidance and a 22-gauge right radial arterial line is placed. The octreotide infusion is maintained at 25 mcg/hr. The operation is complicated by a significant amount of **adhesions** and massive blood loss. The patient requires continuous transfusions of packed red blood cells, fresh frozen plasma, cryoprecipitate, and platelets. Intraoperative electrolytes, blood gases, glucose, lactate, and hematocrit are monitored with bedside portable laboratory testing. Coagulation studies are sent stat to the lab and point-of-care **thromboelastogram** is used to guide intraoperative transfusion management.

A calcium chloride infusion is started to keep **ionized calcium** levels above 1.1 mmol/L. Intermittent boluses of bicarbonate are necessary to correct metabolic acidosis associated with increased lactate levels. Glucose and potassium levels remain within normal limits until the anhepatic phase. After liver revascularization, there is hemodynamic instability requiring **epinephrine** (adrenaline) and **norepinephrine** (noradrenaline) infusions to be run at 0.2 mcg/kg/min and 0.4 mcg/kg/min, respectively. Ventilation becomes more difficult, requiring an increase in peak inflating pressure from a baseline of

15 to 40 cmH$_2$O. Central venous pressure (CVP) is maintained between 5 and 10 mmHg with transfusion of blood products, albumin, and crystalloids. Due to hemodynamic instability, the decision is made to delay completion of the biliary anastomosis. The surgeons place a biliary drain and perform a temporary abdominal closure. After 8 hours of surgery, the patient is transferred to the pediatric intensive care unit (PICU). By the end of the operation, he has received 9,930 mL (20 units) packed red blood cells, 15 units cryoprecipitate, 450 mL fresh frozen plasma, 400 mL platelets, 2,500 mL albumin, and 3,500 mL crystalloids. Blood loss is estimated to have been 20,000 mL and urine output 600 mL. The patient gradually stabilizes in the PICU and returns 1 week later for completion of the Roux-en-Y and closure of the abdominal wall without complications.

DISCUSSION

1. What are the different forms of OLT?
OLT is an established therapy in **pediatric end-stage liver disease**. In 1967, Starzl completed the first orthotopic liver transplant, and later the introduction of cyclosporine, steroids, and tacrolimus further revolutionized orthotopic organ transplantation. By improving survival rates, OLT was widely adopted and in 1983 was recognized by the National Institutes of Heath as a valid therapy for end-stage liver disease. The pediatric donor shortage has led to the use of split graft (one liver is surgically divided to provide two transplantable segments), reduced segment (one segment out of a larger donor, discarding the remaining segment), or living donor liver transplantation (the left segment is harvested from a healthy living donor), as well as whole organ OLT.

2. What patient and intraoperative factors contribute to blood loss during OLT?
Contributing factors to blood loss during OLT can be categorized based on factors related to preoperative, intraoperative, and postoperative periods as well as patient factors.

Preoperative patient factors: The pathophysiology of liver failure and coagulopathy is well described for patients with liver disease. Patients with cholestatic liver disease, such as **TPN**-induced liver failure, have *vitamin K-related factor deficiency*. Patients with severe hepatocellular damage, such as acute and fulminant liver failure, exhibit a generalized **thrombocytopenia** from decreased synthesis of thrombopoietin and increased platelet consumption and sequestration due to splenomegaly. Some patients with end-stage liver disease demonstrate *increased fibrinolytic activity*, resulting in low-grade disseminated intravascular coagulation (DIC). The dilutional effect and hypoalbuminemia of liver failure add to the coagulopathy. Management strategies to decrease the risk of intraoperative bleeding include preemptive platelet administration and preoperative correction of factor deficiency. *Esophageal varices* may be a source of significant bleeding preoperatively, and *portosystemic venous collaterals* greatly increase blood loss during the operation. *Subclinical sepsis* often contributes to background DIC. Prior abdominal surgeries with friable tissues and multiple **adhesions** further contribute to bleeding.

Intraoperative factors: Stage I (pre-anhepatic period) begins with dissection of vascular structures and ends with the native hepatectomy. Blood loss in stage I occurs mainly from transection of collateral blood vessels and **adhesions**. As in the case portrayed above, a history of **short gut syndrome** is associated with increased blood loss.

The trauma literature suggest that a 1:1:1 ratio of red blood cells, fresh frozen plasma, and platelets is beneficial to control existing coagulopathy and prevent further escalation of hemorrhage due to dilutional coagulopathy (Kashuk et al., 2008; Holcomb et al., 2008). Starch, gelatin-based, and dextran colloid administrations have all been shown to reduce hemostasis and clot formation. Point-of-care monitoring has gained acceptance in the management of these patients.

CVP monitoring is an important measure to guide the treatment of hemorrhage. There is evidence that a high venous pressure during the dissection and immediate post-reperfusion stages causes increased intraoperative venous bleeding and greater requirements for blood product transfusion. Deliberate lowering of the CVP during liver resection assists in controlling bleeding during dissection.

Infusion of vasopressors helps support hemodynamics in the face of a lower CVP and lessens fluid requirements that lead to dilutional coagulopathy. While **epinephrine** is typically used, the addition of **norepinephrine** or vasopressin can be beneficial without compromising splanchnic perfusion. Vasopressin decreases portal vein pressure and flow in the native liver, thus reducing venous congestion. In the newly transplanted liver, vasopressin may help decrease metabolic overload.

Stage II (anhepatic phase) begins with implantation of the donor liver and ends with reperfusion of the new organ. The *raw cut surface of a split or reduced-size organ* is prone to greater hemorrhage at reperfusion despite techniques for hemostasis on the donor liver prior to its implantation. The argon beam coagulator can be effective in controlling bleeding from a cut surface. Direct application of materials to accelerate clotting, such as oxidized cellulose and fibrin glue, is a common practice. The degree of degradation of factors V and VIII correlates with the transfusion requirements during OLT. Fibrinolysis may be a problem during the anhepatic or post-anhepatic phase of OLT. Alpha-2 antiplasmin, the principal inhibitor of plasmin and plasminogen activity during this phase, is decreased.

Hypothermia, a progressive problem during liver transplantation, acutely worsens with the release of iced flushing solutions into the abdominal cavity and circulation. Hypothermia impairs platelet availability and function, and decreases enzymatic activity of clotting factors, thereby contributing to coagulopathy.

Activation of factors VII, IX, and X requires free calcium to facilitate adequate coagulation. Maintaining sufficient levels of **ionized calcium** in the face of massive transfusion can be difficult due to the chelating effects of preservatives such as EDTA. Calcium is also important for myocardial contractility, especially in children. *Magnesium* levels are also decreased due to citrate toxicity and chelation during the anhepatic phase. Since magnesium has procoagulant activity, its decrease can contribute to altered **coagulation**.

Stage III (reperfusion and post-reperfusion) begins with reperfusion of the grafted liver and ends with completion of the operation. Transplantation of a healthy liver usually restores the patient's clotting function in the operating room. The cause of fibrinolysis in this stage is mostly related to *tissue plasminogen activator* or *DIC*. Platelet trapping and the use of the University of Wisconsin preservation solution may also directly inhibit platelet aggregation, perhaps via adenosine.

Over-transfusion of packed red blood cells and overcorrection of the coagulopathy with blood products may lead to hepatic artery thrombosis, which is the leading cause of graft failure during the immediate postoperative period in the pediatric population. Typical goals are **PTT** more than 60 seconds, **PT** 18 to 20 seconds, **INR** more than 1.5, fibrinogen levels at 100 mg/dL, hematocrit around 30%, and platelet count of 50,000 to 100,000/microliter. Administration of blood products is guided not only by laboratory data but also by discussion of the clinical hemostasis on the field with the surgeon.

3. **What advances are being made in monitoring and treating intraoperative coagulopathy and transfusion practices during OLT?**

Early intervention to control existing coagulopathy and avoiding hypothermia is important, but point-of-care monitoring of **coagulation** is critical. Point-of-care **thromboelastography** is becoming routine in most transplant centers. The thromboelastogram is used to monitor **coagulation**, fibrinolysis, and bleeding time and can assist the anesthesiologist in treating intraoperative bleeding by helping identify the cause. Bedside **APTT, PT, and INR** equipment is also available in many centers, particularly in Europe.

Cell-salvaged blood reduces the volume of donor blood required but does not replace clotting factors, so balanced transfusion of clotting products is still important. Concentrated clotting factors have a place in focused and low-volume correction of specific coagulation defects. Recombinant factor VIIa is a potent coagulant that may lead to thrombosis, but it may be important as a last resort in life-threatening hemorrhage. A study of its use in pediatric OLT found no increase in hepatic artery thrombosis in a case series of 28 patients (Kalicinski et al., 2005).

4. What are the advantages and disadvantages of antifibrinolytics in pediatric OLT? What are their indications?

Antifibrinolytics are drugs that work by inhibiting the binding of plasmin to fibrin and plasminogen to plasmin in multiple ways. Aprotinin, as well as ε-aminocaproic acid and tranexamic acid, has been used in adult OLT. Aprotinin has been associated with renal and other organ failure and was withdrawn from the market in 2007. There are few absolute indications for the administration of antifibrinolytics in liver transplantation apart from demonstrable fibrinolysis on **thromboelastogram** that is unresponsive to reasonable clotting factor replacement strategies. The use of antifibrinolytic agents during pediatric OLT is limited due to the risk of hepatic artery thrombosis.

SUMMARY

1. **Risk factors for bleeding associated with liver transplant can be related to the patient's past medical history (existing coagulopathy, short gut, friable tissue, and adhesions), current illness (portal hypertension with consequent thrombocytopenia, subclinical sepsis) and the use of a split organ.**
2. **Electrolyte abnormalities, namely hypocalcemia and hypomagnesemia, often contribute to coagulation dysfunction.**

3. Lower CVP may help decrease intraoperative blood loss.

4. Target values during the neohepatic phase are PTT more than 60 seconds, PT 18 to 20 seconds, INR above 1.5, fibrinogen levels at 100 mg/dL, hemoglobin 10 to 12 g/dL, and platelet count of 50,000 to 100,000 to avoid hepatic artery thrombosis.

ANNOTATED REFERENCES

- Massicote L, Lenis S. Effect of low central venous pressure and phlebotomy on blood products transfusion requirements during liver transplantation. *Liver Transpl* 2005; 12: 117–123.

  Reduced transfusion of red blood cells and coagulation factors occurred when the central venous pressure was kept below control levels. It demonstrated a viable alternative to decrease blood loss during liver transplantation.

- Molenaar IQ, Warnaar N, Groen H, Porte RJ. Efficacy and safety of antifibrinolytic drugs in liver transplantation: a systematic review and meta-analysis. *Am J Transplant* 2007; 7: 185–194.

  Studies comparing ε-aminocaproic acid, tranexamic acid, and aprotinin were included. The authors analyzed intraoperative blood loss, blood product transfusion, the perioperative incidence of hepatic artery thrombosis, venous thromboembolic events, and mortality with antifibrinolytics. No increased risk for hepatic artery thrombosis, venothrombotic events, or perioperative mortality was observed. Aprotinin has been withdrawn and is no longer available.

- Ozier Y, Le Cam B. Intraoperative blood loss in pediatric liver transplantation: Analysis of preoperative risk factors. *Anesth Analg* 1995; 81: 1142–1147.

This analysis of 14 preoperative risk factors studied in 95 patients undergoing OLT demonstrated that reduced-size liver graft and increased portal pressure were found to be significant risk factors for blood loss. ε-Aminocaproic acid decreased blood loss in patients at high risk.

Further Reading

Holcomb JB, Wade CE, Michalek JE, Chisholm GB, Zarzabal LA et al. Increased plasma and platelet to red blood cells ratios improves outcome in 466 massively transfused civilian patients. *Ann Surg* 2008; 65: 261–71.

Kalicinski P, Markiewicz M, Kaminski A, Przemyslaw HI, Drewniak T, Symczak M, Nachulewicz P, Jezierska E. Single pretransplant bolus of recombinant activated factor VII ameliorates influence of risk factors for blood loss during orthotopic liver transplantation. *Pediatr Transplantation* 2005; 9: 299–304.

Kashuk JL, Moore EE, Johnson JL et al. Post-injury life threatening coagulopathy: Is 1:1 fresh frozen plasma: red blood cells the answer? *J Trauma* 2008; 65: 261–71.

McDiarmid SV. Current status of liver transplantation in children. *Pediatr Clin North Am* 2003; 50: 1335–1374.

Shouten E, Van de Pol A, Shouten AN, Bollen, CW. The effect of aprotinin, tranexamic acid, and aminocaproic acid on blood loss and use of blood products in major pediatric surgery: A meta-analysis. *Pediatr Crit Care Med* 2009; 10: 182–190.

Urwyler N, Staub LP, Beran D, Deplazes M, Lord SJ, Alberio L, Theiler L. Is perioperative point-of-care prothrombin time testing accurate compared to the standard laboratory test? *Thromb Haemost* 2009; 102: 779–786.

Wagener G, Gubitosa G, Renz J. Vasopressin decreases portal vein pressure and flow in the native liver during liver transplantation. *Liver Transpl* 2008; 14: 1664–1670.

28

Craniosynostosis Repair

PETER HOWE

INTRODUCTION

Craniosynostosis is a condition in which one or more of the fibrous sutures in an infant skull fuses prematurely. This may lead to restricted skull and brain growth and elevated intracranial pressure. Many children with craniosynostosis undergo corrective cranioplasty in infancy, an age when the skull is relatively large in proportion to the rest of the body. Depending on the operation, it is common for blood loss to be substantial and exceed the child's estimated blood volume (EBV). Managing this blood loss is challenging and requires careful planning for fluid and blood product administration. Some children also have craniofacial syndromes that are associated with airway obstruction and difficult intubation.

LEARNING OBJECTIVES

1. Decide upon and justify the threshold for initiating blood transfusion.
2. Describe the risks of massive blood transfusion that are particularly relevant in an infant.
3. Understand, recognize, and treat venous air embolism (VAE).

CASE PRESENTATION

An otherwise healthy, 7-month-old boy with sagittal synostosis presents for cranial vault reconstruction. He weighs 7.1 kg. His preoperative hemoglobin (Hb) is 10 g/dL, equivalent to a hematocrit (Hct) of 30%. His blood volume should be 70 mL/kg, or 500 mL. The child is anesthetized, and two large-bore peripheral intravenous lines are inserted. Monitoring includes a radial arterial line, a femoral central venous catheter (CVC), a urinary catheter, and a rectal temperature probe. The child is carefully placed in the prone position, pressure areas are padded, the endotracheal tube is secured, and the child is kept warm.

His allowable blood loss to reach a Hb of 7 g/dL (Hct 21%) is 3/10 × 500 mL, or 150 mL. The plan is to give three times this volume as Hartmann's sodium lactate solution and thereafter to use a mixture of red blood cells and colloid solutions.

Bleeding is minimal at first but increases once bone is incised. Once 450 mL crystalloid has been given, the Hb is 8 g/dL (Hct 24%). He is transfused with packed cells plus albumin in a 1:1 ratio. Bleeding increases further as bone flaps are removed. Once blood loss reaches 500 mL, Hb, platelets, and clotting parameters are checked. Thereafter, he receives packed cells and fresh frozen plasma in a 1:1 ratio.

*Suddenly, the end tidal CO_2 falls from 37 to 15 mmHg and the mean blood pressure falls from 45 to 30 mmHg. Venous air embolism (VAE) is suspected. The sevoflurane is immediately discontinued and the inspired oxygen fraction (FiO_2) is increased to 1.0. Fluid is given as a bolus, the **table is tilted** so the patient is **head-down**, and the surgeon **floods the operative field** with saline.*

*After the patient's condition stabilizes, the surgeon removes the last bone flap and controls the bleeding. The operation proceeds uneventfully thereafter, with the patient in a slight **Trendelenburg** position.*

DISCUSSION

1. **What is the lowest acceptable Hct/Hb in an otherwise healthy infant undergoing cranioplasty?**

There is little clinical evidence to guide transfusion triggers that is directly relevant to healthy infants undergoing acute, massive blood loss. Most guidelines are based on basic physiology and clinical studies of adults and critically ill patients. The crucial issue is maintaining adequate oxygenation to vital organs. The quantity of oxygen made available to the body is known as the *oxygen delivery*. Oxygen delivery is determined by the product of Hb concentration, cardiac output, and the arterial oxygen saturation. As the Hb falls, oxygen delivery to the tissues is maintained by increasing cardiac output. When cardiac output reaches a maximum then any further fall in Hb will result in insufficient delivery to meet tissue demand and tissue hypoxia occurs. Accepting a lower-than-normal Hb should be considered *only if the patient's cardiac output and oxygen saturation are satisfactory.*

Under conditions of isovolumetric hemodilution, healthy resting adults can tolerate a Hb of 5 g/dL without evidence of inadequate oxygen delivery, but myocardial oxygen supply at these levels is borderline and may become inadequate if the subject's activity level or heart rate increases (Weiskopf et al., 1998). In a study of healthy children undergoing repair of idiopathic scoliosis, patients were hemodiluted to Hb 7 g/dL before the start of surgery. The volume state was closely monitored with arterial and pulmonary arterial catheters, and the FiO_2 remained 1.0 throughout anesthesia. Blood was not re-transfused until the end of surgery unless the intraoperative mixed venous oxygenation fell below 60%. This occurred in only one patient, who developed transient ST-segment depression at a Hb of 2.2 g/dL (Fontana et al., 1995). This small study suggests that if circulatory volume and oxygenation are closely monitored, otherwise healthy children may be able to tolerate low levels of Hb without apparent harm.

During a critical illness, many of the compensatory mechanisms for anemia are impaired. Despite this, data in both adult and pediatric critical care have not shown that a liberal transfusion strategy (target Hb 10–12 g/dL) is associated with a better outcome than a restrictive strategy (target Hb 7–9 g/dL).

However transfusion strategies in the critically unwell intensive care patient may not translate to acute blood loss in the OR.

A recent Cochrane review of transfusion thresholds concluded that "for most patients, blood transfusion is probably not essential until hemoglobin levels drop below 7.0 g/dl" (Hill et al., 2000). This threshold has been applied broadly in the craniofacial surgical context; however, to avoid "getting behind" or the need for rapid transfusion, a higher threshold may be justified at stages of the operation where sudden bleeding is anticipated or most likely.

2. Which risks of blood transfusion are particularly relevant to an otherwise healthy infant undergoing cranioplasty?

Clinical error leading to the transfusion of the wrong blood is the most common cause of adverse events related to transfusion. This risk may be higher amid the anxiety and haste created by uncontrolled hemorrhage. Where possible, check blood products before major bleeding starts. Potassium levels in stored blood increase in proportion to the duration of storage, and in old blood they may be greater than 18 mEq/L. One unit of old stored blood is unlikely to cause hyperkalemia when transfused to an adult, but in an infant, one unit may represent half the circulating blood volume and if transfused rapidly may precipitate arrhythmias. If fresh blood is unavailable, older blood can be washed in a cell saver to reduce the potassium concentration.

3. What information from the arterial line trace suggests that the infant requires more intravenous fluid?

The mean arterial pressure (MAP) is considered the driving pressure for perfusion of most vital organs. When MAP falls below the lower limit of autoregulation (LLA), regional blood flow becomes linearly dependent on MAP. The cerebral LLA in adults is generally considered to be a MAP of 60 mmHg. Although there are no conclusive data regarding the lowest MAP that patients can tolerate without neurologic sequelae, a sustained intraoperative MAP below 60 mmHg is generally considered undesirable.

In children, the cerebral LLA is not clearly known. Baseline MAP is lower in children than in adults, and it is thus often assumed that the LLA is also lower in children, but there are few data to support this assumption.

MAP will fall when a child is significantly hypovolemic, but it is preferable to detect hypovolemia before a fall in MAP. The arterial pressure trace can assist detecting hypovolemia. The arterial pressure trace varies with the respiratory cycle. During the inspiratory phase of positive-pressure ventilation, ventricular preload decreases and stroke volume falls, causing a decrease in both pulse pressure and systolic pressure. A large change in pulse pressure (ΔPP) indicates that the cardiac output is likely to increase in response to fluid. A variation of more than 10 mmHg in the peak systolic pressure during the respiratory cycle of a patient on positive-pressure ventilation is indicative of at least a 10% reduction in circulating volume.

Although the appearance of the waveform may differ between patients due to damping, trends in the same patient may be useful. The slope of the systolic upstroke gives some indication of the contractile state of the myocardium. The diastolic downstroke is a combination of forward pressure from the heart and reflected pressure from the circulation. The slope of the diastolic decay indicates resistance to outflow; a slow fall is seen in vasoconstriction. A flat or low dicrotic notch is seen in hypovolemia. The general pattern is shown in Fig. 28.1.

4. Describe the pathophysiology, diagnosis, and initial management of VAE.

VAE occurs when air at a pressure higher than venous pressure comes into contact with the venous circulation. During cranioplasty, air may enter the circulation either through an open dural venous sinus or through exposed cancellous bone. Air emboli are potentially fatal, both from mechanical obstruction of the right ventricular outflow tract and pulmonary arterial tree, and from platelet aggregation, inflammation, and pulmonary edema. As the right heart obstructs, left ventricular filling decreases and

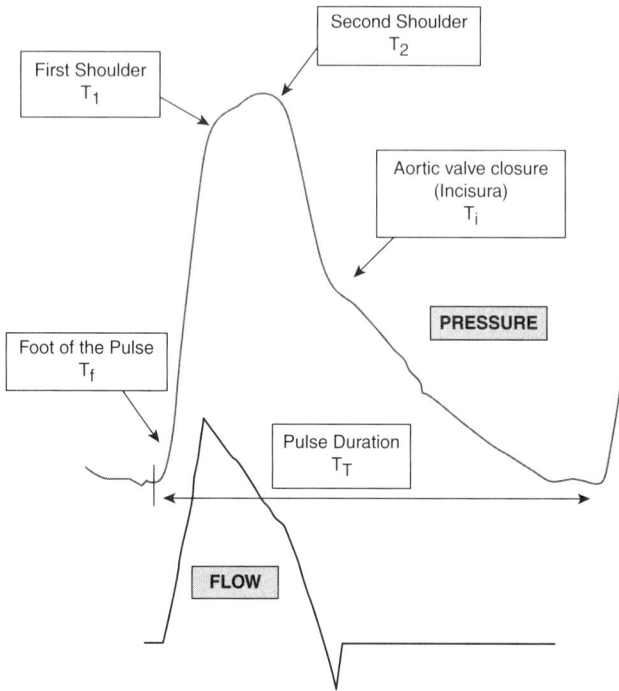

FIGURE 28.1 Arterial waveform.

cardiovascular collapse may ensue. Air may also pass through intracardiac shunts and occlude systemic arteries, leading to focal ischemia.

In an anesthetized patient, physical signs of VAE include raised central venous pressure, tachycardia, **hypotension**, and signs of ventilation–perfusion mismatch, resulting in a **fall in** both **end-tidal CO$_2$** and **arterial oxygen saturation**. Pulmonary artery pressure may be elevated or decreased, depending on the site of obstruction. Bronchoconstriction may cause airway pressures to rise. The mill wheel murmur, a loud, continuous slapping noise heard best at the left sternal border, is probably attributable to the right ventricle beating against subpulmonic air. *These signs may be difficult to differentiate from low right ventricular* *output due to sudden, major blood loss,* especially if central venous pressure is not being monitored. In pediatric cranioplasty, both VAE and massive hemorrhage may occur, especially when cranial bone flaps are raised. They may also occur simultaneously.

If VAE is suspected, the first priority is to prevent further air entry by **repositioning** the patient and **flooding** the **surgical field**. Both **Trendelenburg tilt** and placing the patient in the left lateral position have been shown to divert air from the right ventricular outflow tract. The patient is ventilated with **100% O$_2$** and the *circulation is supported with fluid, vasopressors, and external cardiac massage* as appropriate. External cardiac massage has improved survival in animal studies, presumably by breaking up large intracardiac bubbles. 100% O$_2$ helps to reabsorb nitrogen from smaller bubbles. Aspirating air from a central venous line has been more successful in animal studies than in humans and is probably best considered a last resort. A fluid bolus should always be considered because VAE is not only often associated with major blood loss, but may be difficult to differentiate from major blood loss.

SUMMARY

1. A transfusion threshold of Hb 7 g/dL is justifiable in a hemodynamically stable, well-oxygenated infant.
2. Check the blood in advance. If fresh blood is unavailable, consider washing red cells before transfusion.
3. Major bleeding may occur suddenly and may be difficult to distinguish from VAE. The initial management of both conditions is similar.
4. Keys to the diagnosis of VAE are an at-risk situation (dural venous sinus or cancellous bone open to air); a sudden drop in ETCO$_2$, oxygen saturation, and/or blood pressure; and possibly elevated central venous pressure and elevated airway pressure.

5. Emergency management of VAE is as follows: Inform the surgeon, flood the operative field, place the patient head-down. Call for help. Provide 100% O_2, intravenous fluid, vasopressors, and cardiac massage as indicated. Consider left lateral position.

ANNOTATED REFERENCES

- Barcelona SL, Thompson AA, Cote CJ. Intra-operative pediatric blood transfusion therapy: a review of common issues. Part I: hematologic and physiologic differences from adults. *Pediatr Anesth* 2005; 15(9): 716–726.
- Barcelona SL, Thompson AA, Cote CJ. Intra-operative pediatric blood transfusion therapy: a review of common issues. Part II: transfusion therapy, special considerations, and reduction of allogenic blood transfusions. *Pediatr Anesth* 2005; 15(10): 814–830.

  A succinct but thorough guide to understanding the complications of blood transfusion (Part I) and the management of massive transfusion in the operating room (Part II).
- Reiles E, Van der Linden P. Transfusion trigger in critically ill patients: has the puzzle been completed? *Critical Care* 2007, 11: 142.

  A helpful summary of studies that have compared restrictive and liberal transfusion strategies in critically ill adults and children.
- Weiskopf RB, Viele MK, Feiner J, et al. Human cardiovascular and metabolic response to acute, severe isovolemic anemia. *JAMA* 1998; 279(3): 217–221.

  A remarkable paper that explores the effects of acute hemodilution on conscious healthy adults at rest.

Further Reading

Fontana JL, Welborn L, Mongan PD, Sturm P, Martin G, Bünger R. Oxygen consumption and cardiovascular function in children during profound intra-operative normovolemic hemodilution. *Anesth Analg* 1995; 80(2): 219–225.

Hill SR, Carless PA, Henry DA, Carson JL, Hebert PC, McClelland DB, and Henderson KM. Transfusion thresholds and other strategies for guiding allogeneic red blood cell transfusion. *Cochrane Database System Rev* 2000; Issue 1. Art. No.: CD002042. DOI: 10.1002/14651858.

Orebaugh SL. Venous air embolism: Clinical and experimental considerations. *Crit Care Med* 1992; 20(8): 1169–1177.

van Woerkens, ECSM, Trouwborst A, van Lanschot JJB. Profound hemodilution: What is the critical level of hemodilution at which oxygen delivery-dependent oxygen consumption starts in an anesthetized human? *Anesth Analg* 1992; 75: 818–821.

Vavilala MS, Lee LA, Lam AM. The lower limit of cerebral autoregulation in children during sevoflurane anesthesia. *J Neurosurg Anesth* 2003; 15(4): 307–312.

29

Kidney Transplant

IAN SMITH

INTRODUCTION

Renal transplantation is the preferred treatment for pediatric patients who have end-stage renal disease. A successful transplant improves intellectual and behavioral development, quality of life, and survival, with the survival at 10 years being as high as 83% (Kim et al., 1991). We can optimize the chance of success by understanding the pathophysiology involved and applying this knowledge to guide our management of perioperative fluid balance, electrolyte anomalies, anemia, blood pressure control, and comorbidities. Also critical is an appreciation of the effects and consequences of the various immunosuppressive agents that are used. Close communication is required between the pediatrician, surgeon, and anesthesiologist.

LEARNING OBJECTIVES

1. Appreciate the key points in the preoperative assessment.
2. Understand the practical aspects of monitoring during anesthesia.
3. Review the management principles of intraoperative hemodynamic instability and develop a strategy for managing perioperative electrolyte abnormalities.
4. Consider how to optimally manage postoperative analgesia.

CASE PRESENTATION

*A 6-year-old boy with anuric **end-stage chronic renal failure** (CRF) secondary to severe reflux nephropathy is scheduled for a living related renal transplant. It is his first transplant and he is admitted the day prior to surgery for dialysis through a long-term subclavian central venous catheter. He has been undergoing hemodialysis for the previous year. Medications include irbesartan (an angiotensin receptor antagonist), oral vitamin D, calcium, and intermittent erythropoetin. On examination he is a pale, thin child with a post-dialysis weight of 20.4 kg, HR 92 bpm, BP 132/82, SpO2 96%. Cardiorespiratory examination is otherwise normal and he is afebrile. Blood tests show Hb 8 g/dL (white cell count and platelets are normal), Na$^+$ 140 mEq/L, K$^+$ 4.8 mEq/L, Ca^{2+} 2.6 mEq/L, PO$_4^{2-}$ 1.26 mEq/L, Mg$_4^+$ 0.89 mEq/L, urea 29.1 mg/dL (10.4 mmol/L), creatinine 6.48 mg/dL (573 micromol/L), and albumin 3.7 g/dL. Chest x-ray and ECG are normal. **Echocardiography** shows **mild left ventricular hypertrophy** with **good biventricular systolic function** and no evidence of a **pericardial effusion**. He is cross-matched for 2 units of blood. A cannula is in situ from the previous day's overnight hydration and infusion of anti-T-cell antibodies. His usual antihypertensive medication is given on the morning of surgery.*

*Anesthesia is induced with propofol and atracurium and maintained with sevoflurane in an O$_2$/air mixture. In a sterile manner, the "heparin lock" is aspirated from the hemodialysis catheter, which is then connected to a pressure transducer. The **central venous pressure** (**CVP**) is 4 mmHg. A urethral catheter is inserted. Fentanyl 5 mcg/kg and antibiotics are given before a right lower quadrant skin incision. IV hydration (10 mL/kg saline 0.9% and 10 mL/kg albumin 4%) is given prior to donor graft revascularization. This increases the CVP to 13 mmHg. A venous blood gas shows the Hb has fallen to 6.2 g/dL. Warmed, irradiated packed red cells (10 mL/kg) are transfused; this increases the CVP to 15 mmHg. The Hb increases to 88 g/L and the K$^+$ is 5.2 mmol/L. The ECG shows no changes suggestive of hyperkalemia throughout surgery. Methylprednisolone 10 mg/kg is administered on release of the venous anastomosis. Following reperfusion, urine* *production is confirmed by inspection of the ureter from the donor kidney (before its connection to the bladder). At this stage the blood pressure target is in the "low normal" adult pressure range. Following extubation, an **infusion of morphine** (10–40 mcg/kg/hr) provides early postoperative analgesia; this is supplemented by oral acetaminophen (paracetamol). Monitoring with ECG, oximetry, and hourly urine output is continued for 2 days. The hemodialysis catheter remains in situ for 6 weeks in case of graft failure.*

DISCUSSION

1. What are the key pathologies to consider in the preoperative assessment?

Once active infection is excluded (a contraindication to transplantation), the preoperative assessment concentrates on cardiorespiratory comorbidity, fluid status, and laboratory results. Cardiac causes are responsible for up to 50% of deaths in children requiring dialysis (McDonald & Craig, 2004) and 15% of deaths in pediatric transplant recipients (NAPRTCS, 2008). A hypertensive cardiomyopathy may be present; this can be manifested by a reduction in exercise tolerance. A preoperative **echocardiogram** is required to look for **ventricular hypertrophy** and dilatation and systolic and **diastolic ventricular dysfunction** and to **exclude a uremic pericardial effusion**. Coronary artery calcification is not expected in childhood. Continuation of antihypertensive medications before surgery is recommended and may prevent rebound hypertension. However, intraoperative hypotension may occur, especially with angiotensin converting enzyme inhibitors, and angiotensin receptor antagonists (Smith & Jackson, 2010).

Current volume status is best assessed by reference to the child's weight. Children may be hypovolemic after dialysis. Mild anemia is often present but is well tolerated. Severe azotemia with a BUN above 80 mg/dL may be associated with pericardial and pleural effusions. Platelet dysfunction may also occur and may influence the decision to place an epidural catheter. Common electrolyte anomalies include hypernatremia, hyperkalemia, hypocalcemia, and hypermagnesemia. Severe hyperkalemia should be treated by dialysis before surgery.

The underlying cause of **renal failure** could influence the assessment and perioperative management; for example, Takayasu's vasculitis may affect the coronary circulation, systemic lupus erythematosus (SLE) has protean manifestations, and high-dose steroid therapy given for glomerulonephritis may require perioperative steroid coverage.

2. What level of intraoperative monitoring is appropriate?

Close perioperative monitoring provides the data to optimize perfusion to the donor kidney. Routine intraoperative monitors would include five-lead ECG, SpO_2, $EtCO_2$, and core temperature. Noninvasive blood pressure via an automated measuring device is usual. Placing the blood pressure cuff on the upper limb is preferable in the event that the great vessels need to be clamped during the procedure. Arteriovenous (AV) fistulas are not generally surgically constructed until after the patient is about 12 years of age; however, if one is present, the arm should be carefully wrapped and clearly marked "*not for taking blood or blood pressure readings*." Intra-arterial BP would be reserved for small children undergoing an anastomosis of the allograft directly to the great vessels or when cardiac dysfunction is present (e.g., severe hypertensive cardiomyopathy). Avoidance of the brachial vessels is prudent as damage to these may preclude the future construction of AV fistulas. Central venous pressure (**CVP**) may be monitored by using an existing long-term central venous dialysis catheter or a freshly inserted internal jugular or subclavian line. A multilumen catheter is usually chosen because peripheral intravenous access is often difficult. Careful asepsis is required during line insertion and access due to the child's immunosuppression. Intraoperative transthoracic (TTE) or transesophageal echocardiography (TEE) may be indicated if severe coexisting heart disease is present.

3. What are the intraoperative stages of a renal transplant?

See Table 29.1. The technical aspects of surgery depend on a number of factors. For example, the size of recipient and donor kidney as well as the size of recipient blood vessels will determine the position of graft implantation. The incision is usually in the right lower quadrant; however, in smaller children a large live donor kidney may be too big to insert extraperitoneally. In this case a midline incision may be performed and the kidney inserted into the right paravertebral gutter. Depending on the cause of **renal failure**, the diseased kidney may also need to be removed (e.g., nephrotic syndrome, severe hypertension, or polycystic kidneys).

4. What is the management of intraoperative hypotension?

Guided by the CVP, it is appropriate to fluid load the patient with an isotonic fluid that has no added potassium (e.g., 0.9% saline). The aim is to have the patient "well filled" before unclamping the renal vein and artery. Note that the IV fluids may lead to a dilutional anemia. This may in turn lead to a lower blood pressure for a given cardiac output secondary to the reduction in blood viscosity. If the hemoglobin is less than 7g/dL (70 g/L), then consider blood transfusion. It is useful to wash the packed cells with a cell saver before infusion to reduce the K^+ concentration. Failing this, blood should be as fresh as possible, ideally less than 7 days old. Alterations in heart rate or rhythm need to be addressed on their own merits; however, given the propensity for electrolyte disturbance, obtaining an urgent electrolyte profile would be important. Intraoperative TEE or TTE provides a rapid, noninvasive assessment of cardiac filling and function. Always consider other causes of hypotension, including cardiac tamponade (from a pericardial effusion) and anaphylaxis. In this context, the latter is most likely to occur with neuromuscular blockers, antibiotics, or the immunosuppressive drug basiliximab (monoclonal anti-IL-2Rα receptor antibody). Inotropic support of the circulation is sometimes required to maintain the systemic blood pressure in the target range after anastomosis of the graft vessels.

Table 29.1

INTRAOPERATIVE STAGES, TIME COURSE, AND METHOD OF OPTIMIZING THE PHYSIOLOGY DURING PEDIATRIC RENAL TRANSPLANTATION

Event	Duration	Comments
Induction	40 minutes	Avoid long-acting neuromuscular blockers (e.g., pancuronium).
Incision/ dissection vessels	2 hours	Perioperative antibiotics and immunosuppressive medications
Cross-clamp vessels	N/A	Heparin (as per surgical request)
Vascular anastomosis	30 minutes	IV fluids to raise CVP to 12–15 mmHg
Unclamping vein and artery	N/A	Maintain intravascular volume mannitol/furosemide as per protocol
Ureter anastomosis to bladder	30 minutes	Initial urine output from the graft can be observed in the surgical field.
Closing	30 minutes	Maintain intravascular volume. Monitor urine output. Replace urine output (ml for ml) with a balanced salt solution (e.g., 0.9% saline).
Extubation	15 minutes	Ensure adequate (low normal adult) perfusion pressure and neuromuscular blockade reversal. Ensure patient is warm.

5. What is the management of intraoperative hypertension?

The first question to ask is, "What is the patient's usual blood pressure?" This blood pressure might be acceptable even though it is high relative to an age-matched population without renal failure. Once adequacy of anesthesia and analgesia is confirmed, further pharmacological management is considered. Sodium nitroprusside infusions are hazardous to run without an arterial line but are good from the perspective of their short duration of action. Phentolamine has a slower onset and acceptably short half-life as an alternative. Clonidine and β-blockers may be useful if the heart rate is also high. The ideal situation is to have a fairly short-acting antihypertensive agent so the patient is not left with intractable hypotension following reperfusion of the donor kidney. The target blood pressure following anastomosis may be higher than the child's usual BP.

6. How should one manage intraoperative hyperkalemia?

Hyperkalemia should be considered if the typical ECG changes of peaked T waves, broadening of the QRS complex, and bradycardia occur. There may be associated hypotension. Symptomatic hyperkalemia can occur intraoperatively in association with a blood transfusion. Be aware that a subset of patients presenting for renal transplantation may not have a dialysis catheter, arteriovenous fistula, or a peritoneal catheter *in situ*; the luxury of preoperative dialysis would not be available in this group. Initial management would depend on the severity of clinical features and the degree of suspicion. For example, if there is cardiovascular compromise with suspicion of hyperkalemia, resuscitation needs should be assessed and managed as per the pediatric resuscitation guidelines and treated pragmatically with calcium (as cardiac protection) and K^+-reducing therapy while waiting for the blood K^+ result. The therapies to be considered are in Table 29.2.

7. Which patients should remain intubated at the end of the procedure?

While the vast majority of patients can be extubated, there is a subgroup that may require a period of postoperative ventilation.

Table 29.2

THERAPEUTIC OPTIONS FOR INTRAOPERATIVE TREATMENT OF HYPERKALEMIA

- Increase minute ventilation to decrease $PaCO_2$ (and induce a respiratory alkalosis), which will promote intracellular uptake of K^+.
- Ca^{++} (0.1 mM/kg IV) to protect the myocardium from the arrhythmogenic effects of hyperkalemia. Preferably given into a central vein.
- Sodium bicarbonate IV: Dose (mEq/L) = Base excess (mEq/L) × Weight (kg)/6
- IV insulin (0.1 unit/kg IV) with 2 mL/kg dextrose 50% to increase the intracellular uptake of K^+
- Low-dose epinephrine (adrenaline) infusion (0.02 mcg/kg/min) to stimulate β_2-receptor–mediated cellular uptake of K^+
- Nasogastric calcium polystyrene sulfonate: Dose = 0.6 g/kg to absorb K^+.
- Intraoperative hemofiltration or dialysis. This will take time to implement and extra help will be required.
- Extracorporeal membrane oxygenation (ECMO) if severe cardiovascular instability is present and the hyperkalemia is refractory to treatment

Small patients (<12 kg) often require postoperative ventilation because the implantation of a large adult kidney into the abdomen may severely reduce pulmonary compliance. Patients with severe coexisting heart disease may also benefit from a period of postoperative ventilation because the efforts to maintain the perfusion pressure in the setting of limited cardiac reserve may result in pulmonary edema.

8. What are the options for postoperative analgesia?

Systemic analgesics supplemented with local anesthesia (wound infiltration with local anesthetic, epidural infusions, or wound irrigation catheters) form the basis of initial postoperative analgesia.

Systemic **infusions of** fentanyl or **morphine** are appropriate. Although morphine itself does not accumulate in renal failure, its active metabolites, morphine-6-glucuronide and the neuroexcitatory morphine-3-glucuronide, do. Increased levels of morphine-6-glucuronide may cause increased sedation and respiratory depression. Some practitioners avoid morphine and hydromorphone (which also accumulates active metabolites in renal failure) until renal function is ensured. Ketamine infusions may be a useful adjunct specifically to decrease the amount of opioid infused.

Epidurals are not absolutely contraindicated; however, some anesthesiologists express concern over the high incidence of mild coagulation disturbance in CRF. An epidural catheter with a low-concentration local anesthetic infusion can be run with or without an opioid in the same solution.

Meperidine (pethidine) is **not** used because the metabolite normeperidine may have reduced clearance in this setting and can cause convulsions. NSAIDs are contraindicated as the prostaglandin inhibition may reduce renal glomerular perfusion pressure.

Acetaminophen and tramadol are useful co-analgesics. It is advisable to wait for satisfactory renal function in the graft kidney before starting tramadol. When oral intake is established, an opioid analgesic such as oxycodone is appropriate. Ideally a dedicated pediatric pain service can assist in the management of the patient's analgesic needs.

SUMMARY

1. The preoperative assessment should focus on cardio-respiratory comorbidity, fluid status, and electrolyte balance.
2. Carefully consider the method and type of invasive and noninvasive monitoring.

3. Optimize perfusion of the donor organ; consider the patient's usual BP and give fluids as guided by the CVP. Remember the likely causes of hemodynamic instability.
4. Have a high index of suspicion for electrolyte abnormalities.
5. Analgesia should be multimodal. Consider the individual's needs and renal function and the type of incision.

ANNOTATED REFERENCES

- Coupe N, O'Brien M, Gibson P, de Lima J. Anesthesia for pediatric renaltransplantation with and without epidural analgesia—a review of 7 years experience. *Pediatr Anesth* 2005; 15(3): 220–228.

  An excellent article comparing and contrasting the experience of an Australian tertiary pediatric center, with particular reference to perioperative epidural anesthesia and hemodynamic stability.

- Della Rocca G, Costa MG, Bruno K, Coccia C, Pomei L, Di Marco P, Pretagostini R, Colonello M, Rossi M, Pietroaoli P, Cortesini R. Pediatric renal transplantation: anesthesia and perioperative complications. *Pediatr Surg Int* 2001; 17(2–3):175–179.

  An in-depth article looking at the outcome of 75 pediatric patients receiving a renal transplant in a European center. The sample size allows for an idea of the magnitude of the perioperative complications that occur in this group of patients.

- Lucile Salter Packard Children's Hospital. 2001. *Guidelines for Anesthesia for Pediatric Renal Transplantation.* Accessed Feb. 4, 2011, from http://pedsanesthesia.stanford.edu/down loads/guideline-renal.pdf

Concise and relevant, this excellent short article addresses all the major issues involved with anesthesia for pediatric renal transplantation.

Further Reading

Goodman WG, Goldin J, Kuizon BD, et al. Coronary-artery calcification in young adults with end-stage renal disease who are undergoing dialysis. *N Engl J Med* 2000; 342: 1478–1483.

Kim MS, Jabs K, Harmon WE. Long-term patient survival in a pediatric renal transplantation program. *Transplantation* 1991; 51(2): 413–416.

McDonald SP, Craig JC. Long-term survival of children with end-stage renal disease. *N Engl J Med* 2004; 350:2654–2662.

NAPRTCS Annual Report 2008. Accessed Nov. 10, 2010. http://www.naprtcs.org.

Royal Children's Hospital, Melbourne. 2010. *Acute Pain Management*. Accessed Feb. 4, 2011. http://www.rch.org.au/anaes/pain/index.cfm? doc_id=2384#1.

Shann F, ed. *Drug Doses*, 15th ed. Melbourne: The Royal Children's Hospital Publications, 2010.

Smith I, Jackson I. Beta-blockers, calcium channel blockers, angiotensin converting enzyme inhibitors and angiotensin receptor blockers: should they be stopped or not before ambulatory anaesthesia? *Curr Opin Anaesthesiol* 2010; 23(6): 687–690.

PART 6

CHALLENGES IN CONGENITAL

HEART DISEASE

30

Children with Congenital Heart Disease for Non-cardiac Surgery

MICHAEL CLIFFORD

INTRODUCTION

It is estimated that up to 1 million children in the United States have congenital heart disease (CHD). These children range from those who are essentially normal functionally with anatomically repaired hearts, and hence minimal impact for anesthesia, to those that have had complex and numerous surgical procedures with significant residual abnormalities in circulation and cardiac function, and a range of comorbidities. These latter children have many issues that will affect anesthesia for non-cardiac surgery. When presented with a child with CHD for non-cardiac surgery, the general pediatric anesthesiologist should be able to perform a tailored cardiac preoperative evaluation and plan an appropriate anesthetic with suitable anesthetic techniques, agents, and monitoring. Not every child with CHD has a single ventricle with all its complexity (see Chapter 31), but every child with CHD will offer challenges for the pediatric anesthesiologist.

LEARNING OBJECTIVES

1. Know that children with CHD may have either unre-paired or post-repair problems.
2. Identify the key questions in a cardiovascular evalua-tion that must be answered.
3. Describe the key principles in anesthetic manage-ment for the child with CHD presenting for non-cardiac surgery.
4. Review current management recommendations for endocarditis prophylaxis and for the child with a pacemaker.

CASE PRESENTATION

An 11-year-old, 40-kg boy with **trisomy 21** *presents from the emer-gency department for an appendectomy. He underwent repair of an* **atrioventricular (AV-septal or AV canal) defect** *at 3 months of age. The surgery was complicated by* **complete heart block (CHB)** *neces-sitating a* **permanent pacemaker**.

Outpatient notes from 3 months ago document "moderate" ongo-ing residual **left-sided atrioventricular valve (LAVV) regurgita-tion,** *left atrial enlargement, and elevation of his estimated pulmonary artery pressures to approximately one third of his systemic pressures. His pacemaker is functioning well, and a 12-lead ECG demonstrates CHB with an atrial rate of 100 bpm and an underlying (broad com-plex) ventricular rate of 45 bpm.*

His current medications are lisinopril 10 mg daily, furosemide 10 mg three times daily, and thyroxine 100 mcg daily. His previous episodes of hospitalization have rendered him "anxious" and "needle phobic" and he will "fight the mask." He is allergic to penicillin.

For premedication, the child receives midazolam 0.5 mg/kg and ketamine 5 mg/kg mixed with lemonade with good effect. A 24-gauge *intravenous cannula is inserted, followed by smooth intravenous induction. He is intubated with a size 5.5 mm cuffed endotracheal tube. No leak is noted at 20 cmH$_2$O, so the cuff is left deflated and a prophylactic dose of dexamethasone (0.6 mg/kg) is given to reduce the risk of post-extubation stridor.* **Clindamycin 20 mg/kg is administered** *30 minutes prior to the skin incision and the hospital cardiac technologist* **reprograms his pacemaker from a DDDR to a DOO mode***.*

Following discussion with the surgeon (who thinks the boy may have had a delayed diagnosis and a perforated appendix), the decision is made to insert an arterial line and internal jugular central venous catheter (CVC). A **nitric oxide** *cylinder is attached to the anesthesia machine "just in case."*

His surgery is uncomplicated. Prior to emergence, the boy's pacemaker is reset to his preoperative settings. He begins to spontaneously ventilate and his muscle relaxation is reversed with neostigmine 2.5 mg and glycopyrrolate 400 mcg. He is extubated without evidence of upper airway obstruction and recovers uneventfully.

DISCUSSION

1. What are specific concerns in anesthetizing a patient with CHD?

The underlying pathophysiology of the unrepaired lesion will give an insight into the anticipated problems after repair. Before anesthetizing a child with CHD, one should know what was the underlying condition and what has been done: in other words, *Where does the blood go?* Understanding the anatomy is crucial to understanding the likely impact of anesthesia. This child had an **atrioventricular septal defect** (AVSD) or "canal," a defect that is commonly associated with trisomy 21. The defect in the septum primum can combine with one of the membranous ventricular septum and variable abnormalities of a common atrioventricular valvular apparatus. There are no true "mitral" and/or "tricuspid" valves but rather an oval structure with superior and inferior bridging leaflets spanning the common inlet with variable leaflets on the left and right. The chordal attachments can be complex and can straddle the muscular septum and preclude a biventricular repair. The nature of any residual valvular regurgitation will thus vary with the nature of the original lesion and surgical outcome, necessitating long-term medical therapy or even further cardiac surgery.

After defining the anatomy, the next questions are: *Are there any obstructions to flow (dynamic or static)?* and *Are there any rhythm disturbances*? Children with CHD, both before and after repair, may have stenoses or obstructions to flow that may be fixed or dynamic (for example, the unrepaired tetralogy of Fallot; see Chapter 32). This child has no obstructive lesions. However, if there were a fixed obstructive lesion, it is important to avoid a sudden decrease in systemic vascular resistance, tachycardia, or increases in pulmonary vascular resistance. If there were a dynamic lesion, one should avoid sudden bursts of catecholamine release and hypovolemia.

Surgery or dilated atria may cause conduction abnormalities. In this case, closure of the septal defect affected the atrioventricular bundle (and its left and right branches), resulting in permanent atrioventricular block requiring a permanent pacemaker.

An assessment of cardiac function is vital; in other words, *How well does the heart pump?* Poor function mandates particular care with anesthesia and increases the need for invasive monitoring. In all children with CHD, a recent echocardiographic assessment is invaluable. An important question answered by the echocardiographic assessment is the ventricular function; however, asking about the child's functional capacity to play with siblings and other children may well be more predictive than the best echocardiogram.

In the case presented, other key preoperative concerns are the adequacy of the septal repair and its sequelae, the functional status of the AV valves, and pacemaker evaluation. The echocardiogram enabled an assessment of the severity of **AV valve regurgitation;** remember, however, that such assessment is often subjective and dependent on the technical adequacy of the study. How well these interrogations transpose to the postsurgical trisomic valve is reasonably questioned—although the left atrial and ventricular volume loading, regurgitant jet characteristics, and upstream effects on pulmonary venous flow should correlate with long term functional outcome.

Pulmonary hypertension is a major issue for anesthesia. In any child with CHD, the question should be asked: *Does the child have pulmonary hypertension?* In children with CHD, significant pulmonary hypertension is often indicated by **tricuspid regurgitation**. Children with trisomy 21 are also at increased risk of pulmonary hypertension (see Chapter 62). With pulmonary hypertension, the pulmonary vasculature may be reactive or relatively fixed (see Chapter 35 for details). Reactive vasculature is at greater risk of sudden significant deterioration. Despite the elevation in estimated pulmonary artery pressure, it is unlikely this child will have significant pulmonary hypertension and reactive pulmonary vasculature. Nevertheless, **nitric oxide** should be available in the event of unexplained cardiovascular collapse.

Table 30.1 summarizes the key questions that need to be answered.

2. What are the implications of having a pacemaker?

Pacemakers should be regularly evaluated. The sensing and capture thresholds, battery status, and, particularly for the anesthetist,

---

Table 30.1

CHECKLIST OF PREOPERATIVE PLANNING QUESTIONS

What is the anatomy—where does the blood go?
Are there obstructions, fixed or dynamic?
Is there a risk of rhythm disturbance?
Is there pulmonary hypertension, fixed or reactive?
What is the ventricular function?
What comorbidities exist?

---

the underlying rhythm (hence the degree of pacemaker dependency) should be documented. Any doubt should lead to a consultation with the child's cardiologist.

This child should have his pacing function changed to a **DOO** or VOO mode (to obviate the effects of electrocautery), and routine practices should be adopted to minimize the potential for electrocautery interference. The surgeon should be encouraged to use bipolar rather than unipolar electrocautery. If unipolar cautery is used, the surgeon should apply short, low-energy bursts and the return plate should be placed as far from the heart as possible. The routine use of magnets to manipulate pacemaker function is no longer recommended.

Lastly, transcutaneous defibrillating adhesive pads should be placed before induction (in an anterior–posterior plane), and a defibrillator with pacing function should be connected in monitoring mode. Anticipate the required defibrillating and pacing doses and mark them down for quick reference in case of emergency.

3. What is the role of antibiotics in this case?

Debate rages about the utility of perioperative antibiotics, and recently the role of prophylactic antibiotics for the prevention of *endocarditis* as opposed to *wound infection* has been clarified. The surgeon may well request antibiotics in this case—a potentially contaminated cavity with an increased risk of perioperative infectious complications.

The recently published guidelines from the American Heart Association (which are similar to those from the United Kingdom and Australia) confirm the role of a single perioperative dose of **clindamycin 20 mg/kg** in a child with a penicillin allergy (Wilson et al., 2007). All anesthetists involved in the care of children with CHD should be aware of the latest guidelines for prevention of bacterial endocarditis.

SUMMARY

1. It is vital to understand the anatomy of the circulation and the child's functional status.
2. Review details of the original lesion, previous surgery, and results of recent investigations. From these anticipate residual complications and plan for their implications for anesthesia. If in doubt, contact the child's cardiologist.
3. Have a low threshold for invasive monitoring, and have appropriate inotropes, vasodilators, and pressors immediately on hand.

ANNOTATED REFERENCES

- Andropoulos DB, Stayer SA, Russell IA, Mossad EB, eds. *Anesthesia for Congenital Heart Disease*, 2nd ed. Chichester, West Sussex: Wiley-Blackwell, 2010.

  Brilliant update of a terrific textbook for anyone anesthetizing children with CHD. Highly recommended for pediatric cardiac anesthesiologists and fellows alike.

- Sümpelmann R, Osthaus WA. The pediatric cardiac patient presenting for noncardiac surgery. *Curr Opin Anaesthesiol* 2007; 20: 216–220.

  Wonderful review of each phase of the anesthetic for a child with CHD.

- White MC. Approach to managing children with heart disease for noncardiac surgery. *Pediatr Anesth* 2011; 21(5): 522–529.

  Timely, no-nonsense review of assessment and anesthetic techniques available, with frank discussion of the limitations of the evidence base. Emphasis on preoperative and operative phases and well worth a read.

Further Reading

Jonas R. Complete atrioventricular canal. In RA Jonas. *Comprehensive Surgical Management of Congenital Heart Disease*. London: Hodder-Arnold, 2004.

Lai WW, Mertens LL, Cohen MS, Geva T, eds. *Echocardiography in Pediatric and Congenital Heart Disease—From Fetus to Adult*. Chichester, West Sussex: Wiley-Blackwell, 2009.

Miller-Hance WC. Anesthesia for noncardiac surgery in children with congenital heart disease. In CJ Cote, J Lerman, ID Todres, eds. *A Practice of Anesthesia for Infants and Children*, 4th ed. Philadelphia: Saunders Elsevier, 2009.

Monagle P, Chalmers E, Chan A, DeVeber G, Kirkham F, Massicotte P, Michelson AD. Antithrombotic therapy in neonates and children: American College of Chest Physicians evidence-based clinical practice guidelines (8th ed). *Chest* 2008; 133(6 suppl): 887s–968s.

Practice advisory for the perioperative management of patients with cardiac rhythm management devices: pacemakers and implantable cardioverter-defibrillators: a report by the American Society of Anesthesiologists Task Force on Perioperative Management of Patients with Cardiac Rhythm Management Devices. *Anesthesiology* 2005; 103: 186–198.

Wilson W, Taubert KA, Gewitz M et al. Prevention of infective endocarditis: guidelines from the American Heart Association Rheumatic Fever, Endocarditis, and Kawasaki Disease Committee, Council Cardiovascular Disease in the Young, and the Council on Cardiovascular Surgery and Anesthesia, and Quality of Care and Outcomes Research Interdisciplinary Working Group. *Circulation* 2007; 116(15): 1736–1754.

31

Single Ventricle Physiology

IAN McKENZIE

INTRODUCTION

Congenital cardiac abnormalities in which there is functionally only a single ventricle are a heterogeneous group of conditions. These include patients with marked hypoplasia of one ventricle, usually with hypoplasia or atresia of the inflow of the ventricle, such as in hypoplastic left heart syndrome or conditions where surgical separation of the flow to each ventricle is not possible, such as double-inlet left ventricle. The most common pathway for palliating these conditions will be to use cavopulmonary connections to provide lung blood flow direct from systemic venous return (reliant on systemic venous pressure). The single ventricle pumps to the systemic arterial circulation. Many of these patients will be long-term survivors and present with acute surgical conditions unrelated to their cardiac condition. The safe anesthesia management of patients with single ventricle physiology and cavopulmonary connections involves assessing their cardiovascular reserve and understanding the effects of hypovolemia, anesthesia, positive-pressure ventilation, and the procedure itself on their circulation.

LEARNING OBJECTIVES

1. Understand circulations relying on cavopulmonary connections to provide lung blood flow.

2. Know how to assess the cardiovascular reserve of these patients, identifying risk factors for inadequate reserve.

3. Understand the importance of intravascular volume status and how to prevent and minimize the impact of anesthesia and positive-pressure ventilation.

4. Know that patients with good-quality Fontan palliation who have acute intercurrent illnesses are at significant risk of circulatory collapse at induction of anesthesia and commencement of positive-pressure ventilation.

5. Understand the significance of capnoperitoneum for laparoscopy in patients with Fontan circulation.

CASE PRESENTATION

*A 9-year-old boy weighing 24 kg has a surgical diagnosis of acute appendicitis and is booked for laparoscopic appendectomy. The child has been unwell for 3 days, with **nausea and vomiting for 48 hours** and fever for the past 24 hours. He has **urinated** only once today. The child was born with **hypoplastic left heart syndrome**, eventually palliated with a modified Fontan procedure. He has been attending a normal school and has been able to **participate in sporting activities** but is in the lower percentiles of his peers for exercise tolerance. He has **not been breathless with normal activities** and could walk up two flights of stairs without pausing. His usual pulse oximetry in the cardiology clinic has shown an SpO$_2$ of 95%, and his usual medications have been an angiotensin-converting enzyme inhibitor and aspirin. The surgical team commenced antibiotic treatment with metronidazole, amoxicillin, and gentamicin. A **bolus of 20 mL/kg of 0.9% NaCl** has been given intravenously followed by an infusion of 0.9% NaCl with 5% glucose at 70 mL/hr.*

*On examination his temperature is 38.9°C, **pulse rate is 135 bpm**, **blood pressure is 80/40 mmHg,** and his periphery is warm.*

The abdominal findings are of tenderness and rigidity. He is not cyanotic, with a current pulse oximetry demonstrating an SpO$_2$ of 95% breathing air. His neck veins do not appear distended. There are no cardiovascular murmurs.

DISCUSSION

1. What is the "Fontan pathway"?

This child was born with **hypoplastic left heart syndrome**. This includes very small mitral and aortic valves with associated small left ventricle and ascending and transverse aortic arch. This hypoplasia does not allow significant flow through the left side of the heart.

His first operation (modified Norwood stage 1) in the first week of life involved:

a) Patch reconstruction of the hypoplastic aorta and proximal pulmonary artery anastomosis, "end to side" with the aorta (Damus connection), which provides an unobstructed systemic arterial outflow from the ventricle

b) Atrial septectomy allowing unrestricted access for the pulmonary venous return from the left atrium to the right atrium and thus to the single, now systemic, right ventricle

c) Insertion of a synthetic shunt to provide lung blood flow by connecting the systemic arterial system (innominate artery) to the pulmonary arterial system (modified Blalock-Taussig shunt)

d) Ligation of patent ductus arteriosus (preoperatively the duct was kept open with prostaglandin E$_1$)

The second operation, at 4 months of age, was takedown of the modified Blalock-Taussig shunt and anastomosis of the superior vena cava, "end to side," with the upper surface of the right pulmonary artery ("bidirectional Glenn" cavopulmonary connection), to provide bilateral lung blood flow at low pressure and remove the volume loading of the heart created by the previous systemic arterial-to-pulmonary shunt (Fig. 31.1). This procedure is not done until several months of age because the relatively high venous pressure of the cavopulmonary connection is not tolerated by the newborn.

The third operation, at 4 years of age, was completion of the cavopulmonary connections (modified "Fontan" procedure) with an extracardiac conduit placed "end to side" from the inferior vena cava to the pulmonary artery. The completion of the cavopulmonary connections will allow virtually all systemic venous

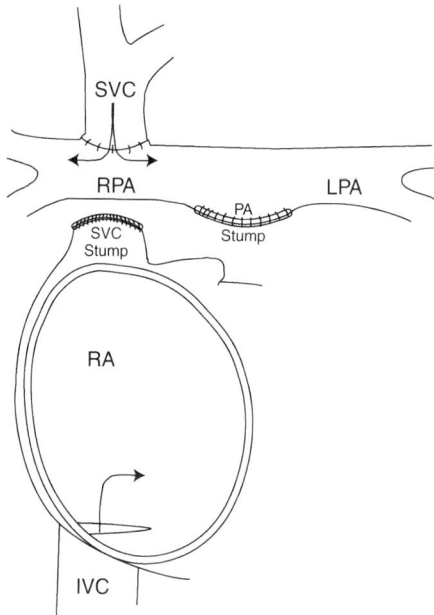

FIGURE 31.1 Cavopulmonary connection: "Bidirectional Glenn." RA. right atrium; SVC, superior vena cava; IVC, inferior vena cava; LPA, left pulmonary artery; RPA, right pulmonary artery; PA, pulmonary artery; ECC, extracardiac conduit.

return to pass through the lungs and be oxygenated, improving systemic arterial oxygenation (Fig. 31.2).

The extracardiac connection in this patient was constructed with a 4-mm fenestration (side-to-side orifice) between the conduit and the common atrium. In a 4-year-old with low pulmonary vascular resistance, the passive venous return of both inferior and superior cavae can usually pass through the pulmonary circuit driven by an acceptably low systemic venous pressure. The fenestration acts as a safety mechanism if resistance to flow through the lungs increases. The fenestration will allow deoxygenated blood to pass from the cavopulmonary circuit into the atrium without passage through the lungs. This will decrease systemic arterial oxygenation but allow maintenance of systemic output and prevent severe rises in systemic venous pressure.

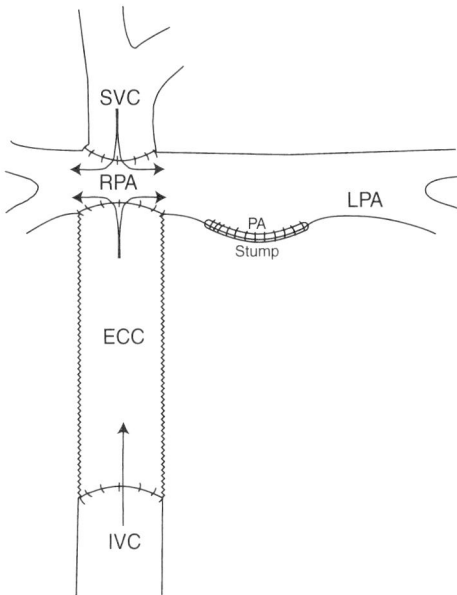

FIGURE 31.2 Complete cavopulmonary connection: "Extracardiac Fontan."

The hypoxia created is better tolerated than the alternative of low cardiac output and very high systemic venous pressure.

2. How can this patient's cardiovascular status be best assessed?

The patient's recent **exercise tolerance** remains the single most important evidence from the history for adequacy of the Fontan palliation and overall cardiovascular reserve. The loss of reserve relating to the current acute appendicitis and peritonitis is difficult to assess, but patients with Fontan circulation tolerate hypovolemia poorly. Evidence of hypovolemia and dehydration should be sought. The **fluid balance history**, **urine output** and concentration, capillary refill time, skin tissue turgor, **pulse rate**, and **blood pressure** may all contribute to this assessment. The jugular venous pulse will not show the usual flickering waves generated in the heart as the superior vena cava is connected to the pulmonary circuit. Venous pressure needs to be high in patients with Fontan circulation as it must provide not only adequate ventricular preload but also a pressure adequate to drive flow across the pulmonary vascular bed, an additional "transpulmonary gradient."

Echocardiography can contribute to the assessment in a number of ways. Adequacy of ventricular filling can be measured and used to assess the adequacy of preoperative resuscitation. Long-term, patients with a Fontan circulation may develop ventricular dysfunction, especially in diastole, often associated with ventricular hypertrophy. Although young for these complications, this patient should be carefully assessed for this potential loss of reserve. Poor myocardial function and atrioventricular valve dysfunction will both require higher atrial pressure for an adequate systemic output, exacerbating the need for the higher-than-normal systemic venous pressures that the Fontan circulation requires.

The status of the fenestration connecting the systemic venous circulation and the common atrium should be assessed. These connections may occlude with time. If present the fenestration may provide some "safety valve" effect should induction of anesthesia and the introduction of positive-pressure ventilation be poorly tolerated.

If there is evidence that the Fontan palliation is poor, such as poor exercise tolerance, low arterial hemoglobin oxygen saturation on pulse oximetry, signs of high venous pressure such as distended veins, peripheral edema, pleural or pericardial effusions or ascites, or protein-losing enteropathy, or evidence of poor myocardial function or atrioventricular valve dysfunction, the situation should be considered very high risk.

3. What is the impact of the acute appendicitis on this patient's circulation?

Hypovolemia is poorly tolerated by patients with a Fontan circulation. Acute appendicitis can cause significant hypovolemia from multiple mechanisms. Generalized sepsis may be associated with systemic vasodilation, decreased tissue oxygen utilization, increased pulmonary vascular resistance, and myocardial dysfunction, all of which will be poorly tolerated by a patient with Fontan circulation. **Tachycardia** may be associated with poor ventricular filling, especially if a patient with Fontan circulation has developed diastolic dysfunction with slow relaxation of the ventricle. Bradycardia may also be poorly tolerated if the ventricle has become noncompliant with hypertrophy. In patients with this complication of the Fontan circulation, the tachycardia associated with fever may worsen cardiac filling more than the potential benefit of increased rate on cardiac output.

4. What are risks of induction of anesthesia in this patient?

This patient will require endotracheal intubation with protection from the risk of aspiration of gastric contents and adequate surgical conditions for intra-abdominal surgery. The usual anesthesia concerns relating to a child with acute appendicitis requiring laparoscopic appendectomy need to be considered in the management of this patient. These issues include adequate resuscitation, prevention of aspiration, and management of the consequences of the surgical capnoperitoneum (such as decreased venous return, diaphragmatic splinting affecting ventilation, and systemic carbon dioxide absorption).

The most significant risk specific to this patient's acute condition combined with Fontan physiology is acute cardiovascular collapse at induction of anesthesia. Loss of reserve due to the factors described above, especially **hypovolemia, should be remedied** where possible before induction. Anesthesia induction agents can further decrease reserve by directly inhibiting myocardial function, by vasodilation, and by decreasing sympathetic drive. Conversion to positive-pressure ventilation is an especially high-risk transition for patients with Fontan circulation, especially with an intercurrent acute illness. Spontaneous ventilation creates intermittent negative intrathoracic pressure assisting venous return. Loss of this assistance and the use of positive-pressure ventilation profoundly impedes the passive venous return that provides pulmonary flow in patients with Fontan anatomy. Inadequate intravascular volume combined with positive intrathoracic pressure in a Fontan patient can lead to catastrophic circulatory collapse due to inadequate filling of the ventricle. Table 31.1 summarizes prevention of cardiovascular collapse under anesthesia.

Table 31.1

TECHNIQUES TO MINIMIZE THE RISK OF CIRCULATORY COLLAPSE

1. Generous intravenous fluid resuscitation to more than "normal" filling of the heart
2. Slow titration of anesthesia agents to minimize excessive peak depressant effects
3. Care to minimize the circulatory effects of positive-pressure ventilation
4. Intensive monitoring of the circulation throughout the sequence

5. **What is an effective approach to intraoperative ventilation in these patients?**

When positive-pressure ventilation is unavoidable, it is important to understand that the emphasis needs to be on maximizing the expiratory time and minimizing expiratory pressure. Minimizing inspiratory pressure is usually NOT helpful, as moderate inspiratory pressure will usually be greater than the pulmonary capillary intravascular pressure so that flow in the capillaries will be stopped by modest inspiratory pressures. Higher pressures will not stop the flow more (like a Starling resistor) and flow will therefore not be reduced further by higher pressures. Higher inspiratory pressures can still increase ventilation, and these units will be perfused during the expiratory phase. Thus, providing low-frequency, high-pressure inflations with long expiratory time and minimal expiratory pressure (a low level of positive pressure in expiration may be needed to prevent atelectasis) is often the best strategy to minimize cardiovascular complications if positive-pressure ventilation is required in this scenario.

6. **What are the implications of changes in pulmonary vascular resistance intraoperatively?**

For successful palliation using cavopulmonary connections to provide lung blood flow, pulmonary vascular resistance must be low. If a patient with Fontan circulation is well, with good exercise tolerance, his or her pulmonary vascular resistance must be low. If a patient has good exercise tolerance and long-term stable Fontan palliation, it would not be expected that the pulmonary vascular system would be especially reactive. This is in contrast to conditions associated with pulmonary hypertension with pulmonary arteriolar changes such as medial muscular hypertrophy, which can create dramatic changes in pulmonary vascular resistance in response to stimuli such as hypoxia or hypercarbia. Even though the vasculature is not especially reactive, care should be taken to prevent any increases in pulmonary vascular resistance in patients with Fontan circulation. Small changes in pulmonary vascular resistance can have significant effects on the circulation.

For the Fontan patient, a rise in pulmonary vascular resistance will be associated with a decrease in cardiac output, an increase in systemic venous pressure, or both. Given that pulmonary vascular resistance is low, even a modest change in resistance may be a proportionally large change and would thus be associated with quite marked changes in cardiac output or systemic venous pressure.

In circumstances where pulmonary vascular resistance is expected to rise (such as conversion to positive-pressure ventilation, or rises with carbon dioxide with spontaneous ventilation under anesthesia), then the circulation should be carefully monitored and the changes responded to, with the aim of maintaining cardiac output with measures designed to decrease pulmonary vascular resistance or increase systemic venous pressure. Laparoscopic surgery may profoundly reduce cardiac output in a patient with Fontan circulation. The associated capnoperitoneum increases the ventilation requirement due to restricted diaphragmatic motion and carbon dioxide absorption. The increased ventilation requirement and any increases in $PaCO_2$ can increase pulmonary vascular resistance and, combined with diminished inferior vena caval return, may jeopardize cardiac output.

There is some scope for increasing cardiac output by improving myocardial function, but this is a less direct approach if poor myocardial function is not the core problem. Improved myocardial function can decrease the preload required, thus decreasing atrial pressure, providing a greater transpulmonary gradient to drive lung blood flow (i.e., cardiac output) for the same systemic venous pressure.

Careful monitoring of the blood pressure and rapid access to cardiovascular resuscitation drugs such as inotropes and vasoconstrictors are important for this patient's management.

SUMMARY

1. **Apparently healthy patients with Fontan palliation with acute conditions such as appendicitis are at**

significant risk of circulatory collapse with induction of anesthesia and commencement of positive-pressure ventilation.

2. Preoperative assessment should include quality of prior cardiac palliation, the effect of the acute condition, and the adequacy of resuscitation.
3. Preoperative resuscitation to adequate systemic venous pressures (and cardiac filling) is vital but difficult to assess in a patient with Fontan circulation.
4. Care must be taken to avoid increases in pulmonary vascular resistance.
5. If positive-pressure ventilation is required, peak inspiratory pressure is usually not a crucial factor. Optimizing expiratory duration and low expiratory pressure is most important for maintaining the circulation in a patient relying on cavopulmonary connections for lung blood flow.
6. The capnoperitoneum associated with laparoscopic techniques may have major circulatory effects in patients with a Fontan circulation.

ANNOTATED REFERENCES

- Leyvi G, Wasnick JD. Single-ventricle patient: pathophysiology and anesthetic management. *J Cardiothor Vascular Anesth* 2010: 24(1): 121–130.

  An excellent up-to-date description of the anatomy and pathophysiology.
- McLain CD, McGowan FX, Kovatsis PG. Laparoscopic surgery in a patient with Fontan physiology. *Anesth Analg* 2006; 103(4): 856–858.

  An excellent summary of the issues.

32

Tetralogy of Fallot

RENEE NIERMAN KREEGER AND
JAMES P. SPAETH

INTRODUCTION

Patients with congenital heart disease are frequently encountered by the pediatric anesthesiologist for non-cardiac surgery. Fortunately, the majority of these patients have already undergone definitive repair of their cardiac lesions and can often be managed using traditional anesthetic methods. However, given the known association of congenital heart disease with other congenital malformations and syndromes, there is a relatively high likelihood that a pediatric anesthesiologist will encounter a situation involving a child with an unrepaired lesion. With the reported increased mortality rate for patients with complex cardiac lesions undergoing non-cardiac procedures (see Chapter 30), an understanding of the pathophysiology and anatomy, as well as the potential effects of the anesthetic medications and techniques chosen, is paramount to their successful care.

LEARNING OBJECTIVES

1. Identify the key physiologic and anatomic derangements present in patients with tetralogy of Fallot (TOF).
2. Devise a method for systematic evaluation of a cardiac patient's preoperative status to allow for optimal planning of intraoperative and postoperative care.
3. Understand anesthetic management principles in patients with TOF.

CASE PRESENTATION

*A 3-month-old boy presents to the emergency department with bilious emesis. The surgical team diagnoses possible malrotation, necessitating urgent surgical intervention. Preoperative anesthetic evaluation reveals a past medical history significant for unrepaired **TOF** and for no prior anesthetics. An emergent echocardiogram demonstrates a gradient across the right ventricular outflow tract (RVOT) of 80 mmHg, an increase over a previous gradient of 40 mmHg. On physical examination, the patient has a distended abdomen and appears slightly cyanotic, with an oxygen saturation of 73% on room air. He was previously being managed at home with a baseline oxygen saturation level of 88% and no history of **hypercyanotic ("Tet") spells**. He is otherwise healthy and has a non-contributory family history.*

*IV access is obtained by the ED staff and preoperative **fluid resuscitation** with 20 mL/kg of crystalloid is initiated. Laboratory tests, including a complete blood count and type and cross, are sent. Following completion of the fluid bolus and review of laboratory results, the patient is brought to the operating room. After standard monitors are placed and the patient is preoxygenated, a rapid-sequence induction with cricoid pressure is performed with 10 mcg/kg of fentanyl and 2 mg/kg of succinylcholine (suxamethonium). Surgery begins and is proceeding without incident when the oxygen saturation suddenly decreases to 65% and the patient becomes hypotensive. Manual ventilation with **100% oxygen is initiated** and a **fluid bolus** is given with minimal improvement. A single dose of IV **phenylephrine** provides prompt return of vital signs to baseline levels. The surgeon reveals that he had inadvertently **compressed** the **inferior vena cava** (IVC) while trying to improve visualization. The remainder of the procedure is uneventful, and the patient is taken to the cardiac intensive care unit for postoperative care.*

DISCUSSION

1. What is TOF?

TOF, first described in 1888, is the most common type of cyanotic heart disease, representing approximately 10% of all congenital heart defects. It is often of unknown etiology, although it is associated with DiGeorge syndrome (chromosome 22q11 deletion) approximately 16% of the time and has been associated with other congenital syndromes such as velocardiofacial syndrome. It is classically described as a group of malformations involving a large, unrestrictive ventricular septal defect (VSD), right ventricular outflow tract (RVOT) obstruction/infundibular stenosis, overriding of the aorta above the RVOT, and right ventricular hypertrophy (RVH). TOF occurs as a result of an abnormality in cardiac embryology involving anteriocranial deviation of the conal septum. The spectrum of disease is wide, encouraging the use of the differentiating clinical terms, "pink Tets" and "blue Tets," to provide a quick means of separating those with clinically less significant disease from those with severe disease. The group known as "pink Tets" have few if any **hypercyanotic episodes ("Tet" spells)** and are generally clinically stable, often being managed at home. Those labeled "blue Tets" often have frequent, severe spells, indicative of more severe disease. These children typically require surgical intervention early in life.

2. What are "Tet" spells?

"Tet" spells are the clinical manifestation of **hypercyanotic episodes** experienced by patients with TOF. These episodes represent an increase in right-to-left cardiac shunting as a result of an imbalance between systemic vascular resistance (SVR) and the resistance to blood flow through the RVOT and into the lungs. A fall in preload brought about by hypovolemia, for example, and/or an increase in the resistance to blood flow to the lungs such as with infundibular spasm are possible causes of these events. They can be spontaneous but are often precipitated by crying, agitation, feeding and pain, and represent an acute increase in catecholamines and cardiac contractility, producing a dynamic infundibular obstruction. If left untreated, they can be fatal in the most severe cases. Older patients will attempt to reverse these episodes by squatting, leading to an increase in SVR, preload, and pulmonary blood flow. Patients with TOF are particularly vulnerable to spells during the induction of anesthesia and during periods of light anesthesia. A treatment algorithm is shown in Fig. 32.1.

3. What drugs and maneuvers can be used in the event of an intraoperative "Tet" spell?

One may mimic a squatting maneuver in a patient by placing the patient in a knee–chest position and/or applying direct pressure to the abdomen. Once IV access is established, **administration of volume** is a first-line intervention to support blood pressure, increase preload, and reduce the RVOT obstruction. If surgery has begun, it is important to ensure that surgical manipulation is not causing an acute reduction in systemic venous return (e.g., **IVC compression** during laparotomy or abdominal insufflation during laparoscopy). **Increasing the FiO$_2$ to 1.0** may help reduce PVR, but pulmonary hypertension is rarely the cause of hypercyanotic spells in patients with TOF. If these maneuvers do not lead to an improvement in arterial oxygen saturation, **phenylephrine** given in IV doses of 0.5 to 3 mcg/kg is useful to increase SVR acutely. The resultant bradycardia is helpful as tachycardia only further contributes to the spell. Increasing anesthetic depth may also help if light anesthesia is thought to be a contributing factor. IV beta-blockade with esmolol will reduce infundibular spasm and has been used effectively to treat hypercyanotic spells. Last-resort rescue maneuvers include surgical opening of the chest with direct aortic compression and extracorporeal membrane oxygenation (ECMO).

4. What should a preoperative evaluation entail for a patient with TOF?

Whenever possible, patients with unrepaired TOF undergoing anesthesia should have an anesthesia consultation initiated well in advance of the procedure to ensure adequate time for optimization of the patient if necessary. The basic pre-anesthetic evaluation should be expanded to include questions that focus on the child's *cardiac history*, including feeding tolerance, frequency of

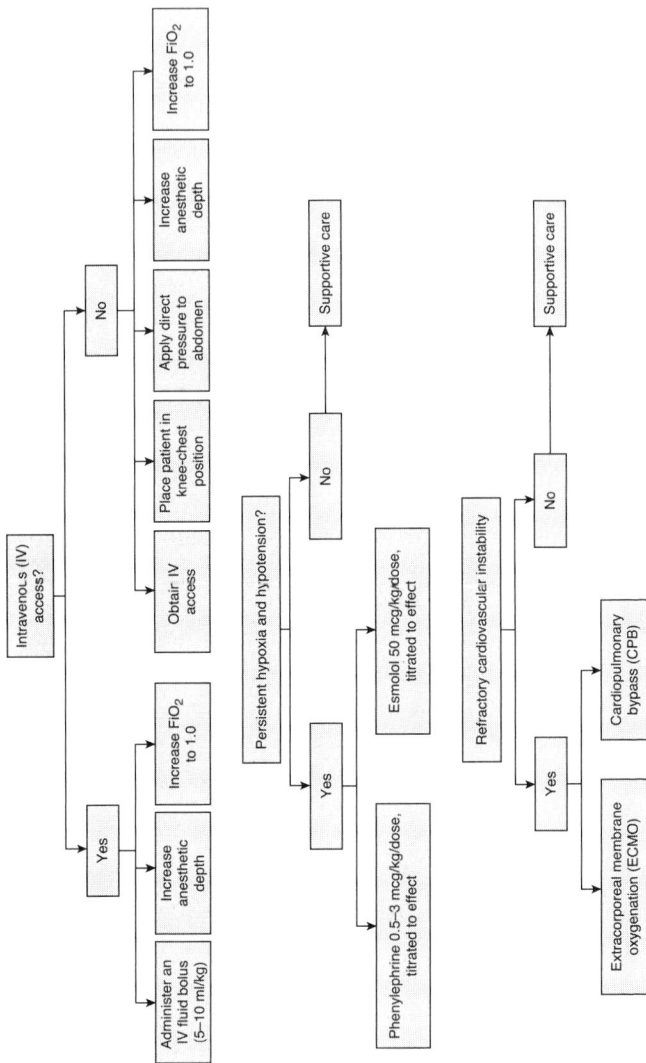

FIGURE 32.1 Treatment of "Tet" spells.

and precipitating factors for **"Tet" spells,** baseline *oxygen satura-tion*, and *medications*. Review of the most recent cardiology evalu-ation, including *echocardiography, electrocardiogram* (ECG), and *cardiac catheterization*, and any *previous surgical intervention* is imperative. The need for infective *endocarditis prophylaxis* should be considered. When possible, the anesthesiologist should com-municate directly with the cardiologist to facilitate care. One should also look for associated *congenital syndromes*, as many patients with TOF have other congenital abnormalities that may complicate the anesthetic or compromise the airway. A hemoglo-bin and hematocrit may be helpful, as well as any other labora-tory studies specific to a patient's particular syndrome if present. In addition, the anesthesiologist should discuss the case with the surgeon, including any concerns with his or her preferred tech-nique, as well as a rescue plan should the need arise. The patient should follow American Society of Anesthesiologists (ASA) guide-lines for preoperative NPO status. The ingestion of clear liquids up to 2 hours before surgery is helpful in preventing dehydration and maintaining preload, which is especially important for patients with TOF.

5. What is the best anesthetic method to use for these patients?

While there is no one right way to anesthetize these patients, it is important that the anesthesia team follow some general principles. Avoidance of known triggers of "Tet" spells such as *hypovolemia* and *abrupt changes in SVR* is of paramount impor-tance. Ideally, a child would come to the operating room with a working peripheral IV catheter in place following IV hydration the night prior to surgery, allowing for a slow, controlled IV induction that maintains the patient's baseline blood pressure. An inhalation induction with carefully titrated sevoflurane can also be done safely in an elective setting. Emergency cases, how-ever, often require the use of a rapid-sequence induction to reduce aspiration risk. In these patients, it is essential that the patients receive **fluid resuscitation preoperatively** to avoid significant hypotension and desaturation that can result from decreased preload on induction. In addition to the typical pediatric emergency drugs, the anesthesiologist should have unit-dose **phenylephrine** and esmolol immediately available, as well as adequate **volume replacement** in the form of crystalloid or colloid for resuscitation. Opioids may be given in divided doses and carefully titrated to effect for pain control. Regional techniques may be preferable for pain management if the child's anatomy and coagulation status permit, thereby avoiding possible opioid side effects. When instituting epidural anesthesia, it is worth slowly dosing the local anesthetic, titrating it against blood pressure, to avoid sudden drops in SVR. Preloading with crystalloid prior to dosing an epidural may be helpful as well. Postoperatively, the patient should be cared for in either the intensive care unit or by an experienced cardiac medical team under careful surveillance. This decision should be a multidisciplinary one with consideration of the patient's preoperative physical status, intraoperative tolerance of anesthesia and surgery, and extent of surgical intervention.

SUMMARY

1. The preoperative evaluation should comprise a basic anesthesia preoperative evaluation with particular attention to cardiac history and current physical status; a thorough review of cardiology data, including echocardiography, ECG, cardiac catheterization, and previous surgical intervention; and review of other congenital anomalies or syndromes.
2. "Tet" spell triggers are as follows—physical: crying, agitation, feeding, pain; physiologic: hypovolemia, decreased SVR.
3. Treatments for "Tet" spells include removal of trigger, volume resuscitation, FiO_2 1.0, phenylephrine,

esmolol, deepening anesthetic, knee–chest position, abdominal compression, direct aortic compression, and ECMO.

ANNOTATED REFERENCES

- Hennein HA, Mendeloff EN, Cilley RE, Bove EL, Coran AG. Predictors of postoperative outcome after general surgical procedures in patients with congenital heart disease. *J Pediatr Surg* 1994; 29: 866–870.

This article demonstrates the fragile state of patients with congenital heart disease and underlines the importance of careful evaluation and perioperative care to avoid further increasing morbidity and mortality, especially in children with complex lesions like TOF.

- Litman RS. Anesthetic considerations for children with congenital heart disease undergoing noncardiac surgery: answers to common questions. *Anesth Clin North Am* 1997; 15(1): 93–103.

This reference provides a good general overview of the important principles to consider when anesthetizing a child with congenital heart disease outside of the cardiac operating room.

- Schmitz ML, Ullah S.Anesthesia for right-sided obstructive lesions. In Andropoulos DB, Stayer, SA Russell LA, Mossad EB, eds. *Anesthesia for Congenital Heart Disease,* 2nd ed. Chichester, West Sussex: Wiley-Blackwell, 2010: 419–443.

As the most recent book chapter on the subject of anesthesia for lesions such as TOF, this offers a good review of the literature with excellent clinical information.

Further Reading

Lell WA, Pearce FB. Tetralogy of Fallot. In Lake CL, Booker PD, eds. *Pediatric Cardiac Anesthesia*, 4th ed. Philadelphia: Lippincott Williams & Wilkins, 2005: 344–356.

Levine MF, Hartley EJ, Macpherson BA, Burrows FA, Lerman J. Oral midazolam for children with congenital cyanotic heart disease undergoing cardiac surgery: A comparative study. *Can J Anaesth* 1993; 40: 934–938.

Nicolson SC, Dorsey AT, Schreiner MS: Shortened preanesthetic fasting interval in pediatric cardiac surgical patients. *Anesth Analg* 1992; 74: 694–697.

Prevention of infective endocarditis: Guidelines from the American Heart Association: A Guideline from the American Heart Association Rheumatic Fever, Endocarditis, and Kawasaki Disease Committee, Council on Cardiovascular Disease in the Young, and the Council on Clinical Cardiology, Council on Cardiovascular Surgery and Anesthesia, and the Quality of Care and Outcomes Research Interdisciplinary Working Group. *Circulation* 2007; 116: 1736–1754.

33

Cardiac Catheterization

ERICA P. LIN AND ANDREAS W. LOEPKE

INTRODUCTION

As the management of congenital heart disease evolves, the use of cardiac catheterization, both as a diagnostic and therapeutic tool, has significantly increased. Increasingly complex interventions are being performed on younger and sicker children. Therefore, anesthesia providers in the cardiac catheterization laboratory must have a good understanding of each patient's underlying cardiac physiology, the implications of the anesthetic technique on this physiology, as well as the inherent risks and potential complications of the procedure to be performed.

LEARNING OBJECTIVES

1. Be familiar with the limitations of the cardiac catheterization lab and the risk of radiation exposure.
2. Understand the general goals for cardiac catheterization and the implications of the anesthetic technique.
3. Appreciate the commonly encountered complications in this setting.

CASE PRESENTATION

A 14-month-old, 8.5-kg girl with **hypoplastic left heart syndrome (HLHS)** *presents for cardiac catheterization to evaluate her frequent* *cyanotic spells and poor growth. The patient was born at 35 weeks' gestation with an antenatal diagnosis of HLHS. As a neonate, she underwent a "**hybrid procedure**." At 5 months of age, she underwent a comprehensive stage II procedure that included aortic arch reconstruction, removal of a pulmonary artery band placed soon after birth, and creation of a bidirectional superior cavopulmonary anastomosis (bidirectional Glenn shunt). Her medications include aspirin, furosemide, and enalapril. Her most recent echocardiogram showed no neo-aortic stenosis or insufficiency, a patent bidirectional Glenn shunt, questionable narrowing of distal branch pulmonary arteries (right > left), and low-normal right ventricular function. Baseline hemoglobin is 16.8 g/dL. During an attempt to examine her, she becomes agitated and notably cyanotic. Oxygen saturation at this time drops from a baseline in the mid-70s to the 50s, and supplemental oxygen via nasal cannula is provided. **Oral midazolam** is administered prior to beginning the procedure.*

*In the catheterization laboratory, noninvasive monitors are placed and the patient tolerates an inhalational induction with sevoflurane in oxygen. A peripheral 22g cannula is inserted with some difficulty due to multiple previous attempts. A nondepolarizing muscle relaxant is given to facilitate **tracheal intubation**, and general anesthesia is maintained with sevoflurane, fentanyl, and vecuronium. Body temperature is maintained with a forced-air warmer. Hemodynamic data, obtained while the patient is normoventilated on room air, demonstrate moderate **pulmonary hypertension** with a mean pulmonary artery pressure of 45 mmHg (~60% systemic). Pulmonary angiography reveals several stenotic areas in the peripheral pulmonary arteries. Heparin is administered and the interventional cardiologist dilates the stenotic lesions with repeated balloon angioplasties. During the intervention, the patient experiences transient worsening of **hypoxemia** (SpO_2 decreases from 78% to 45%) and **hemodynamic instability** (SBP decreasing from 75 mmHg to 30 mmHg); they improve with removal of the catheter from the pulmonary artery. After hemostasis is obtained at the catheter sites, the* *patient is extubated awake and is transported to the post-anesthesia care unit, where she recovers uneventfully.*

DISCUSSION

1. What are some of the challenges for the anesthesiologist working in the cardiac catheterization laboratory environment?

Catheterization laboratories are often located in remote areas of the hospital, away from the main operating room suite. Furthermore, appropriate recovery facilities may be some distance away, as catheterization laboratories have historically not been designed with anesthesiologists' input. It is imperative that monitoring, oxygen supply, resuscitation equipment and drugs, as well as sufficient personnel be available both during the procedure and also for transport to the recovery area.

Regardless of the physical dimensions of the room, functional space is often limited, with bulky fluoroscopy equipment hindering access to the patient and the airway. Subdued lighting, while necessary for the cardiologist, further impairs the anesthesiologist's ability to visually monitor the patient. Intravenous lines, monitor cables, and breathing circuits often require additional length to reach the patient and must be secured in an organized fashion so as not to be snared by the frequent movement of the procedure table and fluoroscopy arms.

Effective communication among all team members is of the utmost importance to ensure situational awareness of both the progression of the procedure and the hemodynamic state of the patient. When anesthesiologists are working as the sole anesthesia provider in these remote locations, the value of skilled personnel to provide support (assistance with venous access, airway management, and equipment) cannot be underestimated, especially in crisis situations. Serious complications can occur during the procedure, which may necessitate the rapid preparation and administration of potent medications, such as bronchodilators, antiarrhythmic drugs, vasopressors, and inotropes.

2. What is the radiation exposure risk for patients and personnel associated with the catheterization laboratory?

Young children undergoing pediatric cardiac catheterization are potentially at greater risk for radiation-induced injuries compared with older patients because their tissues are more radiosensitive and, given their longer lifespan, they may be more likely to develop subsequent sequelae from radiation exposure. Moreover, reduced body size, smaller cardiovascular structures, and complicated anatomic variations may necessitate lengthy, involved procedures that may result in the higher average radiation dose observed in newborns compared with older patients (Rassow et al., 2000). The repeated catheterization sessions commonly performed in children with complex cardiac lesions can therefore lead to considerable cumulative exposures.

During cardiac catheterization, personnel are also inevitably subject to higher levels of radiation exposure compared with other medical specialties (Venneri et al., 2009). Dosimeters should be worn to track cumulative radiation exposure, and since there is no "safe dose" of radiation, every effort should be made to minimize occupational exposure. The goal of the ALARA principle (<u>a</u>s <u>l</u>ow <u>a</u>s <u>r</u>easonably <u>a</u>chievable), as advocated by the Centers for Disease Control and Prevention, is to provide the maximal diagnostic and/or therapeutic benefit while using the lowest possible radiation dose during diagnostic procedures involving ionizing radiation (Justino, 2006). To reduce radiation exposure, anesthesiologists should strictly adhere to *three radiation safety principles:* (1) *Maximize the distance* from the radiation source, as radiation dose varies with the inverse square of that distance (i.e., doubling the distance results in a four-fold dose reduction); (2) *Minimize exposure time;* and (3) Always use *proper shielding* (e.g., lead aprons, thyroid collars, acrylic shield, and protective eyeglasses).

3. Should every child undergoing a pediatric cardiac catheterization receive a general anesthetic?

Wide variations exist in the use of general anesthesia in the pediatric cardiac catheterization lab, ranging from 28% to 99% of cases among sites in a recent multicenter survey (Bergersen et al., 2010). Since pediatric cardiac catheterizations can be complicated and lengthy procedures, most children, especially younger ones, require sedation or anesthesia. The decision to use local anesthesia in combination with sedation versus general anesthesia should be determined in relation to the individual patient and the invasiveness of the intended procedure. Regardless of which modality is used, there should be a dedicated practitioner, not involved in the cardiac catheterization itself, managing the patient's sedation or anesthesia. The skill set required includes the ability to manage the continuum from sedation to general anesthesia, to understand the cardiac pathophysiology, to securely manage the airway, and to prevent, recognize, and treat complications related to both the procedure and the anesthesia/sedation. Pediatric cardiac anesthesiologists are specifically trained in this unique skill set; as the complexity of patients and interventions steadily increases, so will the demand for the participation of pediatric cardiac anesthesiologists in cardiac catheterization procedures (Andropoulos & Stayer, 2003).

4. How does one match the anesthetic technique and the procedural goals?

The ultimate goal of a safe cardiac catheterization procedure is to acquire accurate hemodynamic information and to provide therapeutic intervention while maintaining hemodynamic stability and patient comfort. For diagnostic studies, measurements are usually taken with the patient breathing 21% oxygen, while the pH and partial pressure of carbon dioxide are maintained at preoperative levels. Unfortunately, there is no single technique that guarantees this; the choice of anesthetic agent and airway management may considerably affect these variables. For instance, while spontaneous breathing may promote venous return, it risks hypoventilation, hypercarbia, and airway obstruction. On the other hand, **tracheal intubation** and positive-pressure ventilation may decrease venous return, cardiac output, and hemodynamic stability, while providing a secure airway.

Each patient with congenital heart disease has a unique physiologic state, so a thorough preoperative assessment should review current symptoms, previous interventions, and repairs/palliations to determine the safest anesthetic technique. Anxious patients may benefit from **preoperative sedation.** The choice of sedative and anesthetic medications will depend on the patient's hemodynamic status and cardiac reserve. Inhalational and intravenous agents are commonly combined to minimize adverse effects.

5. What are some of the potential complications of cardiac catheterization?

Adverse events occur more commonly during pediatric cardiac catheterization than during pediatric anesthesia in general (Bennett et al., 2005). Overall, there is a higher complication rate among interventional cases compared to diagnostic procedures or myocardial biopsies. Risk factors for complications include lower patient age or size, and interventions other than occlusion of patent ductus arteriosus or atrial septal defects. Severe **pulmonary hypertension**, not infrequently encountered in the cardiac catheterization laboratory, dramatically increases the risk of morbidity and mortality (Carmosino et al., 2007).

Arrhythmias frequently occur during cardiac catheterization examinations and are usually transient. The vast majority result from mechanical stimulation by the intracardiac catheters and respond to cessation of catheter manipulation and correction of any contributing metabolic or electrolyte abnormalities. Nevertheless, pacing capabilities and equipment for defibrillation must be immediately available for treatment of more persistent, potentially fatal dysrhythmias.

The introduction of intraluminal catheters may cause obstruction of blood vessels, impediment of cardiac chambers, or distortion of cardiac valves, thereby potentially reducing pulmonary or systemic blood flow and/or cardiac output, resulting in **hypotension, oxygen desaturation**, or both. These issues are more prominent in smaller patients, as exemplified by the case scenario. Other catheter-related complications include vascular damage and bleeding at the access sites, vascular thrombosis, air

Table 33.1
PROCEDURES CONDUCTED IN THE CARDIAC CATHETERIZATION LABORATORY

Procedure	Purpose and Comment
Endocardial biopsy	Surveillance, assessment for rejection after cardiac transplant Diagnosis of myocarditis and cardiomyopathy
Valvotomy	Balloon dilation of stenotic aortic, pulmonary, mitral, or bioprosthetic valves
Angioplasty	Treatment of stenosis in native blood vessels (aorta, pulmonary artery) and surgical conduits
Endovascular stents	Applied to pulmonary artery stenosis, systemic venous stenosis, aortic coarctation
Closure of shunts	Patent ductus arteriosus, aortopulmonary collaterals, coronary artery fistulas, arteriovenous malformations: helical wire coils Atrial septal defect, ventricular septal defect: umbrella device comprising two discs
Electrophysiology study and ablation	Delineate mechanism of arrhythmia and destroy abnormal pathways and automatic foci, most commonly with radiofrequency energy and cryotherapy
Implantation of pacemakers and defibrillators	Placement of transvenous leads with tunneling to a subcutaneous pocket

embolus, catheter fragment embolus, valvular incompetence, bleeding, pericardial effusion, cardiac tamponade, and perforation or rupture of vessels of the heart. Cross-matched blood products should therefore be available during all complex interventions.

6. What are some of the emerging interventions performed in the catheterization laboratory?

By definition, **hybrid procedures** are a combination of open surgical and interventional catheterization procedures. Many institutions are setting up their catheterization laboratories to carry out both interventional as well as sterile, surgical procedures (Table 33.1). Emerging techniques to perform minimally invasive neonatal palliation for **hypoplastic left ventricle syndrome (HLHS)** in the cardiac catheterization laboratory, for example, include the placement of bilateral pulmonary artery bands via median sternotomy and stenting of the ductus arteriosus via a transcatheter approach through the right ventricular outflow tract (Galantowicz et al., 2008). The appeal of this hybrid procedure includes the avoidance of cardiopulmonary bypass and a lengthy surgical procedure during the neonatal period as well as the reduction in exposure to blood products and sensitization in children whose treatment path may eventually culminate in cardiac transplantation. With continued experience and availability of newer devices, this hybrid approach may expand to other cardiac lesions.

SUMMARY

1. Preparation, clear communication, and situational awareness in the remote environment of the cardiac catheterization lab are essential.
2. Radiation exposure must be minimized for both the patient and providers.

3. The anesthesia team must be prepared to recognize and immediately treat serious complications related to cardiac catheterization, including arrhythmias, hypotension, hypoxia, and bleeding.
4. Complex therapeutic cardiac catheterization procedures will increasingly replace open surgical procedures in younger, smaller, and higher-risk patients.

ANNOTATED REFERENCES

- Arnold PD, Holtby HM, Andropoulos DB. 2010. Anesthesia for the cardiac catheterization laboratory. In Andropoulos D, Stayer S, Russell I, Mossad E, eds. *Anesthesia for Congenital Heart Disease,* 2nd ed. Chichester, West Sussex, UK: Blackwell Publishing, 521–545.

  A thorough overview of anesthetic considerations in the cardiac catheterization laboratory. Sections are organized based on type of procedure (i.e., diagnostic, endocardial biopsy, interventional, electrophysiologic).
- Bergersen L, Marshall A, Gauvreau K, et al. Adverse event rates in congenital cardiac catheterization—a multi-center experience. *Catheter Cardiovasc Interv* 2010; 75: 389–400.

  This article highlights adverse event rates in congenital cardiac catheterization laboratories at six different institutions. Events are presented by case type (diagnostic vs. interventional vs. biopsy) and classified by severity level. Interventional procedures have a significantly higher incidence of adverse events.
- Justino H. The ALARA concept in pediatric cardiac catheterization: techniques and tactics for managing radiation dose. *Pediatr Radiol* 2006; 36: 146–153.

  This article provides a list of strategies to improve radiation safety in the pediatric cardiac catheterization lab.

Further Reading

Andropoulos DB, Stayer SA. An anesthesiologist for all pediatric cardiac catheterizations: luxury or necessity? *J Cardiothor Vasc Anesth* 2003; 17: 683–685.

Bennett D, Marcus R, Stokes M. Incidents and complications during pediatric cardiac catheterization. *Pediatr Anesth* 2005; 15: 1093–1088.

Carmosino MJ, Friesen RH, Doran A, Ivy DD. Perioperative complications in children with pulmonary hypertension undergoing noncardiac surgery or cardiac catheterization. *Anesth Analg* 2007; 104: 521–527.

Galantowicz M, Cheatham JP, Phillips A, et al. Hybrid approach for hypoplastic left heart syndrome. *Ann Thorac Surg* 2008; 85: 2063–2071.

Rassow J, Schmaltz AA, Hentrich F, Streffer C. Effective doses to patients from paediatric cardiac catheterization. *Br J Rad* 2000; 73: 172–183.

Reddy K, Jaggar S, Gillbe C. The anaesthetist and the cardiac catheterization laboratory. *Anaesthesia* 2006; 61: 1175–1186.

Venneri L, Rossi F, Botto N, et al. Cancer risk from professional exposure in staff working in cardiac catheterization laboratory: insights from the National Research Council's Biological Effects of Ionizing Radiation VII Report. *Am Heart J* 2009; 157: 118–124.

34

Cardiac MRI

NICHOLAS MARTIN

INTRODUCTION

Magnetic resonance imaging (MRI) is an important tool for investigating congenital cardiac conditions. It provides excellent images of the cardiac anatomy and is unrivalled in its ability to illuminate the pulmonary vessels. Conservation of femoral vessels and absence of ionizing radiation gives it an advantage over cardiac catheterization. Apart from the challenges of anesthetizing a child with an uncorrected congenital heart condition, the MRI environment presents some unique challenges to the anesthesiologist. It is usually remote from the main operating suite, and the permanent strong magnetic field requires specialized equipment and precautions.

LEARNING OBJECTIVES

1. Understand the key issues involved in working within the magnetic field.
2. Know how to plan for cardiac MRI procedures.

CASE PRESENTATION

A 4-month-old boy with the diagnosis of hypoplastic left heart syndrome had a Norwood procedure (reconstruction of the hypoplastic aorta and creation of systemic-to-pulmonary shunt) on day 2 of life.

He is booked for cavopulmonary shunt surgery next week and needs an MRI to define the extracardiac thoracic vasculature, particularly the size and shape of the pulmonary arteries.

He last had a bottle of formula feed at 0930 in anticipation of a 1330 start. He is breathing room air with a SpO$_2$ of 75%. The breathing pattern is comfortable at a rate of 40. He is 5 kg. The parents state that he feeds well. Prior to anesthesia the child is checked for metal objects.

Anesthesia is induced in a room adjacent to the scanner outside the **5 Gauss line**, thus allowing the use of standard anesthetic equipment. Electrocardiograph (ECG) monitoring wires and a pulse oximeter probe are applied and a gradual inhalation induction is performed using sevoflurane and oxygen. Once the anesthesia is deep enough, an intravenous cannula is placed in the left saphenous vein and the patient is given 2 mg of atracurium and 50 mL of warmed crystalloid. The patient is intubated with a 3.5-mm endotracheal tube (ETT). He is then transferred to a mobile "MRI-safe" scanning bed and wheeled into the scanner. Anesthesia is continued with oxygen, air, and sevoflurane on a circle system with intermittent positive-pressure ventilation (IPPV) using an **MRI-compatible anesthesia machine** outside the 350 Gauss line. MRI-compatible SpO$_2$ and ECG monitors are then placed. The anesthesiologist places **ear-protecting headphones** on the child and himself and positions himself next to the anesthesia machine to see the monitor, child, and the radiology staff through a window. The headphones allow voice communication with the radiology staff.

After some initial localizing scans the procedure requires multiple **breath holds** of up to 20 seconds to prevent movement artifact during the ECG gated scans. This is accomplished by the anesthesiologist stopping the ventilator intermittently. A **gadolinium-based contrast** is given as a rapid bolus IV when indicated by the radiography staff. The scan (Fig. 34.1) takes 1 hour.

At the end of the scan the neuromuscular block is reversed and the patient is transferred to the induction area for extubation and recovery. The patient is later transferred to the cardiac ward for routine observation overnight.

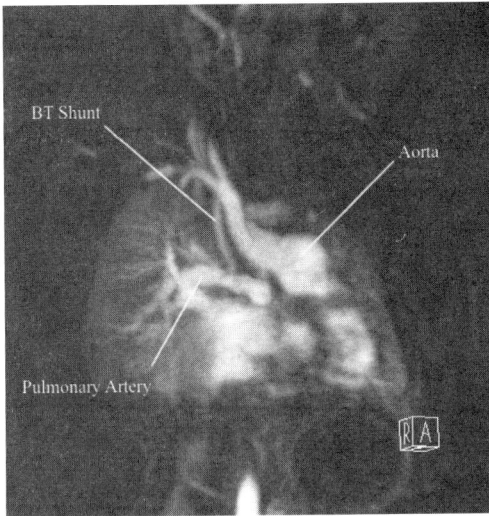

FIGURE 34.1 Gadolinium-enhanced MR angiogram of patient after under-going Norwood procedure. Note good exposure of pulmonary arteries and Blalock-Taussig (BT) shunt.

DISCUSSION

1. **What are the key points in preparing this patient for expo-sure to the magnetic field?**

The strength of the magnetic field is usually measured in Gauss (G) or Tesla (T) units, where 1T = 10,000G. Clinical scanners range up to 3T, while the Earth's magnetic field is about 0.5G. The scan room door is usually placed at the **5 Gauss line** and represents the point at which magnetic effects start to become significant.

Specific attention must be paid to the risks of exposure to a magnetic field. Metallic objects in or attached to the patient can become loose, move, or heat up; this includes ferrous bodies in the eye or neurovascular clips. Additionally, electronic devices themselves can be damaged and cease to function properly (e.g., pacemakers and cochlear implants). Information about specific devices and compatibility with MRI can be found in published texts and online (e.g., www.mrisafety.com). Importantly, the patient should be free from jewelry and the clothing must be free from metal. Some fixed objects are safe (e.g., sternal wires); however, any metal in the field can still cause artifacts on the scan.

The 2007 American College of Radiology Guidelines for MRI (Kanal et al., 2007) classify all objects into three categories: MR-safe, MR-conditional, or MR-unsafe. Any metallic or partially metallic object entering the scanning room must be assessed beforehand and labeled appropriately. If data on the device cannot be found, the staff can use a 1,000G handheld magnet to test the device's potential ferromagnetism.

- *MR-safe* devices are completely non-magnetic, non-electrically conductive, and non-radiofrequency (RF) reactive, eliminating all of the primary potential threats during an MRI procedure.
- *MR-unsafe* devices are significantly ferromagnetic and pose a clear and direct threat to persons and equipment within the magnet room.
- *MR-conditional* devices may contain magnetic, electrically conductive, or RF-reactive components that are safe for operations in proximity to the MRI, *provided the conditions for safe operation are defined and observed.*

Screening for metallic objects is best done by the radiology staff using a checklist. Naturally, these conditions apply equally to all staff and patient's guardians entering the scanner. Anesthetic equipment should have undergone such an assessment and should be clearly marked accordingly.

Lastly, because the scanner is noisy during active scanning (>100 dB), **hearing must be protected** with soft earplugs and over-ear covers.

2. Is gadolinium-based contrast a concern for the anesthesiologist?

Contrast reactions with **gadolinium**-based agents are much rarer than with iodinated agents. The incidence of allergic reactions is estimated to be about 0.04% in pediatrics, with the majority being mild or moderate (Dillman et al., 2007). However, patients with severe renal insufficiency risk developing nephrogenic systemic fibrosis after **gadolinium** exposure, so it should not be used in those patients.

3. What are the key points for preparing this patient for anesthesia?

Any child with congenital heart disease requires a detailed preoperative examination. In this case the history and examination were focused on looking for heart failure, as evidenced by failure to thrive, poor feeding, respiratory embarrassment, or signs such as hepatic enlargement. Previous anesthetic records and cardiology investigations were reviewed.

Avoiding prolonged starvation is a priority with this patient because of the deleterious effects dehydration will have on the shunt flow. Hence, the last bottle feed was given 4 hours before the scan. Consideration was given to placing an intravenous cannula and starting fluids on the ward preoperatively. The anesthetist decided not to do this in this case to avoid bruising the veins through failed awake cannulations, which would make the intravenous access under general anesthesia harder. Vitally, the anesthesiologist communicated with the parents and the ward and the MRI staff to ensure that fasting times were kept to a minimum. Routine use of intravenous warmed crystalloid is recommended for intraoperative hydration.

Anesthetic management is centered on maintaining the balance between pulmonary vascular resistance (PVR) and systemic vascular resistance (SVR). The child has a "balanced circulation"; depending on a number of factors, the blood can flow preferentially to systemic or pulmonary circulations. Painful stimulation or light anesthesia can cause an elevated PVR and hence acute oxygen desaturation from inadequate pulmonary blood flow. An elevation of SVR by vasopressors will improve flow through the shunt and reverse this desaturation. Conversely, a less restrictive systemic-to-pulmonary shunt may allow a steal of flow from the systemic circulation should the PVR decrease, leading to systemic hypoperfusion, hypotension, and acidosis. Keys to success are keeping the arterial CO_2 normal and the patient adequately anesthetized. Careful attention to ventilation is needed.

The procedure is not painful, and simple analgesics are sufficient. The use of a muscle relaxant ensures apnea during the breath-holding scans, reducing the volatile needed and hence reduced cardiac depression.

4. Providing anesthesia inside the scanner

Induction may occur within or outside the scanning room. The advantage to starting outside is access to the full range of anesthetic and resuscitation equipment in a standard operating room environment. The disadvantage is related to the transfer of the anesthetized patient, with the inherent interruptions in monitoring, risk of equipment failures, and other logistics. However, if there is no suitable induction environment close to the scan room, the increased risks from a longer transfer from the operating room area need to be considered. The most suitable location for inducing anesthesia should be chosen based on local organization and patient circumstances.

Anesthesia machines are available that function reliably in fields up to 350G. However, some unique problems occur with equipment in the MRI scanner. Strong magnetic fields induce currents in metal wires, which can lead to heating and burns. Thus, fiberoptic cables are used for pulse oximetry. These are more prone to light interference, and hence the sensors may need to be covered to block extraneous light in order to get a signal and often will not give a reading until the patient is still. The capnograph uses side stream sampling and the long tubing results in a delay of signal display that can be several seconds. Most batteries are intensely ferromagnetic, and thus while a laryngoscope using ferromagnetic batteries could be brought into the scanner in emergent circumstances, it must not be put down, and once laryngoscopy is complete the laryngoscope must be passed to another member of staff to take it out of the scanner room. Laryngoscopes with non-ferromagnetic power sources are available and preferable. If a child is being induced in the scanner, it is a good idea to induce the patient on the scanner table at the end furthermost from the magnet to minimize the risks, because the magnetic field increases exponentially towards the scanner. When parents will be present at induction, they will need to complete the magnet safety screening.

5. Particular anesthesia issues for cardiac MRI

The scan will require multiple **breath holds**. To maintain normocapnea the ventilation is increased between breath holds—that is, the average minute ventilation is kept close to normal. Avoidance of hypercapnea will help ensure PVR stability and also reduce the patient's respiratory efforts, which would otherwise have deleterious effects on the scan. The close attention paid to ventilation requires the presence of the anesthesiologist in the scan room, who will need noise-protecting earphones that allow voice communication with the radiology staff to coordinate the breath holds.

6. How does one approach cardiopulmonary resuscitation while in the magnet room?

There is no commercially available defibrillator rated for use in the MRI, so the patient must be removed from the magnet room to allow advanced resuscitation. Summoned emergency medical staff must not enter the magnet room without strict clearance from the radiology staff to prevent entry of metal objects. Common items such as scissors and pens are likely to fly into the scanner at great speed, with obvious dangerous results. Larger objects such as oxygen cylinders and equipment carts are even more dangerous and may even require the magnet to be turned off to be extricated. Restarting a superconductor is expensive.

Remember that rapid initiation of chest compressions is the key to effective resuscitation of cardiac arrest, and this should be started immediately upon withdrawing the patient from the scanner tube. The patient can then be transferred from the scan room to the safe room as quickly as possible to allow all resuscitation equipment to be used. This situation should be planned for and practiced.

7. What would be the concerns if this patient was from the intensive care unit (ICU)?

If this patient was coming from the ICU, one would have to consider the extra equipment attached to the patient. All implants and clips/wires need to be cleared by the radiology staff before leaving the ICU. They can refer to written and online databases for each piece of equipment. Vital drug infusions will have to continue. However, MRI-safe (up to 30G) infusion pumps are not always available. In this case the infusion pumps would have to remain outside the scanner; the infusion lines are extended so they are long enough to pass through a "waveguide" porthole into the scan room. The waveguide's aperture is limited to only a few inches wide to prevent radiofrequency interference.

Generally, the added length of tubing required to move pressure transducers through the porthole to outside of the scan room makes invasive blood pressure readings too damped. If arterial pressure monitoring is vital, it may be acceptable to have the transducers at the foot end of the scanner table (i.e., as far from the scanner as possible). A frequently cycled noninvasive oscillometric blood pressure cuff may be used instead.

Standard ECG electrodes and cables must be removed and may be replaced with MRI-specific ECG leads that under magnetic fields will not generate heating currents and risk of burns. It is important to note that ST segments change during the MRI due to currents induced by aortic flow, rendering ST analysis impossible.

If the patient had a cuffed ETT, then the metal spring-containing pilot balloon valve would need to be taped down to prevent it flying around.

The MRI scanner room has a high airflow. Coupled with transport to the ICU and inability to use active heating, this means patients can become hypothermic very easily. This patient could be transferred on a cot with overhead heating. The patient should be given warmed blankets and warmed fluid also. Though not in common use, fiberoptic temperature probes are available.

SUMMARY

1. All patients and staff must adhere to magnet safety rules.
2. The equipment is different from that in the operating room and requires some familiarization.
3. Prepare a plan for CPR.
4. Consider anesthetizing the patient in a nonmagnetic location and then transferring the patient.
5. Communication with the radiology staff is vital when coordinating the breath-hold and contrast scans.
6. Close attention must be paid to the ventilation and hydration of the patient.

ANNOTATED REFERENCES

• Institute for Magnetic Resonance Safety, Education, and Research: Home page. http://www.imrser.org/2011. Accessed Jan. 12, 2011.
  This is the official website for the Institute of Magnetic Resonance Safety, Education and Research. It contains a link to www.mrisafety.com, another useful MRI safety-related site.
• Kanal E, Barkovich AJ, Bell C, et al. the ACR Blue Ribbon Panel on MR Safety. ACR guidance document for safe MR practices: 2007. *AJR Am J Roentgen* 2007; 188(6): 1447–1474.

These MRI safe practice guidelines from the American College of Radiology are useful when forming local policies. They were produced by consensus of experts from a range of specialties involved with MRI.

Further Reading

Dillman JR, Ellis JH, Cohan RH, Strouse PJ, Jan SC. Frequency and severity of acute allergic-like reactions to gadolinium-containing IV contrast media in children and adults. *AJR Am J Roentgenol* 2007; 189 (6): 1533–1538.

Leyvi G, Wasnick JD. Single-ventricle patient: Pathophysiology and anesthetic management. *J Cardiothor Vasc Anesth* 2010; 24 (1): 121–130.

Peden CJ, Twigg, SJ. Anaesthesia for magnetic resonance imaging. *Cont Ed Anaesth Crit Care & Pain* 2003; 3(4): 97–101.

35

Pulmonary Hypertension

**GEORGE K. ISTAPHANOUS AND
ANDREAS W. LOEPKE**

INTRODUCTION

Pediatric pulmonary arterial hypertension (PAH) is characterized by a pathologically elevated pulmonary artery pressure in children. The etiology of PAH is multifactorial, and while its prognosis is closely related to the reversibility of the underlying disease process, much progress has recently been made in its diagnosis and treatment, significantly decreasing the associated morbidity and mortality.

LEARNING OBJECTIVES

1. Identify etiologies of PAH in young children.
2. Recognize risk factors for exacerbation of PAH.
3. Identify and describe the management of a pulmonary hypertensive crisis.

CASE PRESENTATION

*A 3-month-old, 5-kg girl with a known history of **meconium aspiration** at birth presents for a high-resolution computed tomography scan to evaluate her pulmonary parenchymal disease. Her birth history is significant for respiratory distress. The Apgar scores were 4 and 9 at 1 and 5 minutes respectively. The patient required intubation and conventional ventilation for 1 week.*

The baby is **tachypneic** *on examination and a peripheral pulse oximeter reveal an SpO$_2$ of 86% while on 125 mL/min of oxygen delivered via nasal cannula. Chest x-ray shows* **cardiomegaly** *with no evidence of consolidation or vascular congestion. There is mild/moderate* **tricuspid valve regurgitation** *on echocardiography, with Doppler velocity suggesting an estimated* **right ventricular systolic pressure** *(RVSP) of approximately 120% of measured systemic systolic blood pressure. She has a persistent moderately sized patent foramen ovale (PFO) and a small patent ductus arteriosus (PDA) with bidirectional shunting.*

After preoxygenation, 2 mg/kg of propofol is administered slowly via her preexisting peripherally inserted central catheter (PICC) line and repeated after 2 minutes. Positive-pressure ventilation is initiated by mask to **avoid hypercarbia** *and* **hypoxia***. Intubation with a size 3.5 mm ID endotracheal tube is uneventful and general anesthesia is maintained with 2.5% sevoflurane and 100% oxygen.*

The patient is undressed in preparation for the imaging study. During removal of her shirt, the patient **coughs,** *which is precipitously followed by* **hypoxemia, hypotension, and loss of peripheral pulses***.* **Chest compressions** *are initiated and 10 mcg/kg* **epinephrine (adrenaline)** *is administered twice (in 3-minute intervals) for the pulseless electrical activity. A 24-gauge peripheral intravenous line is started and a 20-mg/kg bolus of normal saline administered. The cardiac rhythm changes to sinus tachycardia and the brachial pulse becomes palpable. The study is canceled and the patient is transported to the pediatric intensive care unit while intubated to allow for* **administration of 100% oxygen** *and 20 ppm of inhaled* **nitric oxide (iNO)***.*

DISCUSSION

1. How is pediatric PAH diagnosed?

As in adults, pediatric PAH is defined as a mean pulmonary artery pressure of (1) higher than 25 mmHg at rest with normal pulmonary capillary wedge pressure, or (2) higher than 30 mmHg during exercise (Carmosino et al, 2007).

Clinically, PAH has to be considered in children with a history of respiratory complications or cardiac abnormalities when hypoxemia is refractory to oxygen therapy or alveolar recruitment strategies (Roberts et al., 1997) or when the neonatal preductal to postductal oxygen gradient exceeds 20 mmHg (Walsh-Sukys et al., 2000). The suspected diagnosis can be confirmed by echocardiography when tricuspid regurgitation is present or by direct measurement of pulmonary artery pressures during cardiac catheterization.

2. Overall, how is pulmonary hypertension classified?

In 2003, the 3rd World Symposium of Pulmonary Arterial Hypertension (in Venice) reclassified pulmonary hypertension from the previous Evian classification of 1998. Causes of PAH in children are shown in Table 35.1.

3. What are the etiologies leading to persistent pulmonary hypertension of the newborn (PPHN)?

PAH is physiologic during fetal life, but pressures decrease to normal adult levels soon after birth. Generally, three types of developmental defects can lead to PPHN that is not associated with congenital cardiac anomalies (Walsh-Sukys et al., 2000).

A. *Underdevelopment* of pulmonary parenchymal tissue, leading to hypoplastic pulmonary vasculature, such as in infants with congenital diaphragmatic hernia, oligohydramnios with obstructive uropathy, cystic malformations of the lungs, or intrauterine growth restriction

B. Peripartum *maladaptation* with constricted pulmonary vasculature due to adverse pulmonary conditions such as infections (especially group B streptococcus), meconium aspiration, or sepsis with respiratory distress syndrome

C. Genetic predisposition leading to maldevelopment of pulmonary parenchyma

---

Table 35.1

OVERALL CLASSIFICATION OF PEDIATRIC PULMONARY HYPERTENSION MODIFIED FROM THE VENICE 3RD WORLD SYMPOSIUM OF PULMONARY ARTERIAL HYPERTENSION

---

1. **Pulmonary arterial hypertension**

   1.1 Idiopathic (IPAH)

   1.2 Familial (FPAH)

   1.3 Associated with (APAH)

   1.3.2 Congenital Systemic to Pulmonary Shunts

   1.5 Persistent Pulmonary Hypertension of the Newborn (PPHN)**

3. **Pulmonary Hypertension associated with lung diseases and/or hypoxemia**

   3.2 Interstitial Lung Disease

   3.3 Sleep-Disordered Breathing

   3.4 Alveolar Hypoventilation Disorders

   3.6 Developmental Abnormalities

** *Incompletely understood; associated with increased muscularization of pulmonary arterial vessels, sepsis, and aspiration syndromes*

Reprinted from Simonneau G, Galiè N, Rubin LJ, Langleben D, et al. Clinical classification of pulmonary hypertension. *J Am Coll Cardiol* 2004; 43(12 Suppl S): 5S–12S, with permission from Elsevier.

4. **What is the significance of increased pulmonary artery pressures, and what factors may precipitate a crisis?**

Pulmonary hypertension is an independent predictor of morbidity in both children and adults with congenital heart disease undergoing non-cardiac surgery. Moreover, the incidence of pulmonary hypertensive crisis (PHC) and cardiac arrest is significantly increased in children with PAH undergoing non-cardiac surgery or cardiac catheterization, and it may occur suddenly without overt warning signs (Carmosino et al., 2007; Morray et al., 2000).

Physiological derangements such as hypoxemia, hypercarbia, acidosis, or increased sympathetic tone can lead to a sudden, dramatic increase in pulmonary vascular resistance (PVR). This increase in PVR will lead to a rise in right ventricular pressure, right-to-left intracardiac shunt, and a decrease in myocardial oxygen delivery, which will further diminish cardiac output and worsen hypoxemia, hypercarbia, and increase PVR, ultimately leading to cardiac arrest (Fig. 35.1).

PAH can be further categorized into its responsiveness to a drug or oxygen challenge (reactive) or lack of response (fixed), which has significant implications for patient outcome (Sarkar et al., 2005).

5. What are the preferred anesthetic agents for patients with PAH?

Adverse events have not been found to be significantly associated with any particular type of anesthetic, procedure, or method of airway management (Carmosino et al., 2007). The overriding goal in the design of an anesthetic for patients with elevated pulmonary artery pressure is the avoidance of sudden increases in pulmonary artery pressures due to sympathetic stimulation.

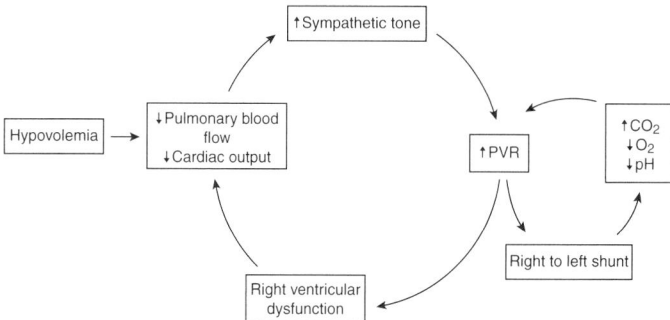

FIGURE 35.1 Cycle of events in pulmonary hypertensive episode.

Anxiolytics help to decrease sympathetic tone, thus avoiding elevated oxygen consumption and arrhythmias. However, combinations of benzodiazepines and narcotics can cause hypotension, producing a reactive increase in sympathetic tone that is counterproductive.

Similarly, inhaled anesthetics can cause a dose-dependent reduction of systemic vascular resistance (SVR) and cardiac contractility, which may lead to an increase in sympathetic tone. However, both isoflurane and sevoflurane have been shown to promote pulmonary vasodilation, whereas nitrous oxide has very little effect on pulmonary hemodynamics in children with PAH.

Opioids are favored in PAH because of their minimal pulmonary and systemic hemodynamic effects and the advantageous blunting of increases in PVR due to noxious stimulation. Propofol has also been used successfully in children with PAH; however, it should be administered with caution as boluses may cause precipitous reduction in cardiac output and SVR. Etomidate provides hemodynamic stability during induction of anesthesia. It also has demonstrated a relaxant effect on pulmonary arteries in normoxic rats (Rich et al., 1994). However, opioids should still be used as adjuncts to etomidate in order to blunt spikes in sympathetic tone, such as during endotracheal intubation. Conversely, ketamine has not been commonly used in pediatric PAH because of concerns about its ability to increase sympathetic tone and PVR (Hickey et al., 1985; Morray et al., 1984). This effect is less problematic when patients are mechanically ventilated and hypoxia and hypercarbia are avoided (Hickey et al., 1985).

6. What are the strategies to treat a pulmonary hypertensive crisis (PHC)?

Avoidance: Avoid factors that may precipitate an increase in PVR, such as hypoxemia, hypercarbia, acidosis, systemic hypotension, and increased sympathetic tone.

Treatment: Prompt diagnosis and treatment of PHC are paramount for successful resuscitation. First in line are the administration of 100% oxygen, treatment of hypercarbia by hyperventilation, and alkalization of blood by administering sodium bicarbonate. Chest compressions and epinephrine may be required if there are signs of significantly diminished cardiac output or cardiac arrest. Muscle relaxants may help in controlling ventilation. Remove any noxious stimulus and consider giving narcotics. Support cardiac output by augmenting preload with fluids and inotropic drugs, such as dobutamine or milrinone, which may also reduce PVR, or dopamine, which will maintain SVR and therefore help to optimize coronary perfusion. Start pulmonary vasodilators.

7. What is the role of pulmonary vasodilators in the treatment of PHC?

Inhaled nitric oxide (iNO): Inhaled nitric oxide is a selective pulmonary vasodilator that activates guanylate cyclase in pulmonary vascular smooth muscle cells and decreases intracellular calcium (Roberts et al., 1997). Its rapid onset and pulmonary selectivity make it the first-line pulmonary dilator therapy during a PHC in children and adults. iNO has also been demonstrated to be safe in the treatment of persistent PAH of the newborn. iNO is inactivated by rapidly binding to hemoglobin, thereby avoiding any systemic effects.

Phosphodiesterase-5 inhibitors: Inhibitors of phosphodiesterase-5, including dipyridamole, zaprinast, pentoxifylline, and sildenafil, lead to vascular smooth muscle relaxation and pulmonary artery vasodilation. Dipyridamole has significant systemic vasodilatory effects and should be used with caution in patients with limited cardiac reserve. Sildenafil has been shown to lead to marked reductions in PVR in neonates and adults and can be used to ameliorate rebound PAH after cessation of iNO. However, it may precipitate severe hypotension when co-administered with iNO. Sildenafil is available in intravenous, oral, and inhaled forms.

Endothelin inhibitors: The smooth muscle mediator endothelin-1 has been implicated in the etiology of PAH because of its potent vasoconstrictive effects. Bosentan is an antagonist at the dual receptors endothelin A and endothelin B (ET_A and ET_B). It is available in oral form with a half-life of 5 hours. Its use in children with PAH has been shown to decrease mean pulmonary artery pressure and PVR and to increase cardiac output.

Calcium channel blockers: Calcium channel blockers have been used in the treatment of PAH due to their pulmonary vasodilatory effects, as well as their ability to reverse smooth muscle cell hypertrophy occurring in PAH. Challenges with this class of drugs are their negative inotropic effects, which are least with nifedipine.

Prostacyclins: Patients with PAH have a reduced capacity for producing vasodilatory prostacyclins in pulmonary arteries. Epoprostenol, the most commonly used prostacyclin analog, leads to improved exercise capacity, hemodynamics, and survival in patients with severe pulmonary hypertension who suffer from symptoms during less-than-ordinary life tasks or at rest (NYHA III and IV) (Badesch et al., 2007). It is used as a continuous infusion due to its extremely short half-life (2–5 minutes) or via a nebulizer into the breathing circuit of ventilated patients.

SUMMARY

1. Risk factors for PAH are hypoxemia, hypercarbia, acidosis, or increases in sympathetic tone that increase PVR.
2. Developmental abnormalities that lead to persistent fetal circulation include underdevelopment of the pulmonary system (e.g., congenital heart disease, polyhydramnios), genetic predisposition leading to abnormally thickened pulmonary arterioles, and events such as aspiration of meconium or premature closure of a patent ductus arteriosus.
3. Signs of PAH include tachypnea, tachycardia, cyanosis, arrhythmias, and cardiac arrest.

4. For management of PAH focus on avoiding or treating hypoxemia, counteracting hypercarbia and acidemia, preventing dehydration/hypovolemia, treating dysrhythmias, and maintaining cardiac output. Avoid increases in sympathetic tone by aggressively treating agitation, noxious stimuli, and pain. Use iNO for direct vasodilation of the pulmonary vasculature, then transition to oral sildenafil.

ANNOTATED REFERENCES

- Carmosino MJ, Friesen RH, Doran A, Ivy DD. Perioperative complications in children with pulmonary hypertension undergoing noncardiac surgery or cardiac catheterization. *Anesth Analg* 2007; 104(3): 521–527.

  A review of medical records of children with PAH who underwent anesthesia or sedation for non-cardiac procedures and cardiac catheterizations. Significant predictor of major complications (cardiac arrest and/or PHC) was baseline suprasystemic PAH but not age, etiology of PAH, or anesthetic type.

- Roberts JD, Fineman JR, Morin FC et al. Inhaled nitric oxide and persistent pulmonary hypertension of the newborn. The Inhaled Nitric Oxide Study Group. *N Engl J Med* 1997; 336(9): 605–610.

  A prospective, randomized, multicenter study of infants with severe hypoxemia and persistent PAH. iNO improved systemic oxygenation and decreased the need for extracorporeal membrane oxygenation when compared to nitrogen without causing systemic hypotension or methemoglobinemia.

Further Reading

Adams JM, Stark AR. Persistent pulmonary hypertension of the newborn. In Garcia-Prats JA, ed. UpToDate. Waltham, MA: UpToDate, 2011.

Badesch DB, Abman SH, Simonneau G, Rubin LJ, McLaughlin VV. Medical therapy for pulmonary arterial hypertension: updated ACCP evidence-based clinical practice guidelines. *Chest* 2007; 131: 1917–1928.

Hickey PR, Hansen DD, Cramolini GM, Vincent RN, Lang P. Pulmonary and systemic hemodynamic responses to ketamine in infants with normal and elevated pulmonary vascular resistance. *Anesthesiology* 1985; 62(3): 287–293.

Morray JP, Lynn AM, Stamm SJ, Herndon PS, Kawabori I, Stevenson JG. Hemodynamic effects of ketamine in children with congenital heart disease. *Anesth Analg* 1984; 63(10): 895–899.

Morray JP, Geiduschek JM, Ramamoorthy C, Haberkern CM, Hackel A, Caplan RA, Domino KB, Posner K, Cheney FW. Anesthesia-related cardiac arrest in children: initial findings of the Pediatric Perioperative Cardiac Arrest (POCA) Registry. *Anesthesiology* 2000; 93(1): 6–14.

Rich GF, Roos CM, Anderson SM, Daugherty MO, Uncles DR. Direct effects of intravenous anesthetics on pulmonary vascular resistance in the isolated rat lung. *Anesth Analg* 1994; 78(5): 961–966.

Sarkar M, Laussen PC, Zurakowski D, Shukla A, Kussman B, Odegard KC. Hemodynamic responses to etomidate on induction of anesthesia in pediatric patients. *Anesth Analg* 2005; 101(3): 645–650.

Simonneau G, Galiè N, Rubin LJ, Langleben D, Seeger W, Domenighetti G, Gibbs S, Lebrec D, Speich R, Beghetti M, Rich S, Fishman A. Clinical classification of pulmonary hypertension. *J Am Coll Cardiol* 2004; 43(12 Suppl S): 5S-12S.

Walsh-Sukys MC, Tyson JE, Wright LL, et al. Persistent pulmonary hypertension of the newborn in the era before nitric oxide. *Pediatrics* 2000; 105: 14–20.

PART 7

CHALLENGES IN

OPHTHALMOLOGY

36

Open Globe Repair

J. FAY JOU AND JUDITH O. MARGOLIS

INTRODUCTION

Ocular trauma in childhood is common and may cause transient or permanent visual impairment. The anesthetic management of children with penetrating eye injuries presents several unique challenges, including potential associated injuries that may take precedence over the treatment of the eye injury, the prevention of aspiration of gastric contents, the regulation of intraocular pressure (IOP), and the prevention of the oculocardiac reflex (OCR). An understanding of the mechanisms and management of these potential problems can favorably influence surgical outcome.

LEARNING OBJECTIVES

1. Be familiar with the determinants of intraocular pressure (IOP).
2. Understand the effects of anesthesia that may increase the risk of vitreous herniation.
3. Discuss contributing factors and management of the oculocardiac reflex (OCR).
4. Grasp the anesthetic management of patients with open globe injury and full stomach.

CASE PRESENTATION

A 7-year-old boy presents to the emergency department after being hit in the right eye with a toy propelled from a slingshot. He weighs 25 kg and is otherwise completely healthy. He had eaten a full meal 1 hour prior to the accident. The patient presents to the operating room for exploration and repair of his ruptured globe.

DISCUSSION

1. What are the determinants of IOP?

Normal IOP is 16 ± 5 mmHg in the upright position and increases by 2 to 4 mmHg when supine. IOP maintains the shape and optical properties of the eye. It is determined by the balance between production and drainage of aqueous humor, change in choroidal blood volume, vitreous volume, and extraocular muscle tone. Temporary variations in pressure are usually well tolerated in normal eyes. However, when the globe is ruptured, IOP is lowered and may be as low as ambient pressure. Any factor that normally increases IOP may decrease the intraocular volume by causing drainage or extrusion of vitreous through the wound. This is a serious complication that can permanently impair vision.

Several cardiac and pulmonary variables affect IOP (Table 36.1). Increase in central venous or systolic blood pressure, hypoxia, hypercarbia, and increased tension within the extraocular muscles all raise IOP. The opposite physiological parameters lower it. Hypoxemia and hypercapnia may increase IOP through choroidal arteriole vasodilatation; sustained hypertension raises IOP by increasing choroidal blood volume. The most significant impact on IOP is *changes in central venous pressure*. Actions that cause congestion in the venous system impede outflow of aqueous humor and increase the volume of choroidal blood. Coughing, straining, bucking on the endotracheal tube, vomiting, excessive cricoid pressure, and the Valsalva maneuver can all elicit a dramatic elevation in IOP, as high as 30 to 40 mmHg.

Table 36.1

EFFECT OF CARDIAC AND PULMONARY VARIABLES ON IOP

Variable	Effect on IOP
Central venous pressure	
Increase	↑↑↑
Decrease	↓↓↓
Arterial blood pressure	
Increase	↑
Decrease	↓
PaO_2	
Increase	0
Decrease	↑
$PaCO_2$	
Increase (hypoventilation)	↑↑
Decrease (hyperventilation)	↓↓

↓ = decrease (mild, moderate, marked); ↑ = increase (mild, moderate, marked); 0 = no effect

Reprinted with permission from Morgan GE. Anesthesia for ophthalmic surgery. In: Morgan GE, Mikhail MS, Murray MJ, eds. *Clinical Anesthesiology*, 4th ed., pp. 826–836. Copyright The McGraw-Hill Companies, 2006.

2. What anesthetic effects increase the risk of vitreous herniation?

Any anesthetic event that alters the above-mentioned factors can affect IOP. Additionally, external pressure on the eye from a tightly fitted mask, improper positioning, coughing, straining, bucking, vomiting, or retrobulbar hemorrhage may result in extravasation of intraocular contents. Other factors include extraocular muscle spasm induced by depolarizing muscle relaxants, surgical stimulation during light anesthesia, or poorly applied cricoid pressure. Choroidal congestion from hypoxia, hypercapnia, osmotic diuretics, laryngoscopy, intubation, or increases in blood pressure also plays a role.

Most anesthetic agents either lower or have no effect on IOP (Table 36.2). This occurs either directly, by alteration in aqueous

Table 36.2

EFFECT OF ANESTHETICS ON IOP

Drug	Effect on IOP
Inhaled Anesthetics	
Volatile agents	↓↓
Nitrous oxide	↓
Intravenous Anesthetics	
Barbiturates	↓↓
Benzodiazepines	↓↓
Ketamine	?
Opioids	↓
Propofol	↓↓
Muscle Relaxants	
Succinylcholine	↑↑
Nondepolarizers	0/↓

↓ = decrease (mild, moderate); ↑ = increase (mild, moderate); 0/↓ = no change or mild decrease; ? = conflicting reports

Reprinted with permission from Morgan GE. Anesthesia for ophthalmic surgery. In: Morgan GE, Mikhail MS, Murray MJ, eds. *Clinical Anesthesiology*, 4th ed, pp. 826–836. Copyright The McGraw-Hill Companies, 2006.

humor flow or extra- and intraocular muscle tone, or indirectly, by altering cardiovascular parameters. All intravenous induction agents (except ketamine) and inhalational agents reduce IOP by direct effects. Sedative agents such as benzodiazepines and opioids also lower IOP. Lidocaine 2 mg/kg blunts IOP response to laryngoscopy and intubation by attenuating airway response and the cough reflex (Yukioka et al., 1985).

Succinylcholine (suxamethonium) is the muscle relaxant of choice in patients with a full stomach. However, its effect on IOP produces the possibility of ocular content extrusion. Succinylcholine raises IOP by 6 to 8 mmHg by increasing extraocular muscle tension and by contracting orbital smooth muscle, which reduces outflow of aqueous humor. The alteration in IOP begins at 1 minute, peaks at 2 to 4 minutes, and lasts up to 6 minutes. Although two large reviews have shown the safety of succinylcholine with no reports of vitreous herniation (Donlon, 1986; Libonati et al., 1985), the use of succinylcholine in patients with open globe injuries remains widely debated. The decision on whether to use succinylcholine in open globe surgeries should be based on the potential for a difficult airway and the viability of the eye. In the setting of an easy airway, regardless of the patient's aspiration risk and regardless of the viability of the eye, succinyl-choline can be avoided and replaced with the currently available short- or intermediate-acting nondepolarizing muscle relaxants. Ideal intubation conditions can be achieved rapidly with large-dose rocuronium (1–1.2 mg/kg, 60 seconds), vecuronium (0.25 mg/kg, 60 to 90 seconds), or cisatracurium (0.25 mg/kg, 60 to 90 seconds) (Doenicke et al., 1998). *If the airway is difficult and the eye is viable,* succinylcholine may be favored because the nonde-polarizing agents may have a prolonged effect that may result in increases in IOP from mask application, hypercarbia, and a longer time with an unprotected airway. *If the risk of aspiration is consid-ered high,* succinylcholine may be used. It is better to avoid aspira-tion by using succinylcholine than to have aspiration occur and have subsequent increases in IOP from hypoxia and hypercarbia.

Studies that examined techniques to prevent the increase in IOP due to succinylcholine have shown that a greater increase in IOP occurs from the stimulation of laryngoscopy and endotra-cheal intubation (Zimmerman et al., 1996). If succinylcholine is chosen, it is imperative to *blunt the IOP response to laryngoscopy and endotracheal intubation* by ensuring adequate depth of anes-thesia with appropriate induction agents and employing laryn-geal airway reflex suppressants such as opioids or lidocaine.

3. What are the contributing factors to and management of the OCR?

The trigeminovagal OCR is characterized by bradycardia and cardiac dysrhythmias, including ectopy, junctional rhythm, atrio-ventricular block, ventricular fibrillation, and cardiac arrest.

The reflex is induced by mechanical stimulation such as traction on the extraocular muscles (especially medial rectus), pressure on the eye or on the empty orbit, and intraorbital injections or hematomas. OCR is thus frequently encountered during ocular procedures and can be evoked in all age groups. Contributing factors include a light plane of general anesthesia, hypoxia, hypercarbia, and increased vagal tone.

The OCR consists of an initial parasympathetic phase followed by a sympathetic phase. Anticholinergic medication is often helpful in preventing this reflex, but the need for routine prophylaxis is controversial. The hemodynamic response to OCR is of fast onset and short duration. The reflex typically fatigues itself with repeated stimulation. In severe cases of OCR requiring pharmacological intervention, intravenous atropine or glycopyrrolate immediately prior to surgery is more effective than intramuscular premedication. Also, a retrobulbar block is unreliable in preventing OCR and may precipitate OCR, cardiac arrest, or retrobulbar hemorrhage.

Management of OCR includes the following:

- Immediate notification of the surgeon and temporary cessation of surgical stimulation or traction until heart rate increases
- Confirmation of adequate ventilation, oxygenation, and depth of anesthesia
- Administration of intravenous atropine if conduction disturbance persists
- In recalcitrant episodes, infiltration of the rectus muscles with local anesthetic

4. How should one manage patients with an open globe injury and full stomach?

In a child with head trauma, the globe and vision must be evaluated and coexisting injuries ruled out. The goal of management of a patient with an open globe injury and full stomach is to *prevent increases in IOP and to prevent aspiration*. Pharmacological reflux prophylaxis with histamine-2 receptor antagonists, proton pump inhibitors, and nonparticulate antacids may be indicated. Sedative-anxiolytics and opioids should be given judiciously to avoid respiratory depression and hypercarbia, nausea, and vomiting. Appropriate preoperative analgesia and sedation will minimize crying and agitation, thereby decreasing the risk of secondary ocular injury from vitreous herniation.

General anesthesia is the preferred method for the pediatric patient undergoing an ocular procedure. Care should be taken during the preoxygenation period to avoid pressure on the eye by the face mask. If the patient has a full stomach and an easy airway, rapid-sequence induction can be accomplished without succinylcholine using a large dose of nondepolarizing agent after induction with propofol or sodium thiopental and properly applied cricoid pressure. Succinylcholine with its shorter duration of action may be the safer choice if there is doubt about the ability to ventilate and/or intubate the patient, even if the eye is viable. In fasted patients, the use of nondepolarizing muscle relaxants is recommended. For either situation, prior administration of IV opioids and/or lidocaine (2 mg/kg) is recommended to attenuate the hypertensive response to laryngoscopy and intubation.

Intraoperative administration of antiemetic medication and decompression of the stomach may decrease the incidence of postoperative emesis, although they do not guarantee an empty stomach. Intravenous lidocaine (1.5 mg/kg) may be given 1 to 2 minutes prior to extubation to reduce coughing during emergence. Extubation should be delayed until the child is awake and has intact airway reflexes.

SUMMARY

1. Overall anesthetic goals are to avoid increasing IOP and to prevent aspiration.

2. Premedicate judiciously; minimize coughing, crying, and vomiting preoperatively.
3. Succinylcholine has been used safely in patients with a full stomach and open globe injury, but high-dose nondepolarizing muscle relaxants offer an attractive alternative. Consider succinylcholine when the risk of aspiration is high, the eye is not salvageable, or a difficult intubation is anticipated.
4. Administer drugs to minimize postoperative nausea and vomiting, and extubate awake.

ANNOTATED REFERENCES

- Kudlak TT. Open-eye injury. In Yao FF, Malhotra V, Fontes ML, eds. *Yao & Artusio's Anesthesiology: Problem-Oriented Patient Management*, 6th ed. Philadelphia: Lippincott Williams & Wilkins, 2008: 1007–1024.

    A case-based, problem-oriented overview of the topic with comprehensive practical explanations and references.
- Morgan GE. Anesthesia for ophthalmic surgery. In Morgan GE, Mikhail MS, Murray MJ, eds. *Clinical Anesthesiology*, 4th ed. New York: Lange, 2006: 826–836.

    A solid discussion of basic principles and anesthesia considerations involved in the management of a patient presenting for ophthalmic surgery.
- Yukioka H, Yoshimoto N, Nishimura K, Fujimori M. Intravenous lidocaine as a suppressant of coughing during tracheal intubation. *Anesth Analg* 1985; 64: 1189–1192.

    Coughing was suppressed completely when 2 mg/kg of lidocaine IV was given between 1 and 5 minutes before intubation compared with partial cough suppression with 1- and 1.5-mg/kg doses.

Further Reading

Allen SL, Duncan E. Open globe injury. In Atlee J, ed. *Complications in Anesthesia*, 2nd ed. Philadelphia: Saunders, 2007: 745–746.

Chidiac EJ. Succinylcholine and the open globe: questions unanswered. *Anesthesiology* 2004; 100: 1035–1036.

Doenicke AW, Czeslick E, Moss J, Hoernecke R. Onset time, endotracheal intubating conditions, and plasma histamine after cisatracurium and vecuronium administration. *Anesth Analg* 1998; 87: 434–438.

Donlon JV Jr. Succinylcholine and open eye injury II [letter]. *Anesthesiology* 1986; 64: 525–526.

Hahnenkamp K, Honemann CW, Fischer LG, Durieux ME, Muehlendyck H, Braun U. Effect of different anaesthetic regimes on the oculocardiac reflex during paediatric strabismus surgery. *Pediatr Anesth* 2000; 10: 601–608.

Libonati MM, Leahy JJ, Ellison N. The use of succinylcholine in open eye surgery. *Anesthesiology* 1985; 62: 637–640.

Zimmerman AA, Funk KJ, Tidwell JL. Propofol and alfentanil prevent the increase in intraocular pressure caused by succinylcholine and endotracheal intubation during a rapid sequence induction of anesthesia. *Anesth Analg* 1996; 83: 814–817.

PART 8

CHALLENGES IN

NEUROSURGICAL

CONDITIONS AND

NEUROMONITORING

37

Prone Positioning for Posterior Fossa Tumor Resection

MATTHIAS W. KÖNIG,
MOHAMED A. MAHMOUD, AND
JOHN J. McAULIFFE, III

INTRODUCTION

Brain tumors are the second most common malignancy in children. About one third occur in toddlers under the age of 3, and about two thirds are located in the posterior fossa. Resection of posterior fossa tumors is often a lengthy procedure that is commonly performed in the prone position. The prone position is associated with physiological changes and predisposes the patient to certain types of injuries.

LEARNING OBJECTIVES

1. Appreciate the logistic challenges of turning a small patient into the prone position.
2. Be aware of potential complications unique to prone positioning.
3. List strategies to avoid position-related injuries.

CASE PRESENTATION

A 2.5-year-old girl is scheduled for elective resection of a posterior fossa medulloblastoma. She initially presented with nausea, vomiting, *lethargy, and problems keeping her balance. Her weight is 14.2 kg, vital signs are within normal range, and preoperative blood counts, electrolytes, and coagulation studies are unremarkable. Anesthesia is induced through an existing intravenous line, the airway is secured with a cuffed 4.5 endotracheal tube, and a second intravenous line and a radial artery catheter are placed. The procedure proceeds uneventfully and after **almost 5 hours** the patient is turned supine. At this time, **marked swelling is noted in the face**, both eyes are swollen shut; the **tongue appears swollen** and protrudes from the mouth.*

DISCUSSION

1. What are common logistic issues of turning the pediatric patient prone?

The list of potential "mishaps" during the turning maneuver is long, but the anesthesia provider should vigilantly watch for the following issues.

Airway: The endotracheal tube (ETT) needs to be securely taped to prevent dislodging; keep in mind that tape will potentially be exposed to several hours of "drooling" in the face-down position. For that reason, some practitioners use skin adhesives (e.g. tincture of benzoin, Mastisol® liquid adhesive) to make tape stick better to the skin, apply clear tape or Tegaderm® on the cheeks on top of the primary ETT tape, or administer anticholinergics to minimize salivation. Access to the airway will be limited once the patient is turned prone, and a dislodged or kinked ETT will be more difficult to correct. Some practitioners advocate armored/spiral ETTs to reduce the risk of kinking; others intubate nasally. Whatever technique is used, bilateral breath sounds, adequate ventilation, and proper positioning and taping of the ETT must be confirmed after turning into prone position and before surgery commences. During skin prep, ensure the prep fluid does not drip down over the tape securing the tube, as alcoholic prep can dissolve tape adhesive.

The laryngeal mask airway (LMA) is probably the best immediate rescue option if the ETT is accidentally pulled out in the prone position, and should be immediately available.

Prolonged "blackout" period: It is tempting to simplify the turning maneuver by temporarily disconnecting monitors and intravenous and arterial lines to avoid having to disentangle them later. However, this frequently leads to periods of prolonged monitoring "blackout" where the patient's vital signs are not properly monitored. When turning, it is critical for the anesthesia provider to avoid being distracted by other tasks that delay adequate monitoring, ventilation, and provision of anesthesia. Some would argue to keep at least the pulse oximetry probe attached while turning, since it will provide basic information on oxygenation and perfusion. End-tidal CO_2 monitoring should be restored with ventilation once the patient is turned. The shape of the trace should be examined for evidence of airway obstruction or bronchospasm that may have been precipitated by the movement of the child.

Positioning and padding: Numerous devices, tables, and frames are used to keep patients in the prone position. However, some common precautions apply to all of them:

- Bony prominences should be padded to limit and diffuse pressure.
- There should be no direct pressure on genitals and breasts.
- The chest and pelvis are typically supported by foam/gel rolls or pillows to allow the abdomen to "hang" free in order to minimize venous congestion and maximize diaphragmatic excursion.
- Direct pressure to eyes and nose is avoided by using suitably cut-out foam pillows, using commercially available pillows/headrests, or securing the head in a holder with pins. The neck should stay in neutral position.
- Arms can be positioned neutrally alongside the body or be abducted less than 90 degrees to avoid traction on the brachial plexus.

- Before the patient is covered with surgical drapes, make sure that no monitoring or fluid lines are under the patient's extremities or torso, where they may cause pressure points. Likewise, the ETT, anesthesia breathing circuit, and oro/nasogastric tube should not put any pressure on the face.
- Verify proper function of all intravenous and arterial lines and monitoring equipment before the patient is draped. Be sure there is easy access to injection sites and access ports to be able to draw blood samples without competing with the surgeon for space.

Temperature: During line placement, the child is frequently left uncovered, and a significant drop in body temperature may occur. To avoid/minimize hypothermia, the patient's body should be covered as much as is practical during this phase, forced-air warming blankets should be used, and the ambient temperature of the operating room should be raised. For small patients, radiant heat loss is the predominant type of heat loss. Raising the operating room temperature well ahead of surgical start time is important in order to warm the walls and major objects in the room to reduce the heat gradient, which would enhance such losses.

2. What are the effects of the prone position on major organ systems?

The pathophysiological consequences of prone positioning are well researched in adults, but data in small children are not available. However, several points can probably be extrapolated from adult studies (Table 37.1).

3. What are typical position-related injuries during and after prolonged prone positioning for surgery?

Although severe long-term morbidity is fortunately rare as a consequence of prolonged prone positioning, the anesthesia provider must be aware of several uncommon but potentially

Table 37.1

PATHOPHYSIOLOGICAL EFFECTS OF THE PRONE POSITION

Cardiovascular	Respiratory	Central Nervous
Venous return ⇓ Stroke volume ⇓ Cardiac output ⇓ ⇔ Heart rate ⇑ Systemic vascular resistance ⇑; Systolic blood pressure ⇓ ⇔ Mean arterial pressure ⇓ ⇔	Functional residual capacity ⇑; ⇔ Total lung capacity ⇑; ⇔ V/Q mismatch ⇓	Jugular venous flow ⇑; ⇔ Jugular venous resistance ⇓ ⇔ Intracranial pressure ⇑; (if head lower than heart)

This table was published in Rozet I, Vavilala MS. Risks and benefits of patient positioning during neurosurgical care. *Anesthesiology Clinics* 2007; 25: 631–653. Copyright Elsevier, 2007.

disastrous complications. It is good practice to *explain these potential risks when obtaining consent for anesthesia*.

Pressure sores/abrasions: These are usually found overlying bony prominences and are rarely a significant clinical problem. Careful padding can help avoid most of these.

Facial/intraoral swelling: After prolonged face-down position, some degree of facial swelling is common. Seeing their child with the eyes swollen shut after surgery may be distressing to some parents, but usually reassurance is all that will be required in cases of facial swelling. Several cases have been reported where significant **tongue swelling** led to *partial or complete airway obstruction* after extubation. In cases of significant tongue swelling, it may be prudent to delay extubation until the swelling subsides.

Neurologic injury: Peripheral nerve injury, most commonly due to *overstretching of the brachial plexus*, has been described after prone surgeries. Abduction of the arms more than 90 degrees should be avoided, as well as using overly thick padding under the arms in small children, which may stretch the plexus by forcing an abducted arm backwards. Rare cases of vascular *injury to the cervical spinal cord* have been reported, and avoidance of excessive neck flexion and hypotension has been recommended to maintain adequate cord perfusion.

Postoperative visual loss is probably the most feared complication by surgeons and anesthesiologists in this setting. Although mostly reported in posterior spine surgery, it has also been reported in a child undergoing sagittal synostosis repair in the prone position (Lee et al., 2005). The exact pathophysiology is still somewhat elusive, but intraoperative *hypotension, anemia, prone position*, and *duration of procedure (>6 hr)* are the most consistently identified risk factors. Direct pressure on the eye is responsible for only a minority of cases. The most common (~90%) ophthalmologic diagnoses are *anterior and posterior optic nerve ischemia*. Much less common is retinal artery/vein occlusion (the only diagnosis that is related to pressure on the eye) and cortical blindness.

Preventive strategies include:

- Hemodynamic stability
- Adequate hemoglobin/hematocrit
- Avoid excessive crystalloid infusion to minimize risk of edema.
- Meticulous positioning of the head and frequent checks to make sure nothing presses on the eyes

4. Can one perform cardiopulmonary resuscitation (CPR) in the prone position?

Conventionally, CPR is performed in the supine position in all age groups. However, successful CPR in the prone position, including cardiac compressions, has been described in a number of cases, both in operating rooms and intensive care units (e.g. Tobias et al., 1994). There are several considerations when conducting CPR of the prone patient:

Speed: Resuscitation relies on rapid initiation of CPR. Taking the time to pack and cover a wound and flip the patient supine may cause deleterious delays in starting chest compressions. In some cases, the anesthesiologist placed his or her clenched fist under the sternum of the patient while the surgeon gave cardiac compressions. CPR can therefore be started while a stretcher is brought into the operating room so that the patient can be turned supine for ongoing resuscitation.

Protecting intravenous access and invasive monitoring: Turning a patient supine under emergency conditions to perform CPR poses the substantial risk of losing intravenous access and the arterial line when they are needed most.

Contamination of surgical field: Depending on the nature of the surgery, turning the patient supine may risk infection and/or trauma to exposed tissue.

SUMMARY

1. Turning an anesthetized child prone requires the undivided attention of the anesthesia provider to protect the airway and intravenous and arterial access.
2. Reestablishing ventilation and complete monitoring— if it has been disconnected before turning—should have highest priority.
3. Closely attend to padding and positioning; frequently recheck the face and eyes.
4. Avoid hypotension and anemia.
5. Not all facial swelling after long prone surgeries is benign, and airway compromise may occur in cases of tongue swelling.
6. CPR is possible in the prone position and may be safer than hastily turning the patient.

ANNOTATED REFERENCES

- American Society of Anesthesiologists Task Force on Perioperative Blindness: Practice advisory for perioperative visual loss associated with spine surgery. *Anesthesiology* 2006; 104: 1319–1328.

  Summary of the current knowledge and expert/evidence-based recommendations on prevention and treatment of perioperative visual loss.

- Edgcombe H, Carter K, Yarrow S. Anaesthesia in the prone position, *Br J Anaesth* 2008; 100: 165–185.

  Excellent and comprehensive review of physiological effects of the prone position and potential complications.

- Tobias JD, Mencio GA, Atwood R, Gurwitz GS. Intra-operative cardiopulmonary resuscitation in the prone position. *J Pediatr Surg* 1994; 29: 1537–1538.

  Case report of successful CPR in a 12-year-old in the prone position after cardiac arrest during posterior spine surgery.

Further Reading

Lee J, Crawford MW, Drake J, Buncic JR and Forrest C. Anterior ischemic optic neuropathy complicating cranial vault reconstruction for sagittal synostosis in a child. *J Craniofac Surg* 2005; 16(4): 559–562.

Martínez-Lage JF, Almagro MJ, Izura V, Serrano C, Ruiz-Espejo AM, Sánchez-Del-Rincón I. Cervical spinal cord infarction after posterior fossa surgery: a case-based update. *Child's Nerv Syst* 2009; 25: 1541–1546.

Sinha A, Agarwal A, Gaur A, Pandey CK. Oropharyngeal swelling and macroglossia after cervical spine surgery in the prone position. *J Neurosurg Anesth* 2001; 13: 237–239.

38

Spinal Surgery

MOHAMED A. MAHMOUD,
MATTHIAS W. KÖNIG, AND
JOHN J. McAULIFFE, III

INTRODUCTION

The aim of all spine surgery is to achieve surgical correction of a defect without incurring new neurologic deficits. The anesthesiologist caring for children and adolescents who undergo spine surgery must address surgical requirements, the issues associated with prone positioning, optimal conditions required for neurophysiologic monitoring, as well as the pathophysiology related to underlying medical conditions. The anesthesiologist must anticipate potential problems in anesthetizing a patient for complex spinal surgery and be prepared to manage all issues and complications.

LEARNING OBJECTIVES

1. Understand the elements of the anesthetic plan for an adolescent who is scheduled for extensive spine surgery.
2. Be familiar with the effects of different anesthetic agents on different modalities of intraoperative neurophysiologic monitoring.
3. Know the potential risks and complications associated with spine surgery.

CASE PRESENTATION

*A 16-year-old girl with idiopathic kyphoscoliosis presents for anterior thoracic vertebrectomy, posterior spine decompression with instrumentation, and fusion with autologous bone graft. Her past medical history is significant for obesity and back pain. Laboratory tests are within normal limits. She weighs 98 kg and is 165 cm tall. Preoperative HR is 80 bpm and BP 125/72 mmHg. An ECG shows normal sinus rhythm, a right bundle branch block pattern, and a **prolonged** QTc **interval** of 489 ms. She has predonated 2 units of **autologous blood**. Her hemoglobin level 4 days before surgery was 10.2 g/dL. Induction is uneventful and **total intravenous anesthesia (TIVA)** with propofol and remifentanil is used for maintenance. A double-lumen tube is placed to allow one-lung ventilation. The patient is turned to the prone position with one orthopedic surgeon working on the anterior decompression and the other orthopedic surgeon working simultaneously on the posterior fusion part of the procedure. Lung isolation provides the surgeons with excellent access to the surgical field. The estimated blood loss now is 3.5 L, which has been replaced with 2 units of autologous whole blood, 1 unit of homologous blood, 1 L of albumin, and 3,200 mL of lactated Ringer's solution. Her blood pressure is 82/58 mm Hg and her hemoglobin is 8.7 g/dL. The surgeon requests **controlled hypotension** to help control the bleeding. After the surgeon places all the screws, the neurophysiologist announces that there is **a significant decrease in the amplitude of the transcranial motor evoked potentials (MEP)**. The surgeon loosens all the screws, but the neurophysiologist states that the MEP signal is still attenuated. The **mean arterial pressure (MAP) is raised** and a **wake-up test** is performed, during which the patient demonstrates movement of both lower extremities. While the surgeon is closing the wound, the audible pulse oximetry tone disappears. The ECG shows a pattern consistent with **torsades de pointes**, which is corrected rapidly with **defibrillation** and intravenous magnesium. Upon transfer to the ICU, **patient-controlled analgesia (PCA)** is used to manage her postoperative pain. Early in the patient's ICU course, she has a swollen face and complains of tongue pain. An otolaryngology consult is obtained* *immediately and the exam reveals a left anterior* **necrotic tongue lesion** *that requires surgical excision of necrotic tissue after 1 week.*

DISCUSSION

1. What are the goals of preoperative evaluation and the possible intraoperative complications for patients with scoliosis?

An important aim of preoperative evaluation of patients with scoliosis is to detect the presence and the extent of cardiac and pulmonary compromise. Respiratory function should be assessed by a thorough *history* (focusing on exercise tolerance and functional impairment) and *physical examination*. Preoperative pulmonary function tests, especially vital capacity, are important predictors of the need for postoperative ventilation. If preoperative vital capacity is less than 30% to 35% of predicted, postoperative ventilation is likely to be required.

Cardiac dysfunction may occur secondary to scoliosis or as a consequence of a neuromuscular disorder causing the scoliosis. Cardiac conditions that can accompany the diagnosis of scoliosis range from no abnormalities to severe cardiomyopathies, rhythm and conduction abnormalities, cor pulmonale, and pulmonary hypertension. Electrocardiogram and cardiac echocardiography should be performed as indicated. Other preoperative studies include complete blood count, renal and liver biochemistry, and coagulation profile. The patient and her parents should be advised about all possible complications, including massive blood loss, paralysis, peripheral nerve injury, **tongue laceration**, awareness during surgery, postoperative vision loss, prolonged postoperative intubation, deep venous thrombosis, and pulmonary embolism.

2. With regard to blood loss, why is proper prone positioning especially important for spine surgery?

Scoliosis surgery is an extensive operation that is often associated with substantial blood loss and significant oozing from the large area of exposed cancellous bone. The degree of blood loss is positively correlated with the number of spinal levels fused, body weight, and duration of surgical instrumentation. Raised intra-abdominal pressure while in the prone position is also associated with increased blood loss, because shunting of blood can cause the vertebral venous system to dilate. To keep the paravertebral venous pressure low, it is important to *ensure that the abdomen is free in the prone position.*

3. What other positioning considerations are important for the prone position?

Particular attention must be given to securing the endotracheal tube (ETT) to avoid unintended extubation. A wire-reinforced ETT may be considered to avoid tube kinking and occlusion. In case of accidental extubation in the prone position, placement of a laryngeal mask airway offers an effective alternative tool for temporary ventilation and can act as a conduit for fiberoptic reintubation.

All pressure points must be meticulously padded to avoid skin breakdown, especially the face, eyes, chest, hips (which are typically supported with bolsters), and knees. The arms should be carefully positioned to avoid stretch on the brachial plexus.

4. What are different strategies used to reduce intraoperative blood loss in this procedure?

Various strategies to reduce intraoperative blood loss include **moderate controlled hypotension**, alteration of operative position, changes in surgical techniques, and administration of anti-fibrinolytic agents. Strategies aimed at decreasing the use of homologous blood products include intraoperative blood salvage, **preoperative autologous donation**, and acute normovolemic hemodilution. Moderate induced hypotension (reduction of systolic blood pressure 20 mmHg from baseline or lowering mean arterial pressure to 65 mmHg in the normotensive adolescent patient) has been shown to decrease blood loss and reduce transfusion requirements. However, induced hypotension is not without risk and has been reported to increase the risk of *spinal cord ischemia and other neurologic deficits, including permanent loss of vision.*

Postoperative visual loss following non-ocular surgery is an infrequent but disastrous complication with an estimated incidence ranging from 0.001% to 0.2%, depending on the type of surgery (Berg et al., 2010). The three recognized causes of postoperative visual loss are ischemic optic neuropathy, central retinal artery or vein occlusion, and cerebral ischemia. A survey of vision loss after spinal surgery has suggested that possible intraoperative risk factors include patient positioning, anemia, and intraoperative hypotension.

Excessive bleeding often occurs during scoliosis surgery and is attributed to numerous factors, including accelerated fibrinolysis. Fibrinolytic inhibitors such as tranexamic acid and aminocaproic acid have been shown to reduce blood loss during scoliosis surgery. The blood loss reduction in children undergoing scoliosis surgery with the high-dose regimen of tranexamic acid (100-mg/kg bolus followed by an infusion of 10 mg/kg/hour) is greater than the lower-dose regimen (10-mg/kg bolus followed by an infusion of 1 mg/kg/hour) (Sethna et al., 2005).

5. What precautions should be taken with neuromonitoring techniques?

Volatile anesthetic agents have been reported to **depress motor and sensory evoked potential** amplitudes in a dose-dependent manner. However, some centers routinely use desflurane and remifentanil during spine surgery while monitoring MEPs. A comparison of the delivered energy required to elicit MEPs in patients receiving desflurane versus **total intravenous anesthesia** (**TIVA**) shows that greater charge per pulse and more pulses per train are required in patients receiving desflurane to elicit comparable MEP amplitudes. Consequently, TIVA techniques with propofol as a central component have been advocated to optimize neuromonitoring during spine surgery. **Hypotension** can compromise spinal cord perfusion, which can decrease the amplitude of the MEPs. Maintenance of a constant level of anesthesia and blood pressure during the case helps to minimize the variability of the neurophysiologic signals and facilitates the prompt detection of conditions that may cause neurologic injury.

If TIVA is used, propofol infusion rates should be chosen to achieve a constant effect site concentration. This will minimize the potential for decay of somatosensory evoked potentials (SSEPs) and MEPs due to excessive drug levels. Bolus dosing of propofol after a steady-state concentration is achieved may result in temporary attenuation or loss of MEPs in some patients. Of all the opioids, remifentanil has the least potential to depress MEPs. Ketamine and etomidate are potentially useful in patients who cannot receive propofol; however, adrenal suppression limits the use of etomidate. Transcranial MEPs have the potential to cause serious **tongue injuries**. Dental guards and soft bite blocks are required, and care must be exercised to ensure that strong jaw muscle contractions do not result in this injury.

There should be a procedure in place describing the responsibilities and actions to be taken by each member of the team in the event of **loss of MEPs or SSEPs** during the case. Once acute loss is detected, there is an urgent need to define the cause and if necessary restore adequate perfusion to the spinal cord. The **mean arterial blood pressure should be raised** to 90 mmHg or more unless contraindicated. This may be accomplished by reducing the anesthetic agent, expanding intravascular volume, or using a vasoactive agent. The hematocrit and other physiological factors (temperature, acid–base balance, oxygen and carbon dioxide tensions) should be optimized while the surgeon looks for and corrects surgical causes. Although the use of steroids remains controversial, some centers recommend that a spinal cord injury treatment protocol with steroids be instituted. The recommended protocol is methylprednisolone 30 mg/kg IV as a loading dose, followed by an infusion of methylprednisolone at 5.4 mg/kg/hour for the next 23 hours. Once the physiological parameters, including blood pressure, are brought to normal values, the MEPs and SSEPs are reassessed for improvement. If improvement in potentials is not seen, an **intraoperative wake-up** test is undertaken, as in the case presented. A CT scan may be indicated immediately postoperatively to be sure that no surgically correctable spinal cord injury exists.

6. Can one resuscitate a patient in the prone position?

Conventional teaching has been that when a life-threatening adverse event occurs, the patient should be returned to the supine position for resuscitation to facilitate access to the airway and precordium. The routine use of two tables in the operating room, one to be available for the immediate supination of the unstable patient, has been suggested. In the event of a malignant arrhythmia, turning a patient with an open spine from prone to the supine position to carry out **defibrillation and cardiopulmonary resuscitation** can take several minutes. CPR and defibrillation in the **prone position** have been reported with success (Miranda & Newton, 2001). Presurgical placement of external defibrillation pads is extremely important in patients at higher risk, such as the case here, in which congenital **prolonged QT syndrome** predisposed the patient to **torsades de pointes** as a result of perturbations in electrolytes and the effects of certain medications. Prolonged QT syndrome is discussed further in Chapter 70.

7. What are the current options for postoperative pain control for spinal fusion?

Several recently developed analgesic techniques effectively control pain after major orthopedic surgery. Neuraxial analgesia provided by epidural and spinal administration of local anesthetics and opioids provides the highest level of pain control. However, such therapy is invasive and labor-intensive. Although intrathecal morphine is used as an analgesic in a variety of medical and surgical conditions, little has been published on its use after posterior spine fusion. Intrathecal morphine in doses of 2 and 5 mcg/kg provided potent analgesia in the first 24 hours after spinal fusion in children, as evidenced by low pain scores and little additional use of morphine with **patient-controlled analgesia (PCA)** (Gall et al., 2001). Since the thecal sac is readily available during these procedures, the addition of a single injection of morphine before wound closure can be done with technical ease if the orthopedic surgeon is willing to offer this option. Technical issues, especially a high incidence of epidural catheter dislodgment, have limited the application of epidural opiate/local anesthetic analgesia following spine surgery. PCA is used in many centers because of its ease of use and relative predictability.

SUMMARY

1. Preoperative evaluation must thoroughly assess the patient's cardiopulmonary status.
2. Meticulous intraoperative positioning is critical to prevent complications.
3. Induced hypotension may increase the risk of spinal cord ischemia and vision loss.
4. Fibrinolytic inhibitors have been shown to reduce intraoperative blood loss.
5. Intraoperative neuromonitoring facilitates the detection of potential cord injury but has significant implications for anesthetic management.
6. PCA is an effective and commonly used technique for postoperative pain control.

ANNOTATED REFERENCES

- Miranda CC, Newton MC. Successful defibrillation in the prone position. *Br J Anaesth* 2001; 87: 937–938.

  This case report describes successful treatment of ventricular fibrillation in an adult undergoing complex spinal surgery in the prone position. The discussion includes different approaches to the placement of defibrillator paddles.

- **Sethna NF, Zurakowski D, Brustowicz RM, Bacsik J, Sullivan LJ, Shapiro F. Tranexamic acid reduces intraoperative blood loss in pediatric patients undergoing scoliosis surgery.** *Anesthesiology* **2005; 102(4): 727–732.**

  The study concludes that intraoperative administration of tranexamic acid significantly reduces blood loss during spinal surgery in children with scoliosis.

- **Soundararajan N, Cunliffe M. Anaesthesia for spinal surgery in children.** *Br J Anaesth* **2007; 99: 86–94.**

  This review article provides a comprehensive discussion of the anesthetic issues in children undergoing spine surgery. Table 4 presents complications of the prone position.

Further Reading

Berg KT, Harrison AR, Lee MS. Perioperative visual loss in ocular and nonocular surgery. *Clin Ophthalmol* 2010; 4:531–546.

Gall O, Aubineau J-V, Berniere J, Desjeux L, Murat I. Analgesic effect of low-dose intrathecal morphine after spinal fusion in children. *Anesthesiology* 2001; 94: 447–452.

Sabina D, Schwartz D. Anesthetic management for pediatric spinal fusion: Implications of advances in spinal cord monitoring. *Anesthesiology Clin North Am* 2005; 23: 765–787.

Urban MK, Beckman J, Gordon M, Urquhart B, Boachie-Adjei O. The efficacy of antifibrinolytics in the reduction of blood loss during complex adult reconstructive spine surgery. *Spine* 2001; 26(10): 1152–1156.

39

Awareness and Recall During Anesthesia

ANDREW DAVIDSON

INTRODUCTION

Awareness is being able to freely recall an event that occurred during a general anesthetic. The phenomenon is well described in adults but, until recently, was poorly described in children. Several studies have now found that awareness does occur in children. It occurs more often than in adults but often has different characteristics to the typical awareness described in adults.

LEARNING OBJECTIVES

1. Know the characteristics of awareness in children.
2. Understand the principles of preventing awareness in children.
3. Know the principles of managing awareness and recall in children.

CASE PRESENTATION

*A 12-year-old boy is scheduled for a rigid **bronchoscopy**. In the preoperative evaluations, his mother says that when she told him he needed an operation, and that he would be asleep, he told her that during his last operation he heard people talking.*

*The previous anesthetic was for a femoral osteotomy when the boy was 6 years old. It was an uneventful anesthetic where the record showed the child received a spontaneous ventilation technique, caudal blockade, and close to 0.6 MAC of isoflurane. When asked about his previous **awareness**, his **memory of the event is fragmentary**. He remembered a buzzing feeling and people talking but could not remember what they said. He felt no pain. He was **not particularly worried** by the event and at the time he **did not tell anybody**. He is not anxious about having another operation, although he says he would prefer to be asleep for this one.*

*For the bronchoscopy, the usual anesthetic technique used by the scheduled anesthetist is a **total intravenous anesthetic** with propofol and low-dose remifentanil without neuromuscular blockade. The anesthetist decides not to change his technique but does give a dose of midazolam after induction and uses a **BIS** monitor. The BIS is kept below 50 for the procedure. The procedure is uneventful. After recovery the anesthetist asks the boy how it went and he reports no awareness. The anesthetist calls again a few days later and again the boy reports no memories of the anesthetic, and his parents report he is behaving normally. The anesthetist **leaves his contact details** and suggests the parents call him back him if the boy's behavior changes over the next few weeks.*

DISCUSSION

1. Do children experience awareness?

There is increasing evidence that shows children do report **awareness** with an incidence somewhere between 0.2% and 1.2% (e.g., Blusse van Oud-Alblas et al., 2009; Davidson et al., 2005). This is a rate higher than that reported during routine anesthesia in adults. It is difficult to accurately measure awareness, and accurately detecting awareness may be more difficult in children (Lopez & Habre, 2009). Interviews looking for awareness must be carefully designed to accommodate a child's level of understanding. Both adults and children may confuse recall of intraoperative events with perioperative events. This may be more problematic in children, as their memory consolidation processes are not as well developed. However, in spite of these limitations, children usually do report memories accurately and *if children report awareness, then their reports should be believed* and they should be managed accordingly.

2. What are the characteristics of the awareness reported by children?

While some recall-of-awareness reports in children are detailed, it is more common for children to report **fragmentary memories**. This is consistent with their developing memory encoding and consolidation processes. Like adults, children rarely report the event to medical staff unprompted, though some have reported it to siblings or parents. Again, like in adults, children may report the event some time after the anesthetic, and they describe both auditory and tactile sensations. Some children report pain, and while relatively **few are very distressed,** most children do not like the experience. While the published case series are small, it seems children are less likely to develop severe psychological problems compared to adults. It is important to remember, however, that there are reports of *some children who do develop a post-traumatic stress disorder* after awareness (Osterman et al., 2001).

Most awareness in children does not seem to have an obvious cause. In adult cases, paralysis with neuromuscular blockade is a recognized risk factor for awareness. *Paralysis is not a recognized risk factor in children.* Awareness under paralysis is far more distressing and has a much greater risk of leading to post-traumatic stress disorder. The lower proportion of aware children who were paralyzed may explain the possibly lower incidence of severe psychological distress after awareness in children.

In adults, the risk of awareness is greater in cardiac and obstetric anesthesia, and during bronchoscopy or trauma surgery. In children, high-risk groups have not been identified. While most awareness in children occurs outside the high-risk groups described in adults, there is no reason to think that these high-risk groups would not be at some increased risk of awareness in children. The studies are too small in these groups to determine if children are indeed at high risk in cardiac, bronchoscopy, and trauma surgery, but the mechanisms underlying awareness would be the same so the increase in risk should be the same.

In adults, awareness is often due to error. In children, review of the reported cases does not demonstrate any obvious anesthetic error. There is some evidence that risk of awareness is higher if the patient has had awareness before, or if a family member has had an awareness event. This implies that in some cases there may be a genetic resistance to anesthesia, though this is unproven. A positive previous history should be regarded as a possible increased risk of awareness in children, just as it is in adults.

3. What can be done to prevent awareness in children?

We do not understand the mechanism or cause of awareness in most cases in children. Thus, it is difficult to know exactly how to prevent awareness in children. We do know that children have a higher anesthetic requirement than adults. It may be that children are aware more often because anesthetists simply do not give enough intravenous or volatile anesthetic in children. It could be that they do not give high enough concentrations of volatile or big enough doses of intravenous anesthetics, or they may not wait long enough for the effect site concentration of a volatile anesthetic to be high enough before stimuli such as surgery or laryngoscopy. Thus, the *simplest way to prevent awareness in children is to be sure to give an adequate dose of anesthetic and to be patient and wait for effect site levels to be high enough*. A problem, however, is that our knowledge of the pharmacology of anesthetics in children is still very incomplete. We have a rough idea of how MAC changes with age but there are few data on how MAC-awake changes with age. Similarly, we have little idea of the effect site equilibration times in children.

In adults, it is controversial as to whether or not TIVA increases the risk of awareness. In experienced hands, TIVA probably does not increase the risk of awareness. In children, however, there are far fewer data on the accuracy of TIVA algorithms. Until the algorithms are fine-tuned in children, there will always be a nagging worry that TIVA in children could increase awareness risk. TIVA is often used with a processed EEG monitor to guide delivery (as in this scenario). Although unproven, it is logical to assume that EEG-guided anesthesia delivery for TIVA would help prevent awareness.

Midazolam is occasionally suggested as a way to help prevent awareness. Midazolam is indeed an excellent agent to inhibit memory encoding, and thus in theory should be very useful to prevent memory formation and awareness, but the dose and duration of effect vary. Relying solely on a single dose at or before induction to prevent awareness is very unwise, and giving midazolam should never be seen as an alternative to an adequate dose of general anesthesia for preventing awareness. Nevertheless, many give an extra dose of midazolam on top of their routine anesthetic for those deemed at high risk of awareness.

The processed EEG is increasingly used to guide anesthetic delivery. The **BIS**™, Entropy™, and Narcotrend™ are the most frequently used. *No trials have evaluated the effectiveness of these devices in preventing awareness in children.* There is, however, substantial evidence that these processed EEG devices function in older children in a similar way to how they function in adults. The readout numbers go down as the concentration of anesthetic increases, and they have a fair to good discriminative power differentiating being awake and anesthetized. As in adults, there are occasions where the performance of these monitors may be compromised, such as when ketamine is used as a sole agent, with high-dose opioid anesthesia, or with high concentrations of sevoflurane.

In a well-conducted randomized trial, the BIS reduced awareness in high-risk adults (Myles et al., 2004). The cases are high risk because there is some reason to suspect inadequate anesthetic may be given due to inability to monitor physiological parameters, or the patient has limited capacity to tolerate anesthesia. It can be fairly safely assumed that BIS would reduce awareness in children who fell into the same high-risk groups—where the mechanism of awareness is likely to be similar. Bronchoscopy is a high-risk group in adults, where BIS may reduce awareness, but bronchoscopy is probably high risk due to difficulty in maintaining accurate delivery of volatile anesthesia. If TIVA is used, then it is less clear that bronchoscopy *per se* is an at-risk procedure. In this scenario, BIS is used to guide TIVA delivery in a child who may be at a higher risk due to previous awareness.

Most pediatric awareness cases are not in these high-risk groups, and the mechanism of awareness in these cases is poorly understood. It is thus hard to extrapolate the adult trial data to these cases. While in theory these devices "work" in children, it remains unproven if they would reduce awareness in the majority of pediatric awareness cases where there are no obvious risk factors for inadequate anesthesia delivery.

4. How should one manage awareness with recall in children?

The principles of managing awareness are the same for both adults and children. It is important to listen to the child, *be understanding and empathetic,* and not to be dismissive or unbelieving. The anesthetist should explain why the awareness occurred, although usually this will not be known. While most children do not develop significant psychological disturbance, some do. Therefore, it is important to *provide* some avenue for *support and follow-up*. It should be remembered that after awareness, post-traumatic stress symptoms may be delayed, so follow-up should be extended and the family should be told to watch for signs of withdrawal, flashbacks, heightened anxiety, or sleep disturbance. If these occur, referral to a psychologist is warranted. In cases where the child was paralyzed and or if he or she is clearly distressed at the outset, then a referral for psychological counseling should be made without delay. The family should be told to inform any future anesthetists about the awareness event so the issue can be discussed openly at the time and to allow the anesthetist to consider measures that might reduce the risk.

SUMMARY

1. Awareness does occur in children.
2. Awareness occurs in all types of anesthesia in children, and specific high-risk groups have not been identified.
3. Awareness is usually less distressing in children, though in some children it can lead to severe psychological disturbance.
4. It is unclear why children are aware, but it should be remembered that children have higher anesthetic requirements.
5. In theory, there may be a role for EEG in preventing awareness in children, but it is unproven.
6. Children who describe awareness should be taken seriously.

ANNOTATED REFERENCES

- Davidson AJ, Huang GH, Czarnecki C, Gibson MA, Stewart SA, Jamsen K, Stargatt R. Awareness during anesthesia in children: a prospective cohort study. *Anesth Analg* 2005; 100: 653–661.
  The first recent study to show a high incidence of awareness in children.
- Davidson AJ, Sheppard SJ, Engwerda AL, Wong A, Phelan L, Ironfield CM, Stargatt R. Detecting awareness in children by using an auditory intervention. *Anesthesiology* 2008; 109: 619–624.
  This study found less awareness when a specific measure was used—children were played noises during anesthesia and asked if they recalled hearing anything.

- Lopez U, Habre W, Laurencon M, Haller G, Van der Linden M, Iselin-Chaves IA. Intraoperative awareness in children: the value of an interview adapted to their cognitive abilities. *Anaesthesia* 2007; 62: 778–789.

  The study that first highlighted the difficulties in measuring awareness in children.

- Osterman JE, Hopper J, Heran WJ, Keane TM, van der Kolk BA. Awareness under anesthesia and the development of post-traumatic stress disorder. *Gen Hosp Psychiatry* 2001; 23: 198–204.

  A small case series of people with post-traumatic stress disorder after awareness. Some were children when the awareness occurred.

Further Reading

Blusse van Oud-Alblas HJ, van Dijk M, Liu C, Tibboel D, Klein J, Weber F. Intraoperative awareness during paediatric anaesthesia. *Br J Anaesth* 2009; 102: 104–110.

Davidson AJ. Measuring anesthesia in children using the EEG. *Paediatr Anaesth* 2006; 16: 374–387.

Lopez U, Habre W, Van der Linden M, Iselin-Chaves IA. Intraoperative awareness in children and post-traumatic stress disorder. *Anaesthesia* 2008; 63: 474–481.

Lopez U, Habre W. Evaluation of intraoperative memory and postoperative behavior in children: are we really measuring what we intend to measure? *Paediatr Anaesth* 2009; 19: 1147–1151.

Malviya S, Galinkin JL, Bannister CF, Burke C, Zuk J, Popenhagen M, Brown S, Voepel-Lewis T. The incidence of intraoperative awareness in children: childhood awareness and recall evaluation. *Anesth Analg* 2009; 109: 1421–1427.

Myles PS, Leslie K, McNeil J, Forbes A, Chan MT. Bispectral index monitoring to prevent awareness during anaesthesia: the B-Aware randomised controlled trial. *Lancet* 2004; 363: 1757–1763.

Phelan L, Stargatt R, Davidson AJ. Long-term post-traumatic effects of intraoperative awareness in children. *Paediatr Anaesth* 2009; 19: 1152–1156.

PART 9

CHALLENGES IN PATIENTS

WITH HEMATOLOGIC AND

ONCOLOGIC DISORDERS

40

Sickle Cell Disease

**ALEXANDRA SZABOVA AND
KENNETH R. GOLDSCHNEIDER**

INTRODUCTION

0.2% of African-Americans have sickle cell anemia while, with 8% to 10% have sickle cell trait. This chapter provides an overiew of the etiology, pathophysiology, and treatment of sickle cell anemia as they affect anesthetic management—before, during, and after surgery.

LEARNING OBJECTIVES

1. Understand the etiology and pathophysiology of sickle cell disease.
2. Know the specifics of preoperative evaluation of a sickle cell patient and the indications for preoperative blood transfusion.
3. Be familiar with intraoperative management of patients with sickle cell disease.
4. Understand the issues in postoperative management.

CASE PRESENTATION

*A 10-year-old girl with a history of sickle cell disease (**HbSS**) presents for preoperative preparation for laparoscopic cholecystectomy. She was hospitalized a month ago for gallstone-induced acute pancreatitis.*

*Although generally healthy, the girl was hospitalized one other time for **acute chest syndrome**. She has had her "usual" aches and pains in her legs and low back, but does not usually need more than ibuprofen or a rare dose of a codeine preparation. Her other home medications include folic acid, and she is scheduled to start **hydroxyurea**. She now has IV fluids running and her **baseline hematocrit is 29 g/dL**. The patient's intravenous induction of general anesthesia and endotracheal intubation are uneventful, and a forced-air warming device is used to maintain normothermia. Her IV maintenance fluids are continued. For postoperative analgesia, she receives morphine 0.1 mg/kg at the beginning and ketorolac 0.5 mg/kg at the end of the case. At the end of the uneventful case, the patient's trachea is extubated after she emerges. In the recovery room she receives another dose of morphine of 0.05 mg/kg IV. The recovery room nurses are instructed to continue IV fluids, keep nasal cannula to maintain oxygen saturations more than 95%, and use additional morphine boluses if needed to keep her comfortable. The bedside nurse calls from the recovery room to say that the patient complains of **chest pain**. The nurse gave two additional doses of morphine without significant improvement. The patient's lungs sound coarse on auscultation; she has slightly more labored breathing and a respiratory rate of 45 breaths per minute. Her saturation is 96% on 2 L/min **oxygen via nasal cannula** and her temperature is 35.9°C. An urgently performed chest radiograph reveals **bilateral infiltrates**, and her hematocrit is now 24 g/dL. The girl's hematologist recommends a **transfusion** of packed red blood cells and the patient is transferred to the **intensive care unit** for close monitoring.*

DISCUSSION

1. What is sickle cell disease or anemia, and what are the preoperative concerns for a patient with sickle cell disease?

In this autosomal recessive disease, the normal hemoglobin A is replaced by hemoglobin S. The normal hemoglobin molecule is a tetramer consisting of four subunits—two alpha and two beta.

Hemoglobin S consists of two normal alpha subunits and two abnormal subunits, where valine substitutes for glutamic acid at the sixth position on the beta chain. Sickling occurs due to hemoglobin polymer formation when PaO_2 drops below 20 mmHg in heterozygotes, and below 40 mmHg in homozygous patients. Polymerized hemoglobin increases blood viscosity and obstructs microcirculation. This further increases hypoxia and sickling and a vicious circle results in tissue infarction, release of inflammatory mediators, and pain. Acidosis, cold, dehydration, trauma, infection, fever, and stress predispose to sickling. Protective factors may include the presence of hemoglobin F (fetal hemoglobin—two alpha and two gamma subunits), which has higher affinity for oxygen. Hemoglobin F is the main hemoglobin present at birth, but its levels decrease significantly after 6 months of age. Around this time the symptoms of sickle cell anemia may become apparent. Disease severity can range from mild in sickle cell *trait* (40% hemoglobin S) to severe (and potentially fatal) sickle cell *anemia* (70–98% hemoglobin S). Diagnosis is made by hemoglobin electrophoresis. Table 40.1 presents an overview of the clinical issues in sickle cell disease.

Clinically, sickle cell anemia presents as chronic hemolysis with acute exacerbations (crises). Acute exacerbations themselves can manifest as painful crises (e.g., abdominal pain mimicking surgical diagnosis or musculoskeletal pain), infarctive crisis, sequestration crisis (with blood pooling in the spleen or liver), and aplastic crisis with complete bone marrow suppression. **Acute chest syndrome** is a medical emergency (mortality up to 10%), the cause of which is not fully understood.

2. What are preoperative considerations for patients with HbSS?

It is helpful to think about the perioperative management in terms of a **key factor quartet: oxygenation, hydration, normothermia, and hematocrit**. In some institutions, patients are admitted 12 to 24 hours preceding the surgery for IV hydration. Preoperative transfusion is indicated for patients undergoing

Table 40.1

OVERVIEW OF CLINICAL ISSUES IN SICKLE CELL DISEASE

Causes of Sickling
Hypoxemia
Hypotension
Hypovolemia
Hyperviscosity
Vasoconstriction
Acidosis
Fever
Increases in 2,3-diphosphoglyceride
Shivering or increased metabolic rate

Clinical Syndromes of Sickle Cell Disease
Chronic pain
Painful or vaso-occlusive crises
Aplastic
Sequestration
Hemolysis (chronic or acute)
Acute chest syndrome

Systemic Effects of Sickle Cell Anemia
Constitutional: Delayed growth and development
Immunologic: Infections, sepsis (especially encapsulated organisms)
Cardiac: Congestive heart failure (due to chronic hypoxia, anemia, and hemochromatosis)
Pulmonary: Increased intrapulmonary shunting
Renal: Papillary necrosis (more in sickle trait), concentrating deficiency
Neurologic: Stroke and sequelae
Hematologic: Chronic anemia, aplastic anemia (parvovirus B19 associated)
Genital: Priapism
Gastrointestinal: Cholelithiasis
Splenic: Infarcts, asplenia, acute sequestration
Skeletal: Avascular necrosis, osteomyelitis
Skin: Ulcers (ankle)
Metabolic: Hemochromatosis

intermediate- and high-risk surgery with or without an underlying pulmonary disorder, with a target hemoglobin 10 mg/dL or higher. Preoperative anxiolytics can be used, with attention to preventing respiratory suppression that might lead to oxygen desaturation, which can trigger sickling. Supplemental oxygen in patients receiving preoperative sedatives is reasonable. A forced-air warmer or similar device is helpful to maintain normal body temperature, and applying it prior to induction of anesthesia helps reduce the drop in temperature that results from the pooling of central and peripheral circulatory compartments caused by general anesthetics. As to packed red blood cell transfusions, data suggest that a conservative regimen targeting a total hemoglobin level of 10 g/dL offers the same efficacy in preventing perioperative complications as an aggressive regimen (target HbSS <30% total), but with half of the transfusion-related complications (Vichinsky et al., 1995). Patients with sickle cell trait do not require preoperative transfusion, except before open heart surgery or extensive thoracic surgery.

3. How does hydroxyurea work in sickle cell disease?

The treatment of sickle cell anemia can be divided in two groups: prophylactic and symptomatic. **Hydroxyurea** is used as part of **prophylactic treatment** to prevent crisis and complications related to the disease. **Hydroxyurea** stimulates hemoglobin F production. Higher levels of hemoglobin F diminish the severity of crises by preventing hemoglobin S polymerization (Charache et al., 1995). Other widely used prophylactic interventions include administration of pneumococcal vaccine and antibiotics in febrile illness/acute chest syndrome. Folic acid is prescribed to prevent megaloblastic anemia. Bone marrow transplantation is reserved for patients less than 16 years of age who have had multiple serious complications related to sickle cell anemia and crises.

Symptomatic treatment in painful episodes starts with rehydration. Pain management follows an ascending algorithm beginning with acetaminophen and nonsteroidal anti-inflammatory drugs (NSAIDs). Patients in crisis usually have moved beyond this step by the time they present to the hospital and often have begun oral opioids at home. Advancing the oral regimen or adding IV opioids, either intermittently or via patient-controlled analgesia pump, is appropriate, depending on previous history of chronic analgesic use, severity of pain, and symptoms. Regional and neuraxial analgesia are also good options. For long-term pain management, acetaminophen, NSAIDs, opioids, and adjuncts have been used (e.g., gabapentin for bony pain, the tricyclic antidepressant amitriptyline for abdominal pain and sleep disturbances).

4. What is acute chest syndrome, and how is it managed?

Acute chest syndrome is a medical emergency that is a feared complication in the post-anesthetic phase, with significant morbidity and mortality (mortality up to 10%). Patients present with an acute pain crisis (lower chest), fever, cough, pleuritic **chest pain**, hypoxemia, pulmonary hypertension, and **lung infiltrates** of the lower bases on chest radiograph. Patients with acute chest syndrome may have concomitant rib infarcts. Recurrent episodes progress to pulmonary fibrosis and chronic respiratory insufficiency. The management follows the quartet of key factors: oxygenation, hydration, normothermia, and hemoglobin. Start **supplemental oxygen via nasal cannula** or face mask to maintain normal oxygen saturation. Hydrate the patient—replace deficits first, maintain hydration with close attention to losses (due to sweating, high fever, urine output, vomiting), and treat fever or hypothermia. **Transfusion** may be indicated, either simple or exchange, depending on the severity of symptoms. Inhaled bronchodilators may be indicated in patients with acute chest syndrome if there is a component of increased airway reactivity. There are few data regarding antibiotic administration in patients with acute chest syndrome; the treatment to date is empiric. An infectious etiology can be identified in only 30% of patients, 10% suffer an embolic event (fat embolism from necrotic marrow), but the majority of patients have an unclear etiology. Pain medications—preferably NSAIDs such as ketorolac, or cautious use of opioids (avoid respiratory depression and worsening oxygenation)—and incentive spirometry are frequently indicated.

Epidural analgesia may be helpful for patients whose analgesia is limited by opioid side effects. Patients may require **admission to the intensive care unit** or other unit where they can be more closely monitored, and their hematologist should be consulted.

5. What are the intra- and postoperative concerns for these patients?

If a patient with sickle cell disease has been adequately prepared preoperatively, then the outcome of the anesthetic should be good. Intraoperative management again follows the quartet of key factors—*oxygenation, hydration, normothermia, and hemoglobin*. There is no unique anesthetic selection for sickle cell patients. Regional anesthesia has been successfully used as the primary anesthetic as well as an adjunct to general anesthesia. Cardiopulmonary bypass represents a unique challenge as it is a combination of hypothermia, acidosis, and low peripheral blood flow. Sickle cell disease patients seem to tolerate it without increased risk (Yousafzai et al., 2010). The use of tourniquets during the surgery is discouraged, although not strictly contraindicated.

Postoperatively. maintain the homeostatic quartet through the post-anesthesia care unit (PACU) until the patient has fully emerged and is ready to be discharged from the PACU. Shivering in the PACU should be treated aggressively, as vigorous exertion can trigger sickling. Note that sickle cell patients may require larger quantities of opioids for analgesia than other patients, due to chronic exposure-induced tolerance. The hematology team should be contacted soon postoperatively to coordinate care, especially for patients with a history of stroke, acute chest syndrome, or splenic sequestration.

SUMMARY

1. Consider admission 12 to 24 hours prior to surgery for hydration and transfusion if hemoglobin is less than 10 g/dL.

2. Key intraoperative factors are oxygenation, hydration, body temperature, and hemoglobin over 10 g/dL.
3. Postoperatively maintain oxygenation, hydration, and body temperature; start incentive spirometry early; and consider overnight observation.
4. For postoperative pain management, patients may be opioid-tolerant. The full range of analgesics may be used; regional analgesia can be used for either postoperative pain or that of vaso-occlusive crises.

ANNOTATED REFERENCES

- Charache S, Terrin ML, Moore RD, et al. Effect of hydroxyurea on the frequency of painful crises in sickle cell anemia. Investigators of the Multicenter Study of Hydroxyurea in Sickle Cell Anemia. *N Engl J Med* 1995; 332(20): 1317–1322.

  This double-blind randomized controlled trial tested the efficacy of hydroxyurea versus placebo on the frequency and severity of crises in adult patients. The trial was terminated prematurely due to strong evidence for patient benefit.

- Vichinsky EP, Haberkern CM, Neumayr L, et al. A comparison of conservative and aggressive transfusion regimens in the perioperative management of sickle cell disease. The Preoperative Transfusion in Sickle Cell Disease Study Group. *N Engl J Med* 1995; 333(4): 206–213.

  The landmark randomized controlled trial that showed that an aggressive transfusion regimen (hemoglobin S <30%) was comparable to a conservative regimen (to achieve a hemoglobin level of 10 g/dL) in preventing perioperative complications in patients with HbSS. The conservative approach reduced transfusion-associated complications by 50%.

- Yaster M, Tobin JR, Billett C, Casella JF, Dover G. Epidural analgesia in the management of severe vaso-occlusive sickle cell crisis. *Pediatrics* 1994; 93(2): 310–315.

An early, retrospective study of nine patients admitted with vaso-occlusive crisis who failed to respond to conventional analgesia. Epidural analgesia was effective in treating vaso-occlusive pain without causing sedation, respiratory depression, or limitation on ambulation.

Further Reading

Alhashimi D, Fedorowicz A, Alhashimi F, Dastgiri S. Blood transfusion for treating acute chest syndrome in people with sickle cell disease. *Cochrane Database System Rev* 2010; Issue 1. Art NO.: CD007843. DOI 10.1002/14651858.CD007843.pub2.

de Montalembert M. Management of sickle cell disease. *Br Med J* 2008; 337: a1397.

Frietsch T. Ewen I. Waschke KF. Anaesthetic care for sickle cell disease. *Eur J Anaesth* 2001; 18(3): 137–150.

Marchant WA, Walker I. Anaesthetic management of the child with sickle cell disease. *Paediatr Anaesth* 2003; 13(6): 473–489.

Wethers D. Sickle cell disease in childhood: Part I. Laboratory diagnosis, pathophysiology and health maintenance. *Am Fam Physician* 2000; 62: 1013–1028.

Wethers D. Sickle cell disease in childhood: Part II. Diagnosis and treatment of major complications and recent advances in treatment. *Am Fam Physician* 2000; 62: 1309–1314.

Yousafzai SM, Ugurlucan M, Al Radhwan OA, Al Otaibi AL, Canver CC. Open heart surgery in patients with sickle cell hemoglobinopathy. *Circulation* 2010; 121(1): 14–19.

Hemophilia

REBECCA McINTYRE

INTRODUCTION

Recent advances in the management of patients with hemophilia have led to significantly improved outcomes. Transmission of infectious diseases through blood product administration and severe arthropathies from recurrent joint bleeds are now rare. In the past, hemophilia was considered a contraindication to having some elective surgery such as adenotonsillectomy due to the risk of life-threatening bleeding complications. Nowadays, management of elective surgery in these patients can be straightforward and safe, provided adequate planning and consultation with a hematologist occur.

LEARNING OBJECTIVES

1. Understand the pathophysiology and classification of hemophilia.
2. Be familiar with the classification and methods of diagnosis of hemophilia and other bleeding disorders.
3. Know the principles of management of patients with hemophilia undergoing elective surgery.
4. Understand the adverse effects of therapy for hemophilia.

CASE PRESENTATION

*A 12-year-old boy is booked to have elective adenotonsillectomy and insertion of myringotomy tubes. He has severe **hemophilia A** (factor VIII 0%). He weighs 36 kg.*

*Anesthesia and Hematology were notified of the planned surgery date by the ENT surgeon. **Hematology formulated a plan for factor replacement** that was written in the patient notes for reference on the day of surgery. Otherwise his preoperative assessment was unremarkable.*

*Just prior to induction, 2,000 units (50 units/kg) of recombinant factor VIII (rFVIII) are given via a peripheral intravenous line. A second intravenous cannula (18G) is placed in case of rapid bleeding. Surgery proceeds uneventfully. At the conclusion of surgery, laryngoscopy reveals a dry surgical field, with minimal blood suctioned from the oropharynx. The patient is transferred to the bed and placed in the lateral position. He is extubated when he opens his eyes to command and coughs. He is transferred to recovery, where a further bolus dose of 1,000 units (30 units/kg) of rFVIII is given intravenously. On the ward, the team runs a continuous infusion of 108 units/hr (3 units/kg/hr) for 72 hours. The team also prescribes tranexamic acid 750 mg orally three times a day, to be continued for 14 days. For analgesia, he receives acetaminophen (paracetamol) and oxycodone as required. **Nonsteroidal anti-inflammatory drugs are avoided**. At 72 hours his status is reviewed on the ward by Hematology. As there are no bleeding problems, he is given a further intravenous bolus dose of 1,000 units rFVIII and discharged home. At home, he self-administers 1,000 units of rFVIII intravenously every second day until 10 days after surgery.*

DISCUSSION

1. How does hemophilia affect coagulation?

The current model of coagulation describes a complex network of various elements that are activated by tissue injury. This model describes interactions that occur on two cell types: tissue factor (TF)-bearing cells and platelets. In this model, coagulation can be divided into an initiation phase, an amplification phase, and a propagation phase. Coagulation is initially triggered by low levels of circulating activated factor VII (fVIIa) binding to TF, which is exposed following vessel injury. fVIIa then activates factor X, which then generates small amounts of thrombin. This reaction is inhibited by tissue factor pathway inhibitor (TFPI) and anti-thrombin (AT) until high enough levels of TF generate enough thrombin to overcome this inhibition (amplification). When this occurs, thrombin activates platelets, fV, fVIII, and fXI, which further increases thrombin generation in a positive feedback mechanism (propagation). Propagation occurs effectively only on the surface of platelets and requires sufficient levels of circulating coagulation factors in the blood (Tanaka et al., 2009; Hoffman, 2003).

In hemophilia A (factor VIII deficiency) and hemophilia B (factor IX deficiency), the initiation of coagulation is normal, but the propagation phase at the platelet level, which is dependent on VIIIa and IXa, is severely impaired. This leads to the clinical picture of uncontrolled bleeding.

Hemophilia is classified as mild, moderate, or severe, according to the concentration of plasma factor level measured. A factor level below 1% of normal is classified as severe, 1% to 5% of normal is moderate, and 5% to 40% of normal is mild.

Patients with severe hemophilia are susceptible to frequent and often spontaneous bleeding. This bleeding may be into joints, soft tissues, the CNS, the airway, or the retroperitoneum or around major organs. Patients with mild disease will usually not have spontaneous hemorrhage but will bleed following surgery or trauma. The child in this scenario has severe hemophilia A. Therefore, without treatment he is prone to spontaneous bleeds and will bleed uncontrollably after trauma or surgery. He is dependent on factor VIII injections to prevent and treat bleeding episodes.

2. How is hemophilia diagnosed?

The clinical features of hemophilia A and hemophilia B are identical and, as discussed above, the clinical picture depends on the degree of factor deficiency. In severe disease, bleeding episodes begin at an early age, are frequent, and occur spontaneously or with only minor trauma. In mild disease, bleeding occurs only with major trauma and may not present until later in life. A history of excessive bleeding following minor trauma, or bleeding following dental procedures, or a family history of hemophilia can raise suspicion. As hemophilia A and B are X-linked inherited disorders, males inherit the gene from female carriers (Table 41.1). Carriers may have a mild form of the disease and can also be at risk of bleeding during surgery.

A coagulation screen will show a prolonged aPTT and normal PT. Specific factor level assays confirm the diagnosis and the severity of disease. Other inherited bleeding disorders can be detected by screening blood tests if a history of easy bleeding is elicited. Von Willebrand disease is more common than hemophilia, occurring in 1% to 3% of the population, and is caused by an inherited deficiency of von Willebrand factor. There are more than 20 types of von Willebrand disease, and interpretation of

Table 41.1			
INHERITANCE OF MAJOR BLEEDING DISORDERS			
	Deficiency	*Inheritance*	*Incidence*
Hemophilia A	Factor VIII	X-linked recessive	1 in 10,000 live male births
Hemophilia B	Factor IX	X-linked recessive	1 in 25,000 live male births
Von Willebrand disease	Von Willebrand factor	Autosomal dominant (common forms)	1–3 in 100

laboratory tests in suspected patients is complex. PT and aPTT may be normal, and further evaluation includes measuring ristocetin cofactor activity, vWF antigen levels, factor VIII coagulant activity, and platelet count. Other, less common inherited bleeding disorders include deficiencies of factor II, factor V, factor VII, factor X, factor XI, and factor XIII (Lee, 2004).

3. How should a patient with hemophilia for elective surgery be managed?

If surgery is indicated in a patient with hemophilia, careful planning is important to ensure that the surgery can proceed safely (Table 41.2). The procedure should always be undertaken at a specialist center with hemophilia expertise.

The first step in the preoperative evaluation is to ascertain the type and severity of the hemophilia, as this will guide therapy. The aim is to restore factor levels to normal during the time that bleeding may occur. This is primarily achieved by factor replacement (either plasma-derived or recombinant), which can be given as an infusion or as a bolus. In this case, the patient has severe hemophilia A, so he requires factor VIII replacement to bring his factor VIII level to 100% during and immediately after surgery. In adenotonsillectomy, bleeding may occur up to 14 days after surgery. This patient was therefore given additional factor replacement for 10 days after surgery. As he was able to administer factor VIII at home, and was considered relatively low risk for postoperative bleeding after day two with suitable factor replacement, he was discharged home on day 3. This may not always be possible, and other issues must be considered in making this decision. For instance, the patient must be able to access emergency hospital services promptly in case of a problem at home. Distance from the hospital, social factors, and willingness to comply with treatment at home must all be taken into account.

In some cases of mild hemophilia A, normal factor levels may be achieved using desmopressin (DDAVP) alone. This acts by releasing stored factor VIII (and vWF) into the circulation. If a

Table 41.2
LOGISTICAL EFFECTS OF HEMOPHILIA IN THE OPERATING ROOM

Venous access:
Difficult peripheral access due to scarring
Fear/anxiety about cannulation
Central line infection and clotting risks

Factor administration:
Antibody-mediated inhibitors affect achieving therapeutic levels of factor
Potential allergic response to administration of factor

Positioning and general management:
Arthropathy: contractures may affect positioning
Acquired brain injury from intracerebral bleeding may lead to seizure, behavioral and spasticity considerations

Minor procedures:
Bleeding risk from minor trauma requires judicious placement of nasogastric tubes, regional anesthesia blocks, arterial lines, intramuscular injections

Infection control:
Precautions are advisable (as for all patients) against HIV, hepatitis C and B, Creutzfeld-Jacob disease; all can be acquired via repeated transfusions

patient has been shown to have an adequate response to a DDAVP challenge, this may be the first line of therapy. The dose is 0.3 mcg/kg intravenously.

Antifibrinolytics (such as tranexamic acid and ε-aminocaproic acid) can be useful in preventing and treating mucous membrane hemorrhage (Association of Hemophilia Clinic Directors of Canada, 1995). The patient in the case above was treated with tranexamic acid for 14 days to help prevent bleeding from the oral and nasal mucosa postoperatively.

Intraoperatively the anesthetist should be vigilant for abnormal bleeding. Should bleeding occur despite factor replacement, factor assays should be checked and Hematology consulted. If bleeding occurs despite adequate factor replacement, the likely problem is surgical, though the development of inhibitors should be considered and tested.

Other considerations in managing a child with hemophilia include assessment of any long-term complications of the disease. The life-limiting complications of hemophilia in the past were related to the transmission of infectious diseases such as HIV and hepatitis C, and debilitating arthropathy due to recurrent hemarthroses. Fortunately, with the advent of better blood screening and recombinant factors, blood transfusion-related infections are almost nonexistent (although the potential for prion disease transmission is still unknown). With prophylactic factor replacement used to prevent recurrent hemarthroses, joints are now well preserved. Boys with hemophilia now have a normal life expectancy without severe disability. Treatment costs are high, but the outcomes are excellent.

Children with hemophilia can have difficult problems related to venous access. Those with difficult access who require regular treatments may have a long-term surgically placed central venous catheter in place. These catheters are prone to complications, particularly infection, and must be treated with care when used. Strict asepsis must be adhered to when accessing and using these long-term lines. Patients who do not have a central line may have an established and effective way of managing intravenous access to help make a potentially painful and stressful procedure acceptable to them. Local anesthetic cream, premedication, parental presence, play therapy, and distraction techniques may be used. The patient or parent may also know which veins are the easiest to cannulate. Discussing how the patient prefers to have his veins accessed is the best way to ensure the patient's cooperation and the anesthetist's success.

In general, regional blocks, intramuscular injections, and arterial punctures should be avoided in patients with hemophilia.

Aspirin and nonsteroidal anti-inflammatory drugs should be avoided. Intravenous cannulas should be treated with care and checked frequently to ensure correct placement. If venipunctures are required, firm pressure should be applied for 3 minutes to the site afterwards.

4. What are potential adverse effects of therapy in hemophilia?

DDAVP is useful in patients with mild hemophilia A and can increase factor VIII levels two- to three-fold within 30 to 60 minutes of infusion. However, there have been case reports of severe hyponatremia and seizures related to its use (Francis et al., 1999). Close monitoring of electrolytes and avoidance of hypotonic fluids with the use of DDAVP is prudent.

Replacement of factors in patients with hemophilia with plasma-derived products carries the risk of transmission of viruses, such as HIV and hepatitis C. The development of recombinant factor concentrates as well as improved screening of blood donors has reduced the incidence of virus transmission in this group.

Development of inhibitors is a treatment-related complication of hemophilia. An inhibitor is an antibody directed against exogenously administered factor VIII or IX, which renders factor replacement ineffective. It occurs in about 20% of cases of severe hemophilia A, and in 3% of patients with severe hemophilia B (Lee, 2004). Inhibitors to factor IX can be associated with anaphylaxis.

Treatment of patients with inhibitors can be challenging, but there has been some success in inducing immune tolerance in these patients by exposing them to frequent high doses of factor replacement over a period of time. In acute bleeding episodes in patients with inhibitors, activated recombinant factor VII (rFVIIa) can be used. rFVIIa directly activates factor X, bypassing the need for factor VIII or IX in the clotting cascade. The dose is 90 to 100 mcg/kg every 2 to 3 hours.

SUMMARY

1. Hemophilia A and B (deficiencies of factor VIII and IX) pose severe hemorrhagic risk for boys.
2. Cooperative management with Hematology and aggressive replacement of the appropriate factor are important.
3. Preoperative evaluation of these patients should include looking for vascular access difficulties, infectious sequelae of repeated transfusions, and joint and neurologic sequelae of prior bleeding episodes.

ANNOTATED REFERENCES

- Hoffman M. Remodeling the blood coagulation cascade. *J Thrombosis Thrombolysis* 2003; 16(1/2): 17–20.

  This paper describes a cell-based model of coagulation that, unlike older biochemical models, is better able to explain why hemophiliacs have a bleeding tendency.

- Lee J-W. Von Willebrand disease, hemophilia A and B, and other factor deficiencies. *Int Anesth Clin* 2004; 42(3): 59–76.

  Aimed at anesthesiologists, this practical review of the pathophysiology of the common inherited bleeding disorders outlines recommended perioperative management strategies.

- Tanaka, KA, Key NS, Levy JH. Blood coagulation: hemostasis and thrombin regulation. *Anesth Analg* 2009; 108: 1433–1446.

  This review comprehensively describes the current concepts of coagulation, its regulation, and responses to surgery and bleeding. It also outlines drugs used to modulate the coagulation system to control bleeding and thrombotic complications

Further Reading

Association of Hemophilia Clinic Directors of Canada. Hemophilia and von Willebrand's disease: 2. Management. *Can Med Assoc J* 1995, 153 (2): 147–157.

Conlon B, Daly N, Temperely I, McShane D. ENT surgery in children with inherited bleeding disorders. *J Laryng Otol* 1996: 110: 947–949.

Francis JD, Leary T, Niblett DJ. Convulsions and respiratory arrest in association with desmopressin administration for the treatment of a bleeding tonsil in a child with borderline haemophilia. *Acta Anaesthesiol Scand* 1999; 43: 870–873.

Haberkern CM, Webel N, Eisses MJ, Bender MA. Essentials of hematology. In: CJ Cote, JL Lerman, TD Todres, eds. *A Practice of Anesthesia for Infants and Children*, 4th ed. Philadelphia: Saunders Elsevier, 2009: 188–191.

Prinsley P, Wood M, Lee CA. Adenotonsillectomy in patients with inherited bleeding disorders. *Clin Otolaryngol Allied Sci* 1993; 18(3): 206–208.

Roberts HR, Monahan PE. Pediatric Hemophilia: Diagnosis, Classification, and Management. Medscape CME Pediatrics 2010, retrieved from http://cme.medscape.com/viewprogram/30887

42

Oncology Patient

MARK J. MEYER AND NORBERT J. WEIDNER

INTRODUCTION

The pediatric oncology population presents challenges to the anesthesiologist. Many of these patients undergo multiple lumbar punctures and bone marrow aspirations as part of their treatment protocol. Radiation therapy is another treatment modality that requires the assistance of an anesthesiologist to be successful for younger children. While seemingly minor procedures, they are a source of anxiety for patients and parents. Furthermore, patients can present with a number of physiological derangements such as anemia, coagulopathies, and toxicities from chemotherapeutic agents. Further, these patients are often infants and toddlers who require attention to their developmental level during anesthetic planning.

LEARNING OBJECTIVES

1. Understand the advantages of general anesthesia for common painful procedures for the pediatric hematology/oncology patient.
2. Review the medical problems of oncology patients, including anthracycline-induced cardiac toxicity, anemia, and thrombocytopenia.
3. Discuss the advantages of various anesthetic techniques for the pediatric oncology patient undergoing

lumbar puncture and bone marrow aspiration and biopsy.
4. Outline the challenges of providing anesthesia for the radiation oncology patient.

CASE PRESENTATION

An 11-year-old boy with lymphoma presents for bone marrow aspiration. Two weeks before, he presented with chest pain and **dyspnea**. *CT evaluation revealed a large anterior mediastinal mass with moderate compression of the right main bronchus and compression of the superior vena cava and the right atrium. He required ICU admission for monitoring of his cardiovascular and respiratory status until therapy could be established. After induction therapy for his lymphoma began, his dyspnea resolved, and he was released from the ICU. Prior to discharge from the ICU, however, he underwent a* **bone marrow biopsy with sedation** *and his parents report that he* **fears his next procedure**. *After 2 weeks of therapy, he has responded well to treatment and his symptoms have resolved. Initial plans for* **radiation treatment** *were deferred. His* **platelet count is 35×10^9/L** *and he is mildly* **anemic**. **Echocardiography** *reveals normal anatomy and biventricular function. His chest x-ray is clear, with no evidence of mediastinal mass. He appears* **fearful** *as he enters the preoperative holding area. His vital signs are normal and his examination is remarkable only for signs of an* **upper respiratory tract infection**.

DISCUSSION

1. What are common hematologic derangements in oncology patients? To what extent are they a concern?

Patients with leukemias and solid malignancies present with bone marrow involvement or have poor marrow production from chemotherapy. Therefore, these patients are often coagulopathic and anemic. In patients with leukemia, thrombocytopenia is common at diagnosis and throughout early treatment. For lumbar puncture, **platelet counts above 50 × 10⁹/L** are acceptable in the absence of active bleeding. Platelet transfusion is considered for those below that level to reduce the risk of epidural hematoma formation.

For bone marrow aspiration, the coagulation status of the patient is less important. Oozing stops with pressure whether an anterior or posterior approach is chosen. Though a hematoma may form, these tend to be small and limited and will not compress key structures.

Anemia is a concern, and most patients are transfused based upon their clinical status. Most otherwise healthy patients can tolerate hematocrits in the mid-twenties under general anesthesia. For patients who are physiologically stressed or have concurrent cardiac or pulmonary disease, a higher hematocrit may be necessary.

2. What cardiotoxic effects are seen with chemotherapy?

Leukemia and lymphoma protocols call for the use of anthracyclines that are known to be cardiotoxic above a defined cumulative lifetime dose. For doxorubicin, the lifetime cumulative dose of 550 mg/m² is the threshold above which cardiac toxicity generally occurs. Toxicity can occur immediately following treatment or may be delayed in onset. Acute anthracycline-induced cardiotoxicity manifests as arrhythmias, pericarditis, cardiomyopathy, and heart failure. However, patients are at greater risk for cardiotoxicity as a result of the cumulative dose. Although contemporary chemotherapy protocols for leukemics do not exceed this threshold value, toxicity can develop even with lower doses. Those with relapse may receive doses above this recognized limit.

Above the recognized threshold, toxicity does not appear to be dose-dependent but the incidence is increased. For survivors, the cardiotoxic effects of anthracyclines can be prolonged, affecting patients for years after their treatment. Under general anesthesia, cardiotoxicity presents as myocardial dysfunction and conduction problems. During the preoperative evaluation, it is important to assess the patient's functional cardiac capacity by inquiring about exercise tolerance, **dyspnea** on exertion, and ortho-pnea. Current protocols call for baseline **echocardiography** at the initiation of treatment and re-evaluation as treatment progresses.

3. What are the advantages of general anesthesia for this patient population?

When compared to conscious sedation, general anesthesia offers several benefits to all concerned: patients and their families, the nursing staff, and the oncologist. While children can tolerate these painful procedures with distraction, topical anesthesia, and conscious sedation, the unaddressed suffering from these tech-niques can inflict considerable distress to all those involved. There is evidence that considerable anxiety and behavioral dis-tress occurs as a result of repeated painful procedures.

Children undergoing painful procedures with conscious seda-tion may find them difficult to tolerate. Considerable physical restraint may be necessary, causing further anxiety and fear. As seen in this patient, a failed sedation led to significant **anticipa-tory anxiety**, which will have to be addressed at future proce-dures. Furthermore, in busy, high-acuity centers, failure to complete the procedure results in delayed diagnosis, delayed treatment, and disrupted clinical roadmaps. One study found that when general anesthesia is compared to conscious sedation, physical restraint was required in 94% of the sedation group. 66% required firm restrain and there was a 10% failure to per-form the procedure in the conscious sedation group. Hospital nursing staff are more satisfied with general anesthesia, since restraining a resisting child causes them considerable distress as well. Therefore, general anesthesia offers fewer procedural fail-ures and greater satisfaction from the patient, family, and staff (Crock et al., 2003).

4. Which anesthetic techniques have been demonstrated to be the safest and most effective?

The ideal general anesthetic technique minimizes anxiety on induction, has few side effects, is readily titratable, and permits a rapid wake-up. Most oncology patients have established central venous access, providing an easy route for rapid intravenous induction. Maintenance can be provided with inhalational agents or propofol (as an "intermittent bolus" or "infusion" technique). Intravenous maintenance with propofol results in fewer airway complications such as laryngospasm and lowers the risk of emergence delirium compared to sevoflurane. While lumbar punctures are modestly painful during the needle entrance part of the procedure, bone marrow aspiration and biopsy cause more pain both during and after the procedure. Injection of a local anesthetic prior to bone marrow needle insertion is helpful to anesthetize the periosteum as well as the skin. Additionally, premedicating the patient with intravenous fentanyl (1 mcg/kg) 5 minutes prior to induction and maintenance with propofol reduces propofol usage and recovery times for bone marrow biopsy and aspiration.

Patients with myocardial dysfunction from chemotherapy may not tolerate the vasodilation from a propofol induction. Etomidate can be used as the induction agent and maintenance provided with propofol, carefully titrated as needed.

5. What are the challenges that face the anesthesiologist during radiation therapy?

Safe and effective **radiation therapy** for children requires the patient to remain motionless so that the radiation beams focus only on the pathological tissue or field, minimizing radiation exposure to healthy tissues. Multiple treatments are often required over a period of weeks, each requiring exactly the same position of the patient. Treatments may last from 5 to 60 minutes and regimens may include 1 to 35 treatments, with each treatment occurring on successive days. During the radiation treatment, no one can be present in the treatment room with the child. Many children ages 7 and above can do this awake with proper instruction and encouragement from family and staff, but younger children and older children with developmental delays are not able to hold still without sedation or general anesthesia.

There are many challenges to the anesthesiologist. The radiation oncology environment is hostile for the anesthesiologist.

During the treatment, the patient is isolated in the lead-lined treatment room and the anesthesiologist, who sits outside the treatment room, can only observe the patient via a video monitor (Fig. 42.1). If the patient requires immediate care from the anesthesiologist, the radiation treatment must be interrupted. Therefore, pre-anesthetic planning should include learning the location of the emergency stop button and door releases. One should plan these emergency interventions with the radiation technologist.

In addition, many patient-related factors are problematic. Patients undergoing craniospinal radiation therapy are placed in a rigid mask that covers the patient's face and attaches to the treatment table. This mask ensures exactly the same position of the patient for each of the treatments, but it limits access to the patient's airway. Use of an endotracheal tube or LMA is only

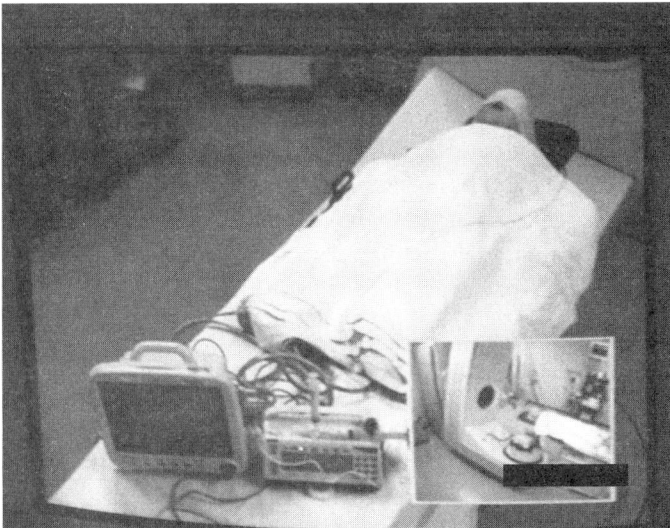

FIGURE 42.1 Patient having radiation therapy. Note head-positioning mask and need for remote video monitoring.

occasionally needed, but it can be awkward to place and maintain it when the positioning mask is in place. In some cases, a poorly fitted mask can contribute to airway obstruction and cause pain. Although seeing a patient daily can make the process seem routine, the patient's airway needs to be reassessed daily. As treatment progresses, mucositis and airway edema can occur and adjustments to airway management may be needed at any time in the series of treatments.

Anesthetic technique for non-emergent treatment involves an intravenous induction with propofol. The airway can be maintained with an oropharyngeal airway or nasopharyngeal airway, using a spontaneous respiration technique. The eyes are taped closed and the patient is monitored with pulse oximetry, ECG, noninvasive blood pressure cuff, and capnography. Maintenance can be accomplished with boluses of propofol for brief treatments and with infusions of propofol for longer treatments. The treatments are not stimulating to the patient, so lower doses can often be used.

ASA guidelines for fasting and intraoperative and postoperative monitoring should be followed for all procedures. Most patients can be effectively managed without intubation, but patients coming for emergency radiation therapy who are not fasted and those who are actively vomiting (usually those receiving chemotherapy) should undergo endotracheal intubation with a rapid-sequence induction.

Not uncommonly, pediatric patients will present with an **upper respiratory tract infection** during the course of their treatment for leukemia or solid tumor. For common elective cases, such as hernia repair, cancellation of the procedure may be prudent; generally there are few medical consequences. In contrast, diagnostic and therapeutic procedures for oncology patients are not elective in nature, and delaying procedures may have serious consequences. Therefore, the decision to proceed with or cancel the anesthetic must be made with careful consideration and discussion with the oncology team.

SUMMARY

1. Pediatric oncology patients often present with serious medical problems related to their cancer as well as to complications of their cancer treatment (e.g., chemotherapy-induced cardiac toxicity).
2. General anesthesia has advantages over conscious sedation for lumbar puncture and bone marrow aspiration/biopsy. It offers fewer procedural failures and greater patient, family, and staff satisfaction.
3. Poorly conducted sedation can result in considerable longstanding harm to children undergoing repeat procedures.

ANNOTATED REFERENCES

- Crock C, Olsson C, Phillips R, Chalkiadis G, Sawyer S, Ashley D, Camilleri S, Carlin J, Monagle P. General anaesthesia or conscious sedation for painful procedures in childhood cancer: the family's perspective. *Arch Dis Child* 2003; 88: 253–257.

    Clearly presents the amount of restraint required for conscious sedation and the disparity in distress created by conscious sedation compared to general anesthesia.
- Hammer GB. Pediatric thoracic anesthesia. *Anesthesiol Clin North Am* 2002; 20: 153–180.

    This article outlines the anesthetic management of children who present with large mediastinal masses.
- Simbre VC, Duffy SA, Dadlani GH, Miller TL, Lipschultz SE. Cardiotoxicity of cancer chemotherapy: implications for children. *Paediatr Drugs* 2005; 15: 187–202.

An important article exploring the acute and chronic manifestation of cardiac toxicity of commonly used chemotherapeutic agents in children.

Further Reading

Maxwell LG, Yaster M. The myth of conscious sedation. *Arch Pediatr Adolesc Med* 1996; 150(7): 665–667.

Meyer MJ. Integration of pain services into pediatric oncology. *Intl Anesth Clin: Frontiers Pediatr Anesth* 2006; 44: 95–107.

Reeves ST, Havidich JE, Tobin DP. Conscious sedation in children with propofol is anything but conscious. *Pediatrics* 2004; 114: 74–76.

Scheiber G, Ribeiro FC, Karpienski H, Strehl, K. Deep sedation with propofol in preschool children undergoing radiation therapy. *Paediatr Anaesth* 1996; 6: 209–213.

Wiesman SJ, Bernstein B, Schecter NL. Consequences of inadequate analgesia during painful procedures in children. *Arch Pediatr Adolesc Med* 1998; 152: 147–149.

43

Opioid-Tolerant Patient

ALEXANDRA SZABOVA AND
KENNETH R. GOLDSCHNEIDER

INTRODUCTION

Caring for patients who are taking chronic opioids may present several challenges for clinicians in the operating room and in the immediate postoperative period. Factors such as **tolerance** and **opioid-induced hyperalgesia** can complicate perioperative pain management.

LEARNING OBJECTIVES

1. Know the difference between tolerance, addiction, and pseudo-addiction.
2. Understand mechanisms of opioid-induced hyperalgesia.
3. Understand mechanisms of opioid tolerance.
4. Review basic principles of opioid rotation (switch).
5. Describe other options to treat the opioid-tolerant patient with acute-on-chronic pain.

CASE PRESENTATION

A 17-year-old, 50-kg girl with a history of tibial osteosarcoma presents for thoracoscopic biopsy of a new lung nodule. She underwent a limb salvage procedure about 10 months ago during which the sciatic nerve was injured. She has had significant neuropathic pain, which is being treated with gabapentin 900 mg three times a day, **methadone 30 mg three times a day,** *and oxycodone 15 mg as needed. Her average pain score with this regimen has been 4–5/10 on a numeric rating scale. She has no other medical problems and has suffered no apparent long-term effects from her chemotherapy. The anesthetic is uneventful, although the resident remarks that the patient requires 4.5% sevoflurane through the case. Fifteen minutes after the patient arrives in the recovery room, the recovery nurse calls to report that the patient has extreme pain and to ask for more rescue pain medications.*

The patient had 10 mg IV morphine in the operating room and an additional 9 mg of IV morphine in the recovery room over the past 30 minutes. She says that she took her gabapentin and methadone with dinner and a last dose of oxycodone before bed but did not take her medications this morning because she was told not to eat or drink before surgery. She reports that her abdomen hurts her, but not because she is hungry. She feels "weird," cold, but sweaty, almost shaking. A **titration** *scheme is established, and the nurse is made aware that the patient is opioid-***tolerant** *and* **will require high doses of opioids** *to become comfortable.*

DISCUSSION

1. How should a patient on preoperative opioids be approached differently from opioid-naïve patients?

When caring for opioid-tolerant patients, it is easy to overlook or underestimate a patient's chronic opioid use. If the patient's dose in the perioperative period does not match his or her daily needs, the patient may face going through withdrawal. It is important to provide equianalgesic doses of oral or parenteral opioid that match the patient's daily dose in 1:1 substitution. Be aware that the total dose required by opioid-tolerant patients may exceed the "usual" dose anywhere from 20% to 300% compared to opioid-naïve patients. **Titrating to effect** is a key whether for IV rescue medications, patient-controlled analgesia, or PO analgesics.

If one opioid is not sufficient for rescue analgesia, clinicians tend to give small doses of several different opioids. They may think that the patient is failing to respond to treatment when, in fact, the treatment has not been maximized and optimized. It is better to **stick to one drug**, repeat loading doses as needed, and titrate to effect. Further, do not rely on opioids exclusively. Consider and give a high priority to regional analgesia, NSAIDs, and muscle relaxants (if indicated). Of note, some patients will present with tolerance due to addiction or abuse of analgesics; in the acute perioperative setting, the clinician's role is to provide comfort and not to treat addiction.

2. What is incomplete opioid cross-tolerance?

As defined in Table 43.1, opioid tolerance is a physiologic response that manifests as the need for an increased drug dose to achieve the same clinical effect. Opioid cross-tolerance is tolerance to all other opioids caused by short- or long-term use of one opioid. Recent research shows that different opioids bind to different sites on the mu opioid receptor—or as newly termed the mu opioid peptide (MOP) receptor. One explanation could be multiple MOP receptor subtypes. Moreover, several different MOP receptor splice variants have been identified. Different binding sites then determine slightly different analgesic effects. This leads to the incomplete opioid cross-tolerance observed clinically. Practically, it translates into the need for lower doses (up to 50% reduction) of the newly initiated opioid compared to the discontinued opioid (following conversion ratios, see below).

3. How does the use of methadone differ from that of other opioids?

Unlike other opioids, where slow-release forms need to be manufactured, methadone possesses innate features as a long-acting pain medication. Methadone has regained popularity recently as a drug for opioid rotation (see below). It is a complex drug and every clinician prescribing it must be aware of its specific issues, especially its **unpredictable pharmacokinetics**. It has a **long**

Table 43.1

SOME KEY TERMS DEFINED

Definitions

Tolerance: Physiologic response to opioid analgesics resulting in a decrease in pharmacologic response following repeated or prolonged drug administration. Can be of two types:

Innate: Predisposition to exhibit drug sensitivity or insensitivity due to pharmacogenetic makeup

Acquired: 3 subtypes:

Pharmacokinetic: Occurs when drug disposition or metabolism is altered as a function of time, frequently a consequence of the drug being an inducer or inhibitor of a specific metabolic enzyme or transporter system

Pharmacodynamic: Occurs when the intrinsic responsiveness of the receptor system diminishes over time

Learned: Occurs when an individual learns to function despite repeated exposure to a drug

Opioid-Induced Hyperalgesia: A paradoxical effect of opioids leading to heightened pain perception

Pseudo-addiction: A term describing a patient with legitimate but undertreated pain who demands more pain medication to achieve relief and comfort

Addiction: A psychophysical condition in which a patient's focus becomes acquisition and use of a drug regardless of physical, psychological, or social harm caused by the use. *Tolerance* is one component of addiction.

Withdrawal: Occurs in the setting of tolerance, with sudden cessation of a medication, leading to a combination of physical symptoms, including abdominal pain/cramping, diarrhea, tachycardia, tremors, sweating, piloerection, anxiety, and/or generalized body achiness

terminal half-life of 7 to 65 hours, causing the potential for sedation with rapid titration. To reach a **steady state** may take **35 to 325 hours** (1.5–13.5 days). Methadone's potential for **significant drug interactions** (either an increase in free methadone plasma levels, or an increase/decrease in the effectiveness of co-administered drugs [e.g., SSRIs, TCAs, fluconazole, ciprofloxacin, doxorubicin, vinblastine]) and **risk of torsades de pointes** (via QT-interval prolongation; it structurally mimics the calcium channel blocker verapamil) cannot be emphasized enough. It also carries a stigma due to its use for opioid addiction management. The main **advantage** of methadone is its **high oral bioavailability** (almost 90%). It is a drug with not only **mu** opioid receptor **agonistic** effect, but also **NMDA antagonistic** properties that provide **slower development of tolerance** and beneficial effects on **neuropathic pain**.

4. How does one execute opioid rotation?

Opioid rotation (or switching) is a change in opioid drug or route of administration with the goal of improving outcomes: analgesia, reduced side effects, and better functioning or quality of life. It is a complex process, and several factors that influence the new drug and dose selection must be taken into consideration: age and race, disease and its treatment, comorbidities, and concomitant pharmacotherapy (Fig. 43.1). The provider executing an opioid rotation must be prepared to deal with withdrawal, acute and protracted (manifesting as dysphoria, fatigue, sleep disturbance).

The dose selection has been based on equianalgesic dose tables. Recently, the assumptions behind the tables have undergone scrutiny, as existing data were found to be limited and numerous gaps were identified. Therefore, equianalgesic dose tables must be viewed as starting points only.

5. What other adjuncts can help in the opioid-tolerant patient?

In caring for patients who are opioid-tolerant, adjunct medications can have a large impact in terms of comfort and side effects.

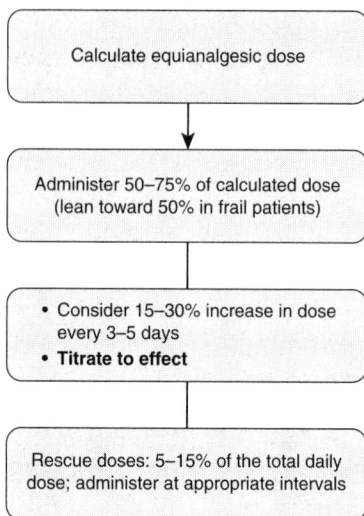

```
┌─────────────────────────────────┐
│    Calculate equianalgesic dose │
└─────────────────────────────────┘
                 │
                 ▼
┌─────────────────────────────────┐
│  Administer 50–75% of calculated dose │
│    (lean toward 50% in frail patients) │
└─────────────────────────────────┘
                 │
┌─────────────────────────────────┐
│ • Consider 15–30% increase in dose │
│   every 3–5 days                 │
│ • Titrate to effect              │
└─────────────────────────────────┘
                 │
┌─────────────────────────────────┐
│ Rescue doses: 5–15% of the total daily │
│ dose; administer at appropriate intervals │
└─────────────────────────────────┘
```

FIGURE 43.1 Guidelines for opioid rotation. (Note that methadone conversion is beyond the scope of this chapter, so these suggestions pertain to other opioids only.)

Ketamine, besides being an anesthetic, works as a noncompetitive antagonist of the phencyclidine binding site of the NMDA receptor. Subanesthetic doses have been used in addition to opioid to attenuate the opioid-induced hyperalgesia (OIH) or opioid tolerance, leading to a 30% reduction in postoperative opioid consumption but no reduction of side effects (except nausea and vomiting). OIH is an interesting phenomenon in which paradoxical increases in pain are seen after administration of opioids, and several approaches to treatment have been tried (Chu et al., 2008). Ketamine appears to reduce central sensitization, which seems to be a component of OIH, and can be useful in patients who are taking large doses of opioids and in preventing the OIH that can be seen with remifentanil use.

Propofol was suggested to modulate OIH via its interactions with GABA-A receptors at the supraspinal level. In subhypnotic doses, propofol had analgesic effects and delayed the onset of remifentanil OIH. However, experimental models suggest that variable effects may be seen in propofol's effect on OIH.

Cyclooxygenase-2 inhibitors (COX-2) have been shown to antagonize NMDA receptors in the CNS. They may have a role in modulation of OIH in humans. Parecoxib was effective in preventing remifentanil-induced hyperalgesia if administered *before* opioid exposure. Many oncology patients are on steroids and have renal compromise, thrombocytopenia, or other reasons to be wary of NSAIDs, so coordination with the primary oncology team is important. As opposed to animal models, where evidence was mixed, several small, human studies suggested that alpha-2 agonists (clonidine, dexmedetomidine) are effective in preventing OIH in the acute setting.

SUMMARY

1. Patients on long-term opioids can have very high opioid requirements in the perioperative period.
2. Tolerance and addiction are not the same, and confusing the two can have adverse effects on patient care.
3. Patients who are not responding well to one medication or in whom side effects limit dose escalation may benefit from opioid rotation.
4. Use of adjunct analgesics is important in limiting side effects of opioids such as sedation and opioid-induced hyperalgesia.

ANNOTATED REFERENCES

- Chu LF, Angst MS, Clark D. Opioid induced hyperalgesia in humans: molecular mechanisms and clinical considerations. *Clin J Pain* 2008; 24 (6): 479–496.

This review highlights the important mechanistic underpinnings and clinical ramifications of opioid-induced hyperalgesia and discusses future research directions and the latest clinical evidence for modulation of this potentially troublesome clinical phenomenon.

- **Dumas EO, Pollack GM. Opioid tolerance development: A pharmacokinetic/pharmacodynamic perspective.** *AAPS Journal* 2008; 10(4): 537–551.

This review article explains some pharmacokinetic and pharmacodynamic aspects of opioid tolerance development. It presents several pharmacodynamic modeling strategies that have been used to characterize time-dependent attenuation of opioid analgesia.

- **Fine PG, Portenoy R. Establishing "best practices" for opioid rotation: Conclusions of an expert panel.** *J Pain Sympt Manage* 2009; 38(3): 418–425.

This is a very practical article, easy to read and understand. It will be helpful for clinicians who do not deal with opioid rotation on a daily basis. It provides helpful and simple rules to follow and factors to consider when attempting opioid rotation.

- **Fredheim OMS, Moksnes K, Borchgrevink PC, Kaasa S, Dale O. Clinical pharmacology of methadone for pain.** *Acta Anaesthesiol Scan* 2008; 52: 879–889.

A useful literature review with a focus on methadone's properties, pharmacokinetics, interactions, pharmacogenetics, and use in cancer and chronic non-cancer pain. It offers switching strategies, equianalgesic dosing, and detailed information on QT-prolongation side effect.

Further Reading

Diatchenko L, Anderson AD, Slade GD, et al. Three major haplotypes of the beta 2 adrenergic receptor define psychological profile, blood pressure, and the risk for development of a common musculoskeletal pain disorder. *Am J Med Genet Part B* 2006; 141B: 449–462.

Nackley AG, Tan KS, Fecho K, Flood P, Diatchenko L, Maixner W. Catechol-O-methyltransferase inhibition increases pain sensitivity through activation of both beta 2 and beta 3 adrenergic receptors. *Pain* 2007; 128: 199–208.

Pasternak G. Incomplete cross tolerance and multiple mu opioid peptide receptors. *Trends Pharmacol Sci* 2001; 22(2): 67–70.

van Rossum D, Hanisch UK, Quirion R. Neuroanatomical localization, pharmacological characterization and functions of CGRP, related peptides and their receptors. *Neurosci Biobehav Rev* 1997; 21(5): 649–678.

44

Mediastinal Mass Biopsy

JON TOMASSON, MOHAMED A. MAHMOUD, AND JAMES P. SPAETH

INTRODUCTION

It has been long recognized that patients with anterior mediastinal masses (AMMs) have a significantly increased risk of adverse perioperative events. Even asymptomatic patients or those with mild clinical symptoms are at risk for cardiopulmonary collapse and even death with induction of anesthesia, thus highlighting the need for careful preoperative evaluation and decision making.

LEARNING OBJECTIVES

1. Understand the presentation and pathophysiology of AMM.
2. Develop a preoperative approach and risk assessment of patients with AMM.
3. Appreciate perioperative management of sedation and anesthesia and their complications in AMM patients.

CASE PRESENTATION

*Late one evening, a previously healthy 6-year-old child presents with the rapid onset of malaise, "head fullness," and **respiratory distress**, which **worsens** when lying **supine**. On examination, the child is anxious and tachypneic and **cannot lie down**; the physical exam is* remarkable for **plethora of the head** and an **enlarged cervical lymph node**. His chest x-ray reveals mediastinal enlargement with a right-sided **pleural effusion**. The admitting physician asks the anesthesia service to facilitate a "quick" chest computed tomography (CT) scan and a cervical lymph node biopsy so definitive therapy can be started. The CT scan is tried without sedation but the child is unable to stay still in the supine position. It is decided to try to avoid general anesthesia and to perform the CT and subsequent lymph node biopsy with local anesthesia and light sedation. An otolaryngologist is called to provide **rigid bronchoscopy**, if urgently needed. Following a dose of ketamine in the supine position, the patient's oxygen saturation drops to 73% and mask ventilation is difficult. The oxygen saturation improves immediately when the patient is moved into the **lateral decubitus** position. The CT is successfully done after placing the patient **prone**, and it reveals a large anterior mediastinal mass compressing the superior vena cava, the trachea, and the right main stem bronchus. The patient is transferred safely to the operating room in the decubitus position and the biopsy is obtained successfully using local anesthesia and a ketamine infusion.

DISCUSSION

1. What is an anterior mediastinal mass and how does it present?

The mediastinum is the interpleural space bound by the sternum anteriorly, the ribs and spine posterolaterally, the thoracic inlet cranially, and the diaphragm caudally. This space is further subdivided into superior, anterior, middle, and posterior mediastinal spaces, based on the location relative to the pericardial sac. Posterior mediastinal tumors are usually of neurogenic origin and generally do not place the patients at high anesthetic risk. AMMs are less common in children but are associated with high perioperative morbidity and mortality.

In the pediatric population, the most common AMMs are of lymphoid source (lymphoblastic lymphomas, and Hodgkin's disease), followed less frequently by thymomas, teratomas, para-thyroid, thyroid, neurogenic, and mesenchymal tumors. Non-neoplastic masses include vascular malformations, granulomas, cysts, and cystic hygromas.

The presentation of an AMM varies greatly depending on its location and size. General symptoms include constitutional tumor effects (fevers, weight loss), chest pain or tightness, and respiratory symptoms such as **dyspnea**, **orthopnea**, stridor, and coughing, which arise from tracheal or bronchial compression. Similarly, cardiovascular function is most commonly affected by compression of the superior vena cava (SVC). This often causes **head, airway,** and **upper extremity edema**, reduced cardiac venous return (SVC syndrome), and headaches. Indirect manifes-tations may include distant **lymph node metastasis** (e.g., neck) and pleural and pericardial effusions.

2. What is the pathophysiology of perioperative cardiorespi-ratory compromise?

As a patient is anesthetized, there is a progressive reduction of the intrathoracic volumes due to reduced chest expansion and a cephalad migration of the diaphragm and abdominal contents. An AMM tends to be highly vascular and engorges when the supine position is assumed, thereby further decreasing venous return. The combination of reduced intrathoracic volume and increased mass from the AMM leads to compression of soft-walled structures such as the airways and blood vessels. Neuromuscular relaxation and loss of spontaneous ventilation leads to further deterioration because the airway stenting from spontaneous ventilation is lost and the intramural muscles that support the airway relax. These changes culminate in severe compression or even total occlusion of a previously patent airway or vascular structure. Large airway gas flow becomes turbulent and further reduces effective ventilation. In summary, the induction of deep sedation or anesthesia may lead to sudden airway collapse that may not be amendable to positive-pressure ventilation, even with endotracheal intubation! Cardiovascular structures are similarly affected by direct tumor compression on the SVC, the pulmonary artery, or the heart itself. A pericardial effusion may additionally compromise cardiac function. These children may initially present with SVC syndrome, right ventricular dysfunction, syncopal episodes, or cardiac arrhythmias.

3. How does one assess risk for general anesthesia in these patients?

Patients with AMM typically present to the anesthesiologist for sedation or general anesthesia for imaging procedures, percutaneous or surgical biopsies, central line placement, or tumor debulking. Due to smaller airway size, children with AMM are inherently at higher risk for airway complications than adults; the incidence of perioperative events has been estimated as high as 7% to 20% (Bechard et al., 2004). One can never assume that an asymptomatic patient is going to experience a safe perioperative course. There is no single physical finding or study that reliably predicts who is at risk; instead, one must determine risk by carefully reviewing the combination of history, physical examination, and diagnostic studies.

Findings on physical evaluation suggestive of higher risk include **orthopnea**, **dyspnea**, coughing, syncope, wheezing, stridor, and reduced lung air entry. One should pay particular attention to whether these findings are position dependent—that is, what position increases symptoms or relieves them (e.g., **worse supine**, improved sitting, prone, or lateral). This information can guide intraoperative positioning. Symptoms suggesting cardiovascular compromise should be sought (syncope, arrhythmias, hemodynamic instability, SVC syndrome, or cardiac tamponade).

All patients need a CT scan of their chest to delineate the anatomy of the tumor and its relation to major intrathoracic structures. Modern fast CT scanners can accomplish this in less than 20 seconds with the patient's torso elevated at 30 degrees if needed. Patients with profound supine symptoms may be scanned in the **lateral or prone position** if that is tolerated better. Prior studies have suggested an increased risk with anesthesia when the tracheal area is less than 50% of normal or one (or both) main stem bronchi are compressed or occluded (Azizkhan et al., 1985; Shamberger et al., 1995).

The classic practice of obtaining flow-volume loop pulmonary function tests has been challenged due to the absence of a tight correlation between abnormal flow-volume loops and findings on chest CT scan. A simplified approach examines the supine peak expiratory flow rate (PEFR) and uses values less than 50% of predicted normal to be an indicator of airway compression. One series showed that pediatric patients with a CT scan tracheal area of more than 50% and a PEFR of more than 50% of normal were able to safely undergo anesthesia (Shamberger et al., 1995), whereas if either of those values (or both) were less than 50%, the risk was increased.

Any patient with cardiovascular compromise should have a transthoracic echocardiogram, preferably in the upright and supine position, to demonstrate whether cardiac or major vessel compression is present. If any compression is apparent, it is useful for the echocardiographer to comment on which positions relieve or worsen the compression. Other findings that have been associated with increased risk are **pleural effusions** and pericardial tamponade. There should be a low threshold for performing a preoperative echocardiogram, as there have been asymptomatic AMM patients who have developed abrupt cardiorespiratory collapse on the induction of anesthesia and subsequently died (Viswanathan et al., 1995).

In summary, in the absence of strong evidence to guide risk assessment in pediatric patients with AMM, one must presume that they are all at risk of severe perioperative adverse events. The only potential exception would be a patient with a small AMM who exhibits no clinical symptoms in the supine position and has no evidence of airway/vascular compression on chest CT scan or echocardiography.

4. What is the perioperative management of these patients?

Expediting preoperative studies is extremely important due to the rapid growth of some of these tumors, yet since perioperative risks are significant, the evaluation must be thorough (Fig. 44.1). Careful collaboration between the different services (including anesthesiology, hematology/oncology, surgery, interventional radiology, and otolaryngology) is imperative. A coordinated plan among the involved services is crucial. Clear communication with the family is likewise important. While a typical informed consent process for a healthy child may or may not include a discussion of death, in this instance the patient and his family should be fully educated about the risks of significant morbidity and mortality.

Generally, sedation unsupervised by an anesthesiologist should be avoided. It is always safest to obtain vascular access prior to the induction of anesthesia in these children. In AMM patients with known SVC syndrome, it is important to place vascular access in the lower extremities to ensure delivery of resuscitative fluids and medications. In patients estimated to be at low risk, it is reasonable to proceed with general anesthesia as long as spontaneous ventilation is initially preserved. Muscle relaxation is deferred until the patient is shown to tolerate positive-pressure ventilation (and preferably relaxation testing, as described below). The anesthesiologist must be ready to respond if the patient begins to develop airway obstruction or cardiovascular collapse.

In patients with uncertain risk or high risk, one must proceed with extreme care. Anesthetics and sedatives should be administered only if necessary. Every effort should be made to obtain the tissue diagnosis using local anesthesia or very limited sedation. That could include getting samples from pleural effusions, bone biopsies, or superficial lymph nodes under local anesthesia. Patients with impending respiratory failure should not be sedated or anesthetized. In these patients, consideration must be given to shrinking the mediastinal mass and improving the associated symptoms with radiation therapy or steroids prior to obtaining tissue biopsy with sedation or general anesthesia.

When anesthesia is still required in the symptomatic patient, venous access should be secured first and then anesthesia should be initiated in the position producing fewest symptoms (in the

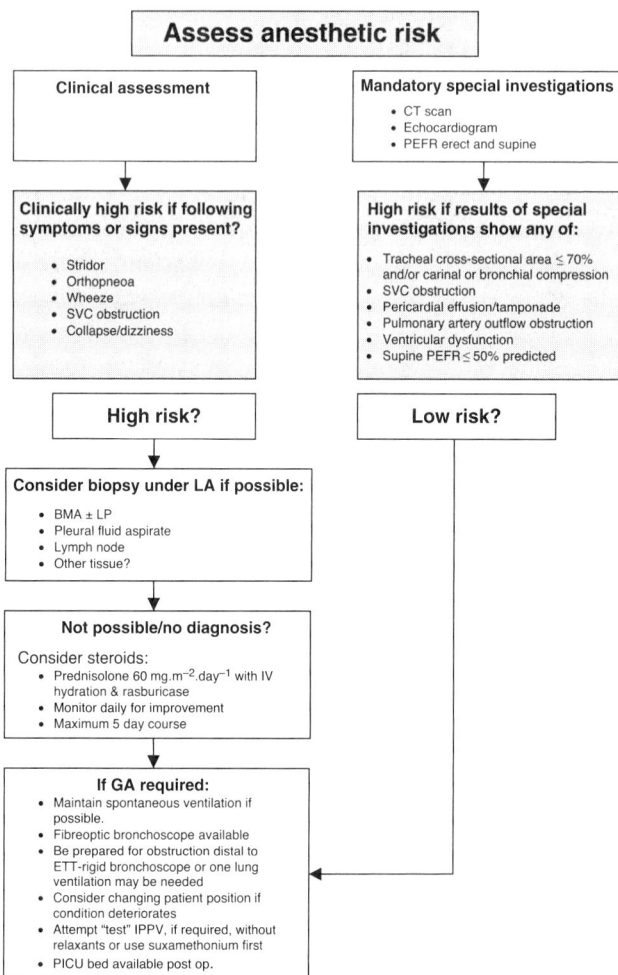

FIGURE 44.1 Preoperative anesthetic guidelines for a child with a mediastinal mass. (Reprinted with permission from Hack HA, Wright NB, Wynn RF. The anesthetic management of children with anterior mediastinal masses. *Anesthesia* 2008; 63(8): 837–846.)

case scenario, the patient should have been anesthetized in a more upright position, since he **could not lie down** when awake). Care is taken to maintain spontaneous ventilation at all costs. This is typically achieved with the use of inhaled anesthetics such as sevoflurane, although intravenous agents have also been used. The combination of dexmedetomidine and ketamine has been used successfully to maintain normal spontaneous ventilation in a patient undergoing a percutaneous mediastinal biopsy under deep sedation (Mahmoud et al., 2008). The airway can be maintained with mask ventilation, a laryngeal mask airway (LMA), or a regular (or reinforced) endotracheal tube (ETT). Lighter levels of anesthesia with spontaneous ventilation help maintain airway patency, and techniques using local anesthetics can reduce the amount of volatile or intravenous anesthetics necessary (e.g., the use of airway regional techniques to facilitate intubation or neuraxial techniques to facilitate surgical anesthesia and postoperative pain control). Large-bore intravenous catheters should be placed when significant bleeding is expected, and an arterial line is placed for patients with large tumors or cardiovascular compromise or when a prolonged procedure is expected.

When ventilation needs to be controlled, the initial approach includes careful hand ventilation to confirm an unobstructed airway. Only then should the anesthetist attempt muscle relaxation with an ultra-short-acting agent (e.g., succinylcholine); if tolerated, it is followed by a relatively short-acting nondepolarizing muscle relaxant such as rocuronium, vecuronium, or cisatracurium. Sugammadex, although not approved for use in the United States, may be helpful in this situation by rapidly reversing the neuromuscular blockade of rocuronium or vecuronium and allowing the patient to quickly return to spontaneous ventilation.

Extubation of the patient with AMM may be just as hazardous as the induction of anesthesia. Depending on the procedure, surgical edema or hemorrhage can further increase intrathoracic pressures and cause airway collapse on extubation. If this is suspected, the patient should be left intubated and transported to the ICU; tumor therapy should be started and extubation attempted only after demonstration of tumor regression (e.g., on a CT scan) in the next few days.

5. What is the approach to acute decompensation in these patients?

An uneventful induction does not preclude complications later on in the case: acute airway or cardiovascular collapse can happen any time during the perioperative course. If collapse occurs then the anesthetic must be lightened or discontinued in an attempt to reestablish spontaneous ventilation, and the patient position must be altered to one that relieved the patient preoperatively. This may mean sitting the patient up or turning him or her to a **lateral decubitus** or **prone position** in an attempt to decompress the airways. The ETT may lose its rigidity during the case and the airway can collapse from the weight of the mass. An armored ETT may decrease this risk. The AMM can compress the trachea distal to the tip of the ETT. In this case, advancing the ETT distally in the trachea or even into a main stem bronchus may reestablish the ability to ventilate the patient. If minor ETT manipulation is unsuccessful in resolving the problem of difficult ventilation, a **rigid bronchoscope** can facilitate reestablishment of ventilation and oxygenation. This necessitates the presence and readiness of a physician in the OR who is trained to perform **rigid bronchoscopy** prior to the initiation of sedation or anesthesia. On rare occasions, even this maneuver has been unsuccessful in saving patients. At this point, immediate surgical airway decompression may be necessary using a median sternotomy. Classically, standby cardiopulmonary bypass or ECMO is recommended, but in this situation it is impractical because of the relatively long time necessary to establish full support. In severe situations, bypass or ECMO would be better initiated prior to induction of anesthesia in the appropriate patient population.

SUMMARY

1. Anterior mediastinal masses can be deadly! Catastrophic events can occur anytime in the perioperative period. Even asymptomatic patients are at risk.
2. Multidisciplinary teamwork with anesthesia, hematology/oncology, otolaryngology, surgery, and interventional radiology is crucial to ensure a safe and effective outcome.
3. For high-risk patients, consider performing the biopsy under local anesthesia (bone marrow aspirate, pleural effusions, lymph nodes). Consider whether preoperative cancer management with radiation or steroid therapy is necessary prior to biopsy.

ANNOTATED REFERENCES

- Cheung SL, Lerman J. Mediastinal masses and anesthesia in children. *Anesth Clin North Am* 1998; 16: 893–910.

  An excellent review of anesthesia implications of AMMs in children. It includes a detailed discussion of the relevant anatomy, pathophysiology, and presentation of AMM in addition to a practical discussion of anesthetic considerations and a management algorithm.
- Erdös G, Tzanova I. Perioperative anaesthetic management of mediastinal mass in adults. *Eur J Anaesthesiol* 2009; 26: 627–632.

  Although this review article focuses mostly on AMM in adults, there is still a detailed description of the pathophysiology associated with AMM and a practical discussion of perioperative anesthesia management.
- Hack HA, Wright NB, Wynn RF. The anaesthetic management of children with anterior mediastinal masses. *Anaesthesia* 2008; 63: 837–846.

This case series describes the experience of a single institution with AMMs over 7 years, including preoperative evaluation, anesthesia management, and outcomes. The discussion contains a good review of pertinent studies looking at preoperative risk assessment in AMM patients, the pros and cons of preoperative cancer management, and an excellent management algorithm.

Further Reading

Azizkhan RG, Dudgeon DL, Buck JR, Colombani PM, Yaster M, Nichols D, Civin C, Kramer SS, Haller JA Jr. Life-threatening airway obstruction as a complication to the management of mediastinal masses in children. *J Pediatr Surg* 1985; 20: 816–822.

Bechard P, Letourneau L, Lacasse Y, Cote CJ, Bussieres JS. Perioperative cardiorespiratory complications in adults with mediastinal mass: incidence and risk factors. *Anesthesiology* 2004; 100: 826–834.

Mahmoud M, Tyler T, Sadhasivam S. Dexmedetomidine and ketamine for large anterior mediastinal mass biopsy. *Pediatr Anesth* 2008; 18: 1011–13.

Shamberger RC, Holzman RS, Griscom NT et al. Prospective evaluation by computed tomography and pulmonary function tests on children with mediastinal masses. *Surgery* 1995; 118: 468–471.

Slinger P, Karsli, C. Management of the patient with a large anterior mediastinal mass: recurring myth. *Curr Opin Anaesthesiol* 2007; 20: 1–3.

Stricker PA, Gurnaney HG, Litman RS. Anesthetic management of children with an anterior mediastinal mass. *J Clin Anesth* 2010; 22: 159–163.

Viswanathan S, Campbell CE, Cork RC. Asymptomatic undetected mediastinal mass: a death during ambulatory anesthesia. *J Clin Anesth* 1995; 7: 151–155.

45

Neuroblastoma Resection

STEFAN SABATO

INTRODUCTION

Neuroblastoma is the most common extracranial solid tumor of childhood, and limited or complete surgical resection is performed in most cases. Anesthesia for these children can be challenging because of the size and location of the tumor, the secretion of vasoactive metabolites from the tumor, and because it involves major surgery in a potentially immunocompromised patient. Adequate preparation for these procedures can avoid intraoperative instability.

LEARNING OBJECTIVES

1. Know how to assess a child with neuroblastoma.
2. Appreciate some of the difficulties of anesthesia for the child with cancer.
3. Understand the principles of management of major blood loss during pediatric surgery.

CASE PRESENTATION

*A previously healthy, 18-month-old, 12-kg boy with a **stage 3 abdominal neuroblastoma** is scheduled for surgical resection of the tumor. On examination, his vital signs were a BP of 75/40 mm/Hg, heart rate of 95, and respiratory rate of 30, and he is afebrile. Routine blood* *tests are normal. A diagnosis of neuroblastoma was made on the basis of CT, and metaiodobenzyl guanidine (MIBG) scanning, **elevated urinary catecholamine concentrations**, and biopsy data. The patient received induction **chemotherapy** consisting of four cycles of carboplatin, etoposide, cyclophosphamide, and doxorubicin over 12 weeks. Repeat CT scanning demonstrated residual disease in the left suprarenal region extending across the midline and encasing the origin of the superior mesenteric artery and the celiac trunk. Post-chemotherapy, echocardiography, chest x-ray, and serum biochemistry) were all normal.*

*In the operating room an intravenous induction is followed by maintenance anesthesia of 3% sevoflurane in oxygen and air (FiO$_2$ = 0.5). **Intravenous access** is obtained for rapid fluid volume replacement with two 20G cannulas. A 22G radial arterial line and a 4 Fr left internal jugular double-lumen central line are placed using ultrasound guidance. A urinary catheter is placed to allow further indirect **assessment of intravascular volume** and organ perfusion.*

*A transverse upper abdominal incision is made and the tumor is exposed. The 7-hour surgery is notable for a prolonged, slow ooze of blood and serous fluid throughout the case. Crystalloid and 4% albumin are initially used to maintain mean arterial pressure, central venous pressure, and urine output targets. A full blood count and coagulation profile is checked every 2 hours and hourly arterial blood gas analysis is used to monitor ventilation, blood sugar, serum electrolytes, and hemoglobin (Hb). Red blood cell transfusions were administered to maintain an Hb of approximately 9 g/dL. When half the **estimated blood volume** had been replaced, platelets and fresh frozen plasma are administered in 10-mL/kg increments to maintain intravascular volume and a normal coagulation profile.*

*The surgeon applies vascular ligatures to the renal and splenic arteries, intermittently obstructing blood flow during the resection of the tumor. This results in decreased urine output, and a metabolic acidosis develops. Postoperatively the patient is transferred to the intensive care unit, where the metabolic acidosis improves. Urine output improves with further fluid boluses, and **intravenous analgesics** are used to provide pain relief.*

DISCUSSION

1. What is the staging system for neuroblastoma? How are patients stratified? How does this affect anesthesia?

In children with neuroblastoma, the **stage of disease** is the most important prognostic indicator. Age at diagnosis is the only other independent risk factor, with an age of less than 1 year associated with higher survival rates (Weinstein et al., 2003). The International Neuroblastoma Staging System (INSS) is the most widely used (Table 45.1).

Each malignancy is stratified into low-, intermediate-, or high-risk categories based on stage, age at diagnosis, histopathology, the presence of MYCN oncogene amplification, and DNA index. Low-risk neuroblastoma with stage 1 disease is most often treated with surgery alone. Intermediate- and high-risk patients are treated with chemotherapy, radiotherapy, and surgery (limited or extensive). It is important to understand the aim of the surgical procedure to provide the appropriate anesthetic. The aim of the initial surgery is to establish or confirm the diagnosis by obtaining tissue, to resect as much tumor as is safely possible, and to stage the tumor by sampling lymph nodes. If the tumor is thought to be unresectable, or if it is easily accessible by percutaneous needle biopsy, then adequate tissue for diagnosis and stratification may be obtained by minimally invasive techniques. After chemotherapy has reduced the disease burden, a second surgical procedure is undertaken. This second operation may be a near-total resection that leaves tumor that is dangerous to remove, or it may aim to remove all remaining disease, including stripping the adventitia off the large arteries to which the cancer is adherent (Kiely, 2007).

2. Who is at risk of hemodynamic instability from circulating catecholamines?

Most patients with neuroblastoma have **elevated urinary catecholamines** and catecholamine metabolites at diagnosis. Dopamine is the most common catecholamine produced by

Table 45.1

THE INTERNATIONAL NEUROBLASTOMA STAGING SYSTEM

Stage	Definition
1	Localized tumor with complete gross excision. Representative ipsilateral lymph nodes negative for tumor microscopically.
2A	Localized tumor with incomplete gross excision. Representative ipsilateral non-adherent lymph nodes negative for tumor microscopically.
2B	Localized tumor with or without complete gross excision. Representative ipsilateral lymph nodes positive for tumor microscopically. Enlarged contralateral lymph nodes negative microscopically.
3	Unresectable unilateral tumor infiltrating across the vertebral column with or without regional lymph node involvement; or, localized unilateral tumor with contralateral lymph node involvement; or, midline tumor with bilateral unresectable infiltration or lymph node involvement.
4	Any primary tumor with dissemination to distant lymph nodes or other organs
4S	Localized primary tumor (Stage 1, 2A, or 2B) in an infant less than 1 year of age with dissemination limited to skin, liver, and/or bone marrow

neuroblastomas, and levels can be assessed quickly from a random urine sample by the ratio of homovanilic acid (its major metabolite) to creatinine. However, in contrast to patients with pheochromocytoma, there are usually no signs or symptoms of excessive circulating catecholamines, and hemodynamic instability as a result of catecholamine release during intraoperative handling of the tumor is fortunately rare. Those at risk of hemodynamic instability may be detected by signs and symptoms of excessive catecholamine production such as sweating, palpitations, diarrhea, tachycardia, hypertension, pallor, diaphoresis, and cardiomegaly on radiographs. If the child is exhibiting clinical signs of excessive catecholamine production it is important to test for epinephrine (adrenaline) and norepinephrine (noradrenaline) from a 24-hour urine collection. These findings warrant preoperative consultation by Endocrinology and Cardiology to guide **preoperative alpha and beta blockade**.

Chemotherapy may decrease the likelihood of encountering hemodynamic instability due to reduced tumor bulk and endocrinologic activity (Creagh-Barry & Sumner, 1992). Thus, the likelihood of catecholamine-induced instability is greater in a primary resection or biopsy prior to chemotherapy than during second operations after chemotherapy. However, there are reports of intraoperative hemodynamic instability during resection of tumors already treated with chemotherapy (Kain et al., 1993). Therefore, intravenous alpha and beta blockers need to be readily available during all surgeries. Finally, the presence of elevated levels of endogenous catecholamines preoperatively does not necessarily predict the need for inotrope or vasopressor administration in the postoperative period, as this is more dependent on the extent and duration of surgery (Ross et al., 2009).

3. What are the practical issues concerning intravenous access and fluid administration in major abdominal surgery?

The patient described here had a tunneled central venous catheter already placed prior to surgery. This line is used for the administration of chemotherapy, but its use in the perioperative setting has limitations. The long thin lumen is not suitable for rapid infusion of IV fluids. Also, measurement of central venous pressure in these lines may be inaccurate. Finally, the tunneled line is placed for long-term access, and therefore all attempts to avoid colonization of bacteria and subsequent line infection should be made. Intraoperatively, many drugs and blood products are given, and they often need to be given rapidly. This makes it difficult to maintain strict asepsis when handling intravenous access devices.

Therefore, in this case, **large-bore peripheral access** was obtained, and a second central venous catheter was inserted. A fluid warmer is necessary to warm blood products, as this patient is prone to hypothermia due to the large degree of exposure from the surgical wound and the large volume of fluid replacement.

In this case, as in most, there was no catastrophic hemorrhage during the operation, but the anesthesiologist still needs to **be prepared for extensive blood loss**, as abdominal neuroblastomas will often surround major vessels. It is important to have all blood products readily available for urgent rapid transfusion. It is helpful to have calculated the patient's **estimated blood volume** (EBV) prior to surgery (in toddlers EBV = 70 mL/kg). The intraoperative Hb (and hence the point at which transfusion may be needed) may be very roughly estimated by considering the observed blood loss. However, observed blood loss is very difficult to accurately quantify, so using serial intraoperative Hb measures is a better method to guide the need for transfusion. When total fluid replacement approaches one blood volume, consider transfusing platelets and clotting factors. In the event of a massive transfusion, it is important to avoid hypocalcemia and hypofibrinogenemia (see Chapter 24).

In this case, the anesthesiologist maintained a Hb concentration of 9 g/dL, even though a lower concentration would otherwise be acceptable. This was to provide a margin of safety given the possibility of sudden bleeding. Even without sudden hemorrhage, there is still often a need for transfusion and fluid replacement over the course of the operation.

Large losses of extracellular fluid occur as well. An exposed abdomen will lose up to 7 mL/kg/hr in evaporative losses alone, and aggressive tumor resection disrupts abdominal lymphatics, resulting in loss of lymphatic fluid. In summary, **large volumes of fluid administration may be required**, and replacement should be guided by the available clinical, laboratory, and invasive and noninvasive measures.

Hypovolemia is not the only cause for poor urine output; ligation of the renal vessels, pressure on the ureters, and even renal infarction should also be considered. Urine output is not always a reliable guide to intravascular volume.

4. What are the anesthetic implications of chemotherapy?

Intense multiagent chemotherapy reduces disease burden and facilitates resection. There are many different chemotherapeutic regimens, and which agents are selected depends on the institution. Many of the toxic effects of an individual drug are common across its class (Table 45.2). Anorexia, nausea, and vomiting are universal adverse effects throughout the duration of treatment. **All patients will be immunosuppressed**, and the utmost precautions against introducing infection must be taken. Thorough assessment by history, examination, and investigation of the cardiac, respiratory, renal, and hematologic systems is necessary prior to anesthesia. Anthracycline-induced cardiomyopathy may occur over a year after completion of therapy. A consultation by Cardiology may be helpful in assessing the cardiac effects of the anthracyclines.

5. Are there specific needs for postoperative analgesia?

There is no single preferred approach to treating postoperative pain in this population. This child had extensive elective surgery with an anticipated long duration and the potential for coagulopathy. The anesthesiologist planned to ventilate the child for the first 12 to 24 hours postoperatively, and therefore an epidural catheter would not have avoided postoperative ventilation. Neither of these two reasons are absolute contraindications to an epidural catheter, and individual/institutional preference varies. Most of the systemic analgesics can be used effectively (see Chapter 43 for potential challenges). Neuroblastoma patients are often too young to directly use patient-controlled analgesia (PCA). Use of PCA by proxy can allow parents to help control their child's pain. Monitoring and family and nursing education are critical if this modality is used. Nonsteroidal anti-inflammatory drugs are generally avoided due to their antiplatelet effect and potential nephrotoxicity.

Table 45.2

COMMON TOXICITIES FROM CHEMOTHERAPY

Drug/Class	Toxicities
Cyclophosphamide/ Alkylating agent	**Immediate**: metallic taste[+], inappropriate ADH, blurred vision, arrhythmias[*], myocardial necrosis[*] **Prompt**: myelosuppression[+], alopecia[+], hemorrhagic cystitis[+] **Delayed**: immunosuppression, gonadal dysfunction, pulmonary fibrosis[+*] **Late**: secondary malignancy[*], bladder fibrosis[*]
Etoposide/ Podophyllotoxin derivative	**Immediate**: hypotension[*], anaphylaxis[*] **Prompt**: myelosuppression, alopecia, peripheral neuropathy[*], stomatitis[*] **Late**: secondary malignancy[*]
Carboplatin/ Heavy metal antineoplastic agent	**Immediate**: metallic taste[*] **Prompt**: myelosuppression, electrolyte disturbance[+], peripheral neuropathy[*], hepatotoxicity[*], renal toxicity[+*], ototoxicity[+*]
Doxorubicin/ Anthracycline antibiotic	**Immediate**: arrhythmias, local ulceration if extravasated, pink urine, anaphylaxis[*] **Prompt**: myelosuppression[+], alopecia[+], stomatitis[+], mucositis[+], hepatotoxicity[+] **Delayed**: immunosuppression, cardiomyopathy (cumulative dose-dependent) **Late**: secondary malignancy[*]

Immediate: Within 1–2 days. Prompt: Within 2–3 weeks. Delayed: Anytime later during therapy. Late: Any time after the completion of treatment. [+] indicates that toxicity may occur later. [*] indicates a rare toxicity.

Source: Baker DL, Schmidt ML, Cohn SL, et al. Outcome after reduced chemotherapy for intermediate-risk neuroblastoma. *N Engl J Med* 2010; 363: 1313–1323.

SUMMARY

1. Staging of neuroblastomas has prognostic value and guides therapy and intervention; therapy may include extensive surgery and chemotherapy.
2. Several of the chemotherapeutic agents have significant physiologic effects, which have both immediate and long-term implications for anesthetic management.
3. It is important to recognize the minority of patients who are at risk of catecholamine-induced hemodynamic instability and formulate a plan for their preoperative and intraoperative care.
4. Intraoperative fluid management is challenging, and adequate venous access is important.

ANNOTATED REFERENCES

- Creagh-Barry P, Sumner E. Neuroblastoma and anesthesia. *Pediatr Anesth* 1992; 2: 147–152.

  A case series that discusses patients at risk of hemodynamic instability.
- Weinstein JL, Katzenstein HM, Cohn SL. Advances in the diagnosis and treatment of neuroblastoma. *Oncologist* 2003; 8: 278–292.

  An excellent review of neuroblastoma from an oncology perspective. Details staging, prognostic indicators, and conventional and novel treatments.

Further Reading

Gupta A, Kumar A, Walters S, Chait P, Irwin MS, Gerstle JT. Analysis of needle versus open biopsy for the diagnosis of advanced stage pediatric neuroblastoma. *Pediatr Blood Cancer* 2006; 47: 875–879.

Haberkern CM, Coles PG, Morray JP, Kennard SC, Sawin RS. Intraoperative hypertension during surgical excision of neuroblastoma: case report and review of 20 years' experience. *Anesth Analg* 1992; 75: 854–858.

Kain ZN, Shamberger RS, Holzman RS. Anesthetic management of children with neuroblastoma. *J Clin Anesth* 1993; 5: 486–491.

Kiely E. A technique for excision of abdominal and pelvic neuroblastomas. *Ann R Coll Surg Eng* 2007; 89: 342–348.

Ross SL, Greenwald BM, Howell JD, Pon S, Rutigliano DN, Spicyn N, LaQuaglia MP. Outcomes following thoracoabdominal resection of neuroblastoma. *Pediatr Crit Care Med* 2009; 6: 681–686.

Sendo D, Katsuura M, Akiba K, Yokoyama S, Tanabe S, Wakabayashi T, Sato S, Otaki S, Obata K, Yamagiwa I, Hayasaka K. Severe hypertension and cardiac failure associated with neuroblastoma: a case report. *J Pediatr Surg* 1996; 12: 1688–1690.

Wagner LM, Danks MK. New therapeutic targets for the treatment of high-risk neuroblastoma. *J Cell Biochem* 2009; 107: 46–57.

PART 10

CHALLENGES IN METABOLIC AND ENDOCRINOLOGIC CONDITIONS

46

Diabetic Patient

MARIO PATINO AND ANNA M. VARUGHESE

INTRODUCTION

Diabetes is the most common metabolic disorder in children, and its incidence is increasing. The rapid development of new, complex regimens for treatment and the availability of many forms of insulin make the management of these patients complex and best conducted in conjunction with a pediatric endocrinologist. Perioperative management of diabetic patients requires knowing the pathophysiology, current treatment, degree of control and compliance with therapy, previous complications, and complexity and duration of the surgical procedure.

LEARNING OBJECTIVES

1. Recognize if metabolic control of a diabetic child is optimal before proceeding to a surgical procedure.
2. Understand the perioperative risks and complications for diabetic patients.
3. Identify goals in the management of these patients and design a perioperative plan to meet these goals.
4. Learn to effectively manage life-threatening complications such as severe hypoglycemia.

CASE PRESENTATION

A 7-year-old, 20-kg girl with a past history of bladder exstrophy is undergoing a bladder augmentation procedure for intractable urinary incontinence. A year ago she was diagnosed with **type 1 diabetes mellitus** *after being admitted with urosepsis and diabetic ketoacidosis. Over the past 9 months she has been managed with a* **continuous subcutaneous insulin infusion (CSII)** *of rapid-acting insulin or insulin lispro (Humalog®) at a* **basal rate** *of 0.3 units/hr with* **prandial boluses** *of 2 to 3 units of insulin lispro. On average, she receives 15 units of insulin lispro per day. Her blood glucose level is checked three or four times a day and is usually below 250 mg/dL (13.9 mmol/L). The patient is scheduled as the first case of the day and is to be admitted after surgery. Complete blood count (CBC) and electrolytes are normal, there is no evidence of ketonuria, and her* **HbA1c** *is 8.5%. A preoperative blood sugar is 275 mg/dL (15.3 mmol/L). Using a* **correction formula** *calculation, an additional 0.6 units of insulin lispro (Humalog®) is administered subcutaneously. The CSII is discontinued, and maintenance fluids are administered with dextrose 5% with half-normal saline. A continuous infusion of* **intravenous** *regular* **insulin** *is started at 0.4 units/hr to maintain an* **insulin-to-carbohydrate ratio (I:C ratio)** *of 1 unit of insulin per 8 g of dextrose. Intraoperative blood glucose levels are measured every hour. Blood glucose levels are between 110 and 180 mg/dL (6.1–10 mmol/L) during the first 2 hours of the procedure, after which they increase to 350 mg/dL (19.4 mmol/L). Two units of rapid-acting insulin (insulin lispro) are administered subcutaneously, and the continuous infusion of insulin is increased by 25% to 0.5 units/hr; over the next hour the blood glucose level dropped to 110 mg/dL (6.1 mmol/L). At the end of the procedure the patient is breathing spontaneously and ready to be extubated, but she is unable to follow commands. There are no residual effects of muscle relaxants or inhalation agents present. The patient is clammy to touch and has an elevated heart rate. Her blood glucose level is 35 mg/dL (1.9 mmol/L).* **The intravenous insulin infusion** *is immediately stopped and* **20 mL of 50% dextrose** *is* *rapidly administered through **the central line**. Shortly after, the patient wakes up and is extubated and transferred to the ICU. In the ICU, maintenance fluids of 5% dextrose with half-normal saline are restarted with a continuous infusion of regular insulin at a rate of 0.4 units/hr. On the second postoperative day the patient is placed on a liquid and soft diet, **CSII** is restarted with her regular settings, and the patient is transferred to a regular ward.*

DISCUSSION

1. How can one determine if a diabetic child is in optimal condition prior to undergoing an elective operation?

Initial assessment should include current regimen and stability, previous complications, and recent evaluations by a pediatric endocrinologist. It is important to identify patients who are at risk for episodes of hyperglycemia or hypoglycemia, such as those with a prolonged fasting time, bowel preparation prior to surgery, steroid therapy, or continuous TPN infusion.

If the patient presents with an acute disease process and uncontrolled blood glucose levels, the presence of acidosis and ketonuria must be evaluated to rule out ketoacidosis (see Chapter 47). A preoperative blood sugar is mandatory, and recent electrolytes should be evaluated. **Glycosylated hemoglobin levels (HbA_{1C})** provide information about the degree of glycemic control in the past 2 to 3 months. The American Diabetes Association (ADA) recommends the following levels as ideal in the management of diabetic children: below 8.5% in children less than 6 years of age, below 8% in children 6 to 12 years of age, and below 7.5% in children older than 12 years. (American Diabetes Association, 2011).

If the patient has uncontrolled diabetes with a *persistent blood glucose level above 250 mg/dL* (13.9 mmol/L), *electrolyte imbalances*, and/or *ketonuria*, an elective procedure should be postponed and preoperative optimization by a pediatric endocrinologist is recommended.

2. **What are the risks and complications of diabetic patients undergoing major and prolonged procedures?**

The response to surgical stress is characterized by an increase in the counter-regulatory hormones (glucagon, cortisol, catecholamines, and growth hormone) that enhance gluconeogenesis, glycogenolysis, and protein and fat catabolism. This makes the control of blood glucose levels more challenging. Also, surgical stress can increase inflammatory cytokines (interleukin-6 and tumor necrosis factor alpha) that impair insulin secretion. Therefore, the perioperative period can be marked by episodes of hyperglycemia due to this increase in counter-regulatory hormones and the insulin deficiency of type 1 diabetes mellitus (or the relative insulin deficiency and insulin resistance of type 2 diabetes mellitus). Patients are also susceptible to episodes of hypoglycemia due to preoperative fasting and the exogenous administration of insulin. Uncontrolled hyperglycemia compromises immune function; this increases the risk of surgical site infection and alters the wound healing process. Also, diabetic patients are at greater risk of developing autonomic dysregulation, with poor compensatory effects for episodes of hypotension. They may have gastroparesis, with a resultant increased risk for aspiration. Insulin overdose can lead to a life-threatening episode of hypoglycemia. Given the susceptibility to fluctuating blood glucose levels during the perioperative period, frequent measurement of blood glucose (every 30 to 60 minutes) is strongly suggested.

3. **What are the goals of perioperative management of pediatric diabetic patients undergoing major procedures? How is insulin therapy optimally managed?**

From the metabolic standpoint, the goal is to maintain a blood glucose concentration between 110 and 180 mg/dL (6.1–10 mmol/L). Intensive glycemic control with a target below 110 mg/dL (6.1 mmol/L) increases the risk of episodes of hypoglycemia and is currently not recommended. Ideally, diabetic children would be scheduled as the first case of the day to avoid prolongation of the fasting time and to facilitate the implementation of an insulin/carbohydrate regimen.

Principles of Management:
Knowing the following terms will aid better understanding of perioperative insulin therapy:

- *Total daily dose (TDD) of insulin:* Number of units given in 24 hours
- *Basal insulin*: Physiological insulin levels produced by the pancreas when not stimulated by glucose. Basal insulin prevents gluconeogenesis and ketogenesis.
- *CSII*: **Continuous subcutaneous insulin infusion** administered via a portable pump
- *Insulin-to-carbohydrate ratio* (**I:C ratio**): Number of units of insulin administered per gram of carbohydrate. During the perioperative period, the I:C ratio is usually 1:5 to 1:8 for the administration of continuous intravenous insulin. The I:C ratio may be modified according to the patient's response. Postpubertal children are more resistant to insulin and may need an I:C ratio of 1:3 to 1:5.
- *Insulin correction factor or insulin sensitivity factor (ICF or ISF):* This is a determination of the expected decrease in blood sugar concentration (in mg/dL) after the administration of 1 unit of insulin. It is calculated by dividing 1,500 by the TDD ("the 1,500 rule").
- *Correction formula (CF):* Knowing the insulin sensitivity factor, this formula is used to estimate the dose of insulin needed to bring a patient's blood glucose level to a target or goal level.

CF = (Patient's blood glucose level – goal blood glucose)/ Insulin sensitivity factor

4. **How does the correction formula factor into perioperative insulin dosing?**
Perioperative insulin management is based on providing the usual pattern of physiological secretion of insulin. However, insulin requirements during the perioperative period increase. Insulin therapy consists of three different elements: **basal**, **prandial**, and *supplemental* administration.

Basal administration of insulin is given by long-acting insulin, by intermediate-acting insulin (NPH [Neutral Protamine Hagedorn]), or by continuous subcutaneous administration of rapid-acting insulin with the use of a portable pump (CSII). Basal administration is equivalent to the physiological insulin levels that avoid gluconeogenesis and ketogenesis. Basal insulin therapy is approximately 50% of the total daily dose and is necessary in type I diabetics independent of the patient's fasting status.

Prandial administration uses rapid-acting insulin, which is determined by the amount of carbohydrates to be consumed (insulin-to-carbohydrate ratio).

Supplemental administration is determined by the level of glucose above the goal. Supplemental administration of insulin is calculated using a **correction formula**. Knowing the insulin sensitivity factor, a correction formula is used to calculate the insulin dose to be administered to maintain a blood glucose level at 150 mg/dL (8.3 mmol/L). Usually 100% of the correction factor is administered, but in prepubertal children and in patients with history of hypoglycemia, 50% or 75% of the correction factor may be administered since prepubertal children are more sensitive to the effects of insulin and have a higher risk of hypoglycemia. Tables 46.1 and 46.2 outline care guidelines for patients undergoing shorter and longer procedures, respectively.

In the case presentation, the insulin daily dose for this patient is 15 units. The insulin *correction factor* or *insulin sensitivity factor* is 1,500/15 = 100. Theoretically, 1 unit of insulin administered subcutaneously to this patient would decrease the blood glucose level by 100 mg/dL (5.5 mmol/L). If this patient's preoperative blood glucose level is 275 mg/dL (15.3 mmol/L) and the perioperative blood glucose goal is 150 mg/dL (8.3mmol/L), then: **Correction formula** = (275 − 150)/100 = 1.25 units. Theoretically 1.25 units of insulin would decrease the blood glucose level to the target level. However, 0.6 units of insulin were administered instead of 1.25 units (50% of the correction formula) to avoid the risk of hypoglycemia in this prepubertal patient.

Table 46.1

MANAGING DIABETIC PATIENTS FOR SHORTER PROCEDURES

Guidelines for management of diabetic children undergoing surgical procedures lasting less than 2 hours

- On the morning of surgery, if the patient is on the conventional therapy (NPH), administer 50% of the NPH insulin (basal insulin requirements) and check preoperative blood glucose level, electrolytes, and ketonuria. If the blood glucose level is <100 mg/dL (5.5 mmol/L), start fluids at maintenance rate with 5% to 10% dextrose. If the blood glucose level is >250 mg/dL (13.9 mmol/L), administer a supplemental dose of rapid-acting insulin SC with the calculation of a correction factor (administer 50% of the correction factor to titrate response).
- If the patient is receiving continuous SC administration of rapid-acting insulin, continue the same basal rate. If the blood glucose level is >250 mg/dL (13.9 mmol/L), administer an additional bolus of SC rapid-acting insulin with 50% of the correction factor.
- If the patient is receiving long-acting insulin (i.e., insulin glargine [Lantus®]) once every 24 hours administered at night, there is no requirement for additional doses on the day of surgery. If a patient is on long-acting insulin every 12 hours, give the full morning dose, since there is no associated peak effect and this will provide the basal insulin needs. For a blood glucose level of >250 mg/dL (13.9 mmol/L), an additional bolus of SC rapid-acting insulin is given according to the correction factor.

4. What are other issues in perioperative management?

Other important considerations in the perioperative management of diabetic patients are the risks of hypokalemia and hyponatremia. Frequent monitoring is required. The risks of surgical site infection should also be considered; appropriate antibiotic prophylaxis must be given prior to the surgical incision, and adequate

Table 46.2

MANAGING DIABETIC PATIENTS FOR LONGER PROCEDURES

Guidelines of management in diabetic children undergoing surgical procedures lasting more than 2 hours

- All morning doses of insulin are held. Start maintenance fluids with 5% dextrose with half-normal saline and continuous insulin intravenous infusion to maintain an I:C ratio of 1 unit of insulin per 8 g dextrose. Insulin is diluted in normal saline to a concentration of 1 unit/mL (or 0.5 unit/mL for younger children). Both insulin and glucose are administered through the same intravenous line. For a blood glucose level >250 mg/dL (13.9 mmol/L), administer a correction factor dose with the administration of SC insulin.
- Intraoperatively, insulin is administered by continuous intravenous infusion to maintain an I:C ratio of 1:8. Consider an I:C ratio of 1:5 in postpubertal children, with a goal to maintain blood glucose levels between 110 and 180 mg/dL (6.1–10 mmol/L).
- Continue maintenance fluids with 5% dextrose with half-normal saline. Administer isotonic fluids to replace the deficit and third-space losses.
- Check blood glucose hourly. After any adjustment to the therapy, check blood glucose every 30 minutes.
- If the blood glucose level is >180 mg/dL (10 mmol/L), administer a correction factor dose (calculated with the 1,500 rule with an ideal blood glucose level of 150 mg/dL [8.3 mmol/L]) with the administration of SC rapid-acting insulin. Considering the biological effect of the rapid-acting insulin given SC, do not administer a correction factor more frequently than every 3 hours.
- For a persistent blood glucose level >180 mg/dL (10 mmol/L), consider increasing the continuous intravenous insulin infusion (20–25%).
- For blood glucose levels >60 mg/dL (3.3 mmol/L) and <110 mg/dL (6.1 mmol/L), decrease the insulin infusion and increase the dextrose infusion. Follow blood glucose levels every 30 minutes.
- For a blood glucose level <60 mg/dL (3.3 mmol/L), discontinue the insulin infusion and administer 0.5 to 1 g/kg of intravenous dextrose.

antibiotic redosing is required. Given the alterations in wound healing, appropriate positioning and padding in these patients is important to avoid any skin breakdown and/or pressure on the skin.

Postoperative care requires adequate pain control to blunt the increase in counter-regulatory hormones and to facilitate the control of blood glucose levels. Maintenance fluids with 5% to 10% dextrose and the administration of intravenous or subcutaneous insulin are continued at the previously titrated insulin dose. Blood glucose should be measured hourly as long as the patient continues on **continuous IV insulin infusion**.

5. How should hypoglycemia be treated?

The patient above developed a serious episode of hypoglycemia at the end of the procedure. Hypoglycemia is a life-threatening situation and requires immediate treatment to avoid a neurologic injury. **25% or 50% dextrose** is recommended, and continuous **infusion of insulin** must be *immediately discontinued*. Although concentrations of dextrose above 10% are considered hypertonic and carry the have risk of causing phlebitis and venous thrombosis, in an emergency situation 25% dextrose can be administered through a peripheral vein. However, **50% dextrose** must always be administered through a **central line**. The recommended dose is 0.5 to 1 g/kg of dextrose. This is equivalent to: 1 to 2 mL/kg 50% dextrose, 2 to 4 mL/kg 25% dextrose, 4 to 8 mL/kg 12.5% dextrose, or 5 to 10 mL/kg 10% dextrose. Another option is the intramuscular administration of glucagon in a dose of 0.25 mg (<5 years of age), 0.5 mg (5–12 years), and 1 mg (>12 years).

SUMMARY

1. **Preoperative evaluation includes blood glucose, HbA$_{1C}$, and electrolytes. Basal insulin requirements and duration of fasting should also be considered.**

2. Perioperative fluxes in blood glucose levels are to be expected; the patient requires close monitoring and manipulation of the insulin and glucose regimen.
3. Hypoglycemia is more dangerous than hyperglycemia and requires rapid intervention.

ACKNOWLEDGMENTS

The authors thank Lawrence Dolan, MD, and Alejandro Diaz, MD, pediatric endocrinologists, for reviewing this chapter and providing guidelines in the management of diabetic children.

ANNOTATED REFERENCES

- Chadwick V, Wilkinson KA. Diabetes mellitus and the pediatric anesthetist. *Pediatr Anesth* 2004; 14: 716–723.
  A slightly different approach to managing diabetic children; experience from the United Kingdom.
- Escobar O, Drash A, Becker D. Management of the child with type 1 diabetes. In Lifshitz F, ed. *Pediatric Endocrinology*. New York: Informa Healthcare, 2007: 101–124.
  In-depth chapter about the management of type 1 diabetes.
- Rhodes ET, Ferrari LR, Wolfsdorf JI. Perioperative management of pediatric surgical patients with diabetes mellitus. *Anesth Analg* 2005; 101: 986–999.
  A hallmark article in the perioperative management of diabetic children.

Further Reading

Ahmed Z, Lockhart C, Weiner M et al. Advances in diabetic management: implications for anesthesia. *Anesth Analg* 2005; 100: 666–669.

American Diabetes Association: Position Statement. Standards of Medical Care in Diabetes—2011 Diabetes Care, 2011; 34(1).

Betts P, Brink S, Silink M, Swift PGF, Wolfsdor J, Hanas R. Management of children and adolescents with diabetes requiring surgery. *Pediatr Diabetes* 2009; 10: 169–174.

Lyles S, Silverton J, Rosenbloom A. Practical aspects of diabetic care. In Lifshitz F, ed. *Pediatric Endocrinology*. 125–154. New York: Informa Healthcare, 2007: 125–154.

Meneghini L. Perioperative management of diabetes: Translating evidence into practice. *Cleve Clinic J Med* 2009; 76: s53–s59.

Rodbard HW, Blonde L, Braithwaite SS, et al. Medical guidelines for clinical practice for the management of diabetes mellitus. *Endocrine Practice* 2007; 13: 1–68.

Shamsuddin A, Barash P, Inzucchi S. Scientific principles and clinical implications of perioperative glucose regulation and control. *Anesth Analg* 2010; 110: 478–497.

Diabetic Ketoacidosis During Appendicitis with Perforation

XIMENA SOLER AND LORI A. ARONSON

INTRODUCTION

Type 1 diabetes mellitus (DM) is a chronic disease of carbohydrate, fat, and protein metabolism caused by a functional lack of insulin. Diabetic ketoacidosis (DKA) involves a combination of hyperglycemia, acidosis and ketosis, and is more often associated with type 1 DM. A child in DKA who presents for emergency surgery may be critically ill and requires expert management of his or her metabolic state to ensure a safe outcome.

LEARNING OBJECTIVES

1. Identify patients at risk for DKA.
2. Understand the pathophysiology of DKA.
3. Discuss perioperative management of acidosis/hyperglycemia in emergent situations with implications for anesthesia.

CASE PRESENTATION

*A 9-year-old boy with **type 1 DM** diagnosed 2 years ago presents to the emergency department with fever and intermittent **abdominal pain** for 10 days and vomiting and diarrhea for the past 3 days.*

His home insulin regimen consists of insulin glargine 10 U at night and insulin aspart for carbohydrate correction (see information on **carbohydrate correction factor** in Chapter 46). His past medical history is significant for attention-deficit/hyperactivity disorder (ADHD), for which he receives lisdexamfetamine and clonidine.

Physical examination reveals an alert, thin, ill-appearing patient. His observations are weight 40 kg, height 150 cm, BP 90/52, RR 34, HR 136, and SpO$_2$ 98%. He has dry mucous membranes and a distended abdomen with rebound tenderness at McBurney's point. Laboratory analysis reveals serum glucose of 421 mg/dL (23.4 mmol/L), Na 134 mmol/L, K 4.5 mmol/L, HCO$_3$ 14 mEq/L, and BUN 27 mg/dL (urea 9.6 mmol/L). Arterial blood gas analysis showed **pH 7.21**, pCO$_2$ 32 mmHg, pO$_2$ 102 mmHg, HCO$_3^-$ 12 mEq/L, and **BE -9**. His urine analysis shows a **glucose >1,000 mg/dL** (55.5 mmol/L) with **elevated ketones**. Complete blood count reveals elevated white blood cells at 16.3 × 10^9/L with 74% neutrophils and HbA1$_C$ of 12. His abdominal CT scan demonstrates a **perforated appendix** with periappendicular abscess.

The **consulting endocrinology service** initiates management with a 10-mL/kg bolus of 0.9% NaCl. Body surface area (BSA m^2) and corrected serum sodium are calculated to start maintenance IV fluids. A continuous IV **insulin infusion** is started to treat the ketonuria and metabolic acidosis. He is not given an initial IV insulin bolus, although he receives his usual home dose of subcutaneous insulin glargine. Bedside glucose is checked every hour and a renal panel is done every 2 hours until the bicarbonate level exceeds 15 mEq/L, and then every 4 hours until the bicarbonate level reaches 20 mEq/L. Serum calcium, magnesium, and phosphate levels are also measured every 4 hours. As the anion gap resolves and the bicarbonate levels reach 18 mEq/L, the continuous insulin infusion is stopped. **Dextrose 5% and 0.45% NaCl** are started as the glucose level corrects to below 400 mg/dL (22.2 mmol/L). To manage the intra-abdominal infection, the boy receives a dose of antibiotics in the emergency room and is scheduled for a periappendicular drain as soon as the laboratory values and dehydration are corrected. The anesthesiologist, in consultation with the endocrinologist, continues the **fluids and glucose control in the operating room**. Eight weeks later the serum glucose is normal, the *ketonuria has resolved, and the HbA1c has improved. The patient returns for an uneventful laparoscopic appendectomy.*

DISCUSSION

1. Which patients are at risk of DKA?

Type 1 DM is the most common metabolic disease of childhood, with a yearly incidence of 15 to 21 cases per 100,000 people younger than 18 years. DKA is frequently the first finding in a newly diagnosed diabetic patient, and the risk increases in children with poor compliance to therapy, poor metabolic control, suboptimal social circumstances, and in insulin pump users. DKA usually takes days to develop, but it can take only hours in children with acute illness or trauma, or those in need of surgery. The metabolic effects may be compounded by the requisite period of starvation that precedes and accompanies surgery. Comorbidities that may be triggering the DKA episode need to be identified. **Abdominal pain** (a typical symptom of DKA) may mask an underlying disease process. Fever is not seen in uncomplicated DKA and should always be investigated.

2. What is the definition and pathophysiology of DKA?

Biochemically, DKA is defined as **hyperglycemia** above 200 mg/dL (11.1 mmol/L), venous pH below 7.3, or bicarbonate below 15 mEq/L (15 mmol/L) with **ketonemia** or **ketonuria**. The severity of DKA is categorized by the degree of **acidosis** as mild (venous pH <7.3 or bicarbonate <15 mEq/L), moderate (pH <7.2 or bicarbonate <10 mEq/L), or severe (pH <7.1 or bicarbonate <5 mEq/L) (Wolfsdorf et al., 2009). The insulin deficiency generates a three-pronged response: lipolysis, increased glycogenolysis/gluconeogenesis, and the expected impaired glucose utilization. The former contributes to the formation of ketone bodies as a byproduct of ATP generation. The other two contribute to hyperglycemia, osmotic diuresis and acidosis. The whole process is framed by an increase in circulating catecholamines and worsening of the cycle.

3. What is the clinical presentation of DKA?

DKA presents clinically with a combination of dehydration, Kussmaul respirations, nausea, vomiting, and abdominal pain (unrelated to surgical pathology) and a progressive decrease in the level of consciousness. The major morbidity and mortality associated with DKA is *cerebral edema* (CE). Most episodes occur 4 to 12 hours after treatment, and mortality can be as high as 23%. It accounts for 70% to 80% of diabetic-related deaths in children under 12 years (Metzger, 2010).

4. What are the risk factors for DKA-cerebral edema (DKA-CE)? What is the treatment?

Important predictors of DKA-CE are younger age, new-onset diabetes, acidosis, abnormalities of sodium, potassium, and urea, and elevated $PaCO_2$. In addition, those who have received early administration of insulin and high fluid volumes are at risk (Metzger, 2010; Edge et al., 2006). Treatment of DKA-CE involves elevation of the head of the bed, decrease in fluid administration, and mannitol (0.5–1 g/kg) or 3% NaCl (3 mL/kg). If the patient is intubated, hyperventilation may help temporarily. A CT scan should be obtained to rule out other potential causes of neurological deterioration, such as thrombosis.

5. What is the clinical management of DKA in pediatric patients?

After obtaining an **endocrinology consult**, DKA management should use standardized pediatric-specific treatment protocols (an example is shown in Table 47.1) and flow sheets to ensure safe correction of metabolic abnormalities while minimizing the high risk of developing CE. The International Society for Pediatric and Adolescent Diabetes published its Clinical Practice Consensus Guidelines for DKA (Wolfsdorf et al., 2009), and these are considered the gold standard internationally.

The primary goals are *slow rehydration,* correction of acid–base and electrolyte imbalance, normalization of serum glucose, and treatment of any precipitating event. Fluid resuscitation

Table 47.1

SAMPLE PROTOCOL FOR DKA MANAGEMENT

Management of DKA

Initial Assessment

<u>Assess ABC and mental status</u>: If altered mental status, document and consider 10ml/kg NS boluses every 30 minutes.

Record last known meal, blood glucose, and home urine ketone measurement if available.

<u>Establish IV access and</u>:

1. <u>Obtain initial labs</u>: Arterial or venous blood gas, glucose by glucometer, renal panel, serum glucose, Ca, Mg, Phos, urinalysis. Hgb A1c, anti-islet cell antibodies (if new onset). Consider TSH and FT4, CBC with differential.

2. Obtain height and calculate BSA (m^2):
$$\sqrt{weight \; (kg) * height \; (cm)/3600}$$

3. <u>Calculate corrected serum Na</u>: Corrected Na = serum Na + ([(serum glucose − 100)/100] × 1.6)

Initial Fluid Therapy

1. <u>Less than 7% dehydration</u>: start maintenance therapy with ½ NS at 3000 mL/m^2/24 hrs.
   Potassium: If serum K< 6.0 mEq/L, begin with 40mEq/L with half as KCl, half as KPhos.
   Note: If initial serum K< 4.0 mEq/L, begin with 60 mEq/L with half as KCl, half as KPhos. With severe hypokalemia (< 3.5 mEq/L), higher concentration of K may be necessary.

2. <u>7-10% dehydration</u>: NS 10 mL/kg IV over 30 minutes, then start maintenance therapy as above.

3. <u>Greater than 10% dehydration</u>: If CV compromise, consider additional infusions of NS until hemodynamically stable prior to initiation of maintenance fluid therapy.

468

Table 47.1 (*continued*)

Initial Fluid Therapy

4. <u>Hypernatremic dehydration</u>: If corrected Na >155 mEq/L, consult Endocrinologist and begin NS at 2000 mL/m^2/24 hours while administering insulin. Goal is to lower serum glucose to target of 200-300 mg/dl over 24 hours with little or no decrease in corrected serum Na. To replace free water deficit, will gradually add more free water with ¾NS to decrease serum Na by 15–20 mEq/L 24 hours over 72 hours.

Plan ahead: order D5%- and D10%-containing solutions to have when needed. Add 5% Dextrose to solution when BG decreases by > 100 mg/dl/hr OR when BG is <400 mg/dl. Have same 10% Dextrose solution on hand.

Remember, you need insulin to correct acidosis. If glucose is dropping too quickly, add glucose to fluids and avoid decreasing insulin drip unless absolutely necessary (eg. new fluids aren't available yet) then turn drip back up ASAP.

Insulin Treatment

1. <u>If ketone positive and bicarb < 15 mEq/L</u>: Begin continuous IV infusion of 0.1 Units/kg/hr of Regular Insulin. No bolus dose of insulin is required. Disconnect the insulin pump for patients on pump. OK to continue to give home Lantus dose Qday for patient on Lantus.

2. <u>If corrected Na >155 mEq/L OR glucose >1000 mg/dl with small-moderate ketones</u>: Consult Endocrinologist, and consider using lower insulin infusion rate (0.01-0.05 Units/kg/hr)

3. <u>If isolated hyperglycemia or ketone positive with bicarb >15 mEq/L</u>: may forego infusion and start subcutaneous rapid acting insulin according to home regimen, with the following supplemental doses added to each home baseline dose:
   a) small urine ketones: 2.5% Total daily dose
   b) moderate urine ketones: 5% TDD
   c) large urine ketones: 7.5% TDD

Continue IV maintenance fluid therapy as above, regardless of chosen insulin treatment

(*continued*)

Table 47.1 (*continued*)

Monitoring

1. <u>Bedside glucoses</u>: Q1 hr while on insulin drip.
2. <u>Renal panel</u>: Q2 hrs until bicarb >15 mEq/L, then Q4-6 until bicarb >20 mEq/L. Consider additional renal panels as needed.
3. <u>Ca, Mag, Phos</u>: Q4 hrs while on insulin drip
4. <u>Urine ketones</u>: Nurses on floor will dip all urine for ketones until negative × 3

Stop Insulin

1. <u>Stop insulin drip therapy when</u>: Pt is hungry and able to take adequate intake by mouth **and:**
   a) anion gap resolved, <u>or</u>
   b) bicarb >18 mEq/L
2. <u>For pts who have not yet received Lantus or Levemir</u>: Give the basal insulin dose 1 hour before discontinuing insulin drip.
3. <u>Initial subcutaneous rapid acting insulin dose</u>: Give first rapid acting insulin dose 10 minutes before discontinuing insulin drip.

Consider PICU management if: pt has altered mental status, pH < 7.1, age less than 2 with pH < 7.25, blood glucose >1000 mg/dl, corrected sodium >160 mEq/L.

Consider giving IV NaHCO$_3$ if: significant metabolic acidosis (pH < 7.0) and shock persist following initial infusion of NS. Administer 1-2 mEq/kg slowly over 2-4 hours to prevent paradoxical CNS acidosis.

Worry about cerebral edema if: Head ache, seizures, anisocoria, hypertension, bradycardia, posturing, or altered mental state develop acutely. Elevate the head of the bed, keep patient calm. Empirically treat by administration of Mannitol 1000 mg/kg/dose over 20-30 min or 3 % NS 3 ml/kg/dose, hyperventilate only if respiratory drive is compromised, transfer to PICU.

should begin with an isotonic solution, typically 10 to 20 mL/kg over 1 hour. If the patient is in shock, the volume can be infused as quickly as necessary; urinary losses should not be added to the calculation of replacement fluid. Mannitol should be readily available and administered for signs of CE. Close monitoring of electrolytes is critical. Low-dose insulin therapy is now the standard of care, with an infusion starting 1 to 2 hours after intravascular volume expansion has begun and continued until resolution of DKA. IV insulin bolus may increase the risk of CE and should *not* be used. IV sodium bicarbonate may be indicated in extreme acidemia, although its use is controversial.

6. What are the anesthetic implications of DKA?

The decision to proceed with surgery before complete correction of DKA must be discussed among the surgeon, endocrinologist, and anesthesiologist. If possible, surgery should be delayed until the glyco-metabolic control is reestablished. In emergent surgical situations, fluid resuscitation and insulin therapy may be undertaken during anesthesia with close monitoring of laboratory data and continuous communication with the endocrinologist.

Severe electrolyte abnormalities and some of the fluid deficit should be corrected prior to surgery. Electrolyte abnormalities and acidosis can impair myocardial function and worsen muscle weakness when combined with intraoperative medications. Close hemodynamic monitoring with arterial or central line access may be indicated. Vasopressors may be necessary to allow for hemodynamic stability in the face of limited fluid resuscitation and the general myocardial depressant effects of many anesthetics. The use of the DKA management protocol in place for the institution must be a part of the anesthetic plan. A baseline head CT scan is recommended if the patient is at high risk for CE, as early signs of CE will be masked in the unconscious surgical patient. The use of regional anesthesia techniques as a sole anesthetic is rarely practical in children but should be considered.

In addition to **insulin**, it is necessary to maintain a **dextrose solution** to avoid hypoglycemia during correction of the acidosis.

Most DKA protocols call for addition of **potassium chloride** to the replacement fluids. Fluids containing potassium must be run via a pump at a set rate and through a separate line from intraoperative volume replacement lines. Electrolytes as well as glucose and serum osmolality need to be monitored hourly. Insensible losses and replacement of intravascular volume caused by blood or other fluid loss should be replaced with an appropriate isotonic solution to preserve intravascular volume. Both IV insulin and glucose infusions should be continued until the glyco-metabolic control is stable and 1 to 2 hours after the patient is able to resume oral feeding without difficulty. If postoperative nausea and vomiting are present, IV insulin and glucose infusion should not be discontinued. All the fluids administered must be accounted for in the deficit calculations.

SUMMARY

1. Risk factors for DKA include new-onset type 1 DM, younger age, insulin pump use, and poor compliance.
2. DKA can mask a significant comorbidity such as urinary tract infection or appendicitis. DKA is characterized by hyperglycemia, ketonemia, and acidosis. Early treatment is critical. Cerebral edema is a severe complication of DKA.
3. DKA treatment protocols now call for slow rehydration, delay of insulin therapy, and close monitoring of electrolytes. The anesthetic management needs to account for the potential fluid deficit during the procedure and the myocardial effects of electrolyte abnormalities.

ANNOTATED REFERENCES

- Glaser N. Cerebral injury and cerebral edema in children with diabetic ketoacidosis: could cerebral ischemia and

reperfusion injury be involved? *Pediatr Diabetes* 2009; 10: 534–541.

Reviews the most frequent, serious complications of DKA, with a focus on cerebral edema in DKA.

- **Metzger DL. Diabetic ketoacidosis in children: An update and revised treatment protocol.** *BC Med J* 2010; 52(1): 24–31.

A succinct application of the ISPAD guideline in clinical practice. Dr. Metzger presents a valuable protocol derived from the conclusion of the consensus.

- **Wolfsdorf J, Craig ME, Daneman D, Dunger D, Edge J, Lee W, Rosenbloom A, Sperling M, Hanas R. International Society for Pediatric and Adolescent Diabetes (ISPAD). Clinical practice consensus guidelines 2009 compendium: diabetic ketoacidosis.** *Pediatr Diabetes* 2009; 10 (supp 12): 118–133.

A thorough review on the pathophysiology, pharmacology, and clinical management of DKA. The new recommendations for fluid management and changes in insulin therapy are described with a nice algorithm.

Further Reading

Cooke DW, Plotnik L. Management of diabetic ketoacidosis in children and adolescents. *Pediatr Rev* 2008; 29(12): 431–436.

Dunger DB, Sperling MA, Acerini CL. ESPE/LWPES consensus statement on diabetic ketoacidosis in children and adolescents. *Arch Dis Child* 2004; 89: 188–194.

Edge J, Jakes RW, Roy Y, Hawkins M, Winter D, Ford-Adams ME Murphy NP, Bergomi A, Widmer B, Dunger DB. The UK case-control study of cerebral edema complicating diabetic ketoacidosis in children. *Diabetologia* 2006; 49(9): 2002–2009.

Rhodes ET, Ferrari LR, Wolfsdorf JI. Perioperative management of pediatric surgical patients with diabetes mellitus. *Anesth Analg* 2005; 101: 986–999.

48

Hypopituitarism

LIANA G. HOSU AND LORI A. ARONSON

INTRODUCTION

Hypopituitarism refers to decreased secretion of pituitary hormones, which can result from diseases of the pituitary gland or hypothalamus. Surgery in the presence of untreated panhypopituitarism is rare. It is important to recognize the presence of hypopituitarism and most importantly adrenal insufficiency, a condition that can result in mortality from adrenal crisis without stress-dose corticosteroid treatment.

LEARNING OBJECTIVES

1. Understand the pathophysiology of hypopituitarism.
2. Recognize the clinical features of hypopituitarism.
3. Know the optimal perioperative management of patients with hypopituitarism.

CASE PRESENTATION

*A 7-year-old girl presents for functional endoscopic sinus surgery. Her past medical history is significant for craniopharyngioma diagnosed at age 5, when she underwent resection and radiation therapy. Since her surgery she has been taking **growth hormone**, **thyroid supplement**, and **desmopressin**.*

*Her perioperative endocrine management is discussed with the endocrinology team and her medications are continued preoperatively. Her preoperative labs show mild hypernatremia (Na 145 mEq/L), increased serum osmolality (310 mEq/L), and a mild **anemia** (hematocrit 29%).*

*After a smooth induction and intubation, the patient becomes hypotensive. A fluid bolus is given with minimal improvement in her blood pressure. A dose of hydrocortisone is administered due to concern about **hypocortisolism**. Intraoperatively, she is noted to have an increased output of dilute urine. Intraoperative labs show significant hypernatremia (Na 159 mEq/L) and increased serum osmolality. In consultation with the endocrine service, the decision is made to administer **desmopressin**. Vasopressin infusion is considered for further management. Based on estimation of water deficit and the level of hypernatremia, a fluid management plan is discussed to correct the hypernatremia slowly and to manage the polyuria. Postoperatively, the patient is admitted to the ICU for further management of her **diabetes insipidus**.*

DISCUSSION

1. What are the hormones of the pituitary gland?

The pituitary gland, situated in the sella turcica at the base of the brain, has two parts: anterior and posterior. The anterior pituitary secretes six hormones, which act on target organs and modulate hypothalamic and anterior pituitary activity: corticotropin, thyrotropin, prolactin, follicle-stimulating hormone, luteinizing hormone, and growth hormone. The posterior pituitary stores vasopressin (ADH) and oxytocin.

2. What is the clinical relevance of hypopituitarism?

Hypopituitarism may be either partial or complete and may result from either pituitary or hypothalamic disease. Cortisol and thyroxine are regulated by corticotrophin and thyrotropin. Cortisol secretion varies with the circadian rhythm, being highest in the morning and with stress, fever, hypoglycemia, and surgery. Surgery is one of the most potent activators of the *hypothalamic–pituitary–adrenal (HPA) axis.* Adrenocorticotropic hormone (ACTH) concentrations increase with incision and during surgery, with greatest secretion during reversal of anesthesia and extubation and in the immediate postoperative period. *Adrenal insufficiency* may result from destruction of the pituitary or adrenal glands, or from long-term administration of exogenous glucocorticoid, such as for treatment of severe asthma. Prednisone or its equivalent in doses of greater than 20 mg/day for longer than 3 weeks suppresses the HPA axis for up to 1 year after cessation of steroids. The HPA axis is not suppressed with doses of less than 5 mg/day of prednisone or its equivalent.

Pituitary or hypothalamic insufficiency can cause secondary hypothyroidism. Patients who are euthyroid on replacement therapy are not at increased risk of perioperative morbidity. However, patients with myxedema coma, those with severe clinical symptoms of chronic hypothyroidism, or those with markedly decreased T3 and T4 levels are at increased risk of having complications during the perioperative period secondary to cardiovascular depression refractory to catecholamine administration, hypothermia, airway difficulties due to generalized edema, and aspiration due to delayed gastric emptying. Elective surgery in symptomatic hypothyroid patients should be postponed until patients are rendered euthyroid.

Diabetes insipidus (DI) reflects the absence of ADH due to destruction of posterior pituitary (neurogenic DI) or failure of renal tubules to respond to ADH (nephrogenic DI). DI is differentiated on the basis of the response to desmopressin, concentrating urine in the presence of neurogenic but not nephrogenic DI. DI that develops during or immediately after pituitary gland surgery is generally transient and due to trauma to the posterior pituitary.

3. What are the risk factors for hypopituitarism?
The prevalence of hypopituitarism is 46 cases per 100,000 individuals, with an incidence of 4 cases per 100,000 per year

(Schneider et al., 2007). Most cases are due to pituitary tumors or their treatment. The mechanisms by which pituitary tumors cause hypopituitarism include mechanical compression of normal pituitary tissue, impaired blood flow to the normal tissue, and interference with the delivery of hypothalamic regulating hormones through the hypothalamic-hypophysial portal system. Reducing the size of the mass may relieve the pressure and restore pituitary function. Patients with brain, head, or neck tumors treated with radiation may have damage to the hypothalamus or pituitary gland resulting in partial or complete hypopituitarism. Since loss of pituitary function can be delayed several years after radiation, hormonal evaluation should be performed every 6 months.

Risk factors for postoperative pituitary deficiency are the size of the tumor, the degree of destruction of adjacent normal tissue, and the ability of the neurosurgeon to remove the tumor without disturbing the normal pituitary tissue. If a total hypophysectomy is performed, panhypopituitarism, including DI, results.

Table 48.1 lists causes of hypopituitarism in children.
Empty sella syndrome refers to an enlarged pituitary fossa resulting from arachnoid herniation through an incomplete sellar

---

Table 48.1

CAUSES OF HYPOPITUITARISM IN CHILDREN

Pituitary adenoma and treatment

Empty sella syndrome

Head trauma

Radiation therapy

Infiltrative diseases (e.g., eosinophilic granuloma)

Sheehan's syndrome (pituitary necrosis after postpartum hemorrhage)

Genetic: congenital and syndrome-associated hypopituitarism

---

diaphragm. 48% of children with either an isolated growth hormone deficiency or a combination of pituitary hormone deficiencies may have empty sella syndrome. Other causes of hypopituitarism include a tumor or cyst in the hypothalamus or infundibulum, infiltrative and vascular disorders, infection, hemochromatosis, granulomatous disease, and trauma (Vance, 1994).

4. How does one recognize hypopituitarism?

The clinical manifestations of hypopituitarism vary depending on the extent and severity of the pituitary hormone deficiency. Damage to the anterior pituitary can occur suddenly or slowly, can be mild or severe, and can affect the secretion of one, several, or all of its hormones. Some diseases, such as pituitary apoplexy (abrupt destruction of the pituitary gland by infarction or bleeding into the gland, usually in the context of an undiagnosed tumor), develop rapidly, causing sudden impairment of ACTH secretion and consequently sudden onset of symptoms of cortisol deficiency. Other insults, such as radiation therapy to the pituitary or hypothalamus, usually act slowly, causing symptoms many months or years later. The presentation of patients with deficiencies of those hormones that control target glands is often similar to the presentation of patients with primary deficiencies of the target gland hormones they control. Patients in whom the hypopituitarism is due to a pituitary or sellar mass may also have symptoms related to the mass: headache, visual loss, or diplopia.

The symptoms of corticotropin deficiency include fatigue, weakness, headache, anorexia, weight loss, nausea, vomiting, abdominal pain, and altered mental status. In its most severe form, cortisol deficiency leads to death due to vascular collapse. Physical examination is notable for lack of the hyperpigmentation that occurs in patients with primary adrenal insufficiency. Orthostatic hypotension is common. Women with longstanding adrenal insufficiency often have loss of axillary and pubic hair. Hyponatremia may occur as a result of increased ADH secretion but the serum potassium concentration is usually normal, since adrenal production of aldosterone is not dependent on corticotropin. In contrast, both hyponatremia and hyperkalemia are common in patients with primary adrenal insufficiency. Normochromic, normocytic **anemia** and eosinophilia may also occur with corticotropin deficiency. Orthopedic manifestations have been seen, and slipped capital femoral epiphysis is associated with endocrinopathies, including panhypopituitarism, in a little over 5% of cases (Bowden & Klingele, 2009).

The clinical presentation of TSH deficiency is exclusively that of thyroxine deficiency and includes fatigue, weakness, cold intolerance, constipation, facial puffiness, bradycardia, and dry skin. Impaired memory or altered mental activity is characteristic of severe hypothyroidism. Physical examination may reveal bradycardia, periorbital puffiness, and delayed relaxation of tendon reflexes.

Growth hormone deficiency in children typically presents as short stature. Prolactin deficiency manifests as inability to lactate after delivery. Deficient secretion of the gonadotropins follicle-stimulating hormone and luteinizing hormone causes infertility and sexual dysfunction in both men and premenopausal women. Pubic and axillary hair is present unless there is concomitant adrenal failure.

Classic manifestations of DI are polydipsia and a high output of poorly concentrated urine despite increased serum osmolarity, volume contraction, and dehydration. A simple calculation of serum osmolality may be helpful (normal 285–295 mOsm/kg or mmol/L).

Serum osmolality (mmol/L) = 2 $[Na^+]$ + 2 $[K^+]$ + Glucose + Urea (all in mmol/L) or

Serum osmolality = $2[Na^+]$ + [Glucose]/18 + [BUN]/2.8 (where [Glucose] and [BUN] are measured in mg/dL).

Without treatment, intravascular volume depletion occurs, cardiac stroke volume decreases, and heart rate increases in an effort to maintain cardiac output. These patients may have weak peripheral pulses, orthostatic hypotension, cold, clammy skin, shallow and rapid breathing, and a reduced level of consciousness. Hypernatremia may manifest as seizures and hyperreflexia.

5. What studies can be performed to confirm hypopituitarism?
Pituitary insufficiency can be confirmed by using endocrine laboratory and imaging studies. Although basal serum hormone measurements may be all that is needed to confirm hypopituitarism, dynamic tests are used if the results of serum hormone tests are equivocal or to diagnose partial deficiencies. Both the target hormone concentration and the pituitary hormone concentration should be measured to assess the appropriateness of both values. After clinical and biochemical diagnosis of hypopituitarism has been made, an imaging study of the hypothalamic–pituitary region should be performed to determine whether a mass is present. The most informative image is an MRI scan. A high-resolution CT scan with contrast administration is an adequate alternative.

6. What is involved in the perioperative management of patients with hypopituitarism?
Management of anesthesia for patients with hypocortisolism includes the administration of exogenous corticosteroid supplementation and a high index of suspicion for primary adrenal failure if unexplained intraoperative hypotension occurs. Selection of anesthetic drugs and muscle relaxants is not influenced by the presence of treated hypocortisolism, with the possible exception of etomidate. Etomidate has been shown to transiently inhibit synthesis of cortisol in normal patients. If surgery becomes necessary, perioperative management must include administration of supplemental corticosteroids and intravenous infusion of sodium-containing fluids. Minimal doses of anesthetic drugs should be administered as these patients may be exquisitely sensitive to drug-induced myocardial depression. Invasive monitoring of systemic blood pressure and cardiac filling pressures may be indicated. Plasma concentrations of glucose and electrolytes should be measured frequently during the perioperative period. In view of skeletal muscle weakness, the initial dose of muscle

relaxant may need to be decreased and the response monitored using a peripheral nerve stimulator.

Elective surgery should be deferred in patients with symptomatic hypothyroidism, although controlled clinical studies have not confirmed an increased risk when patients with mild to moderate hypothyroidism undergo elective surgery. Complications from hypothyroidism and anesthesia may include increased sensitivity to depressant drugs, a hypodynamic cardiovascular system with bradycardia and decreased cardiac output, slow metabolism of drugs, impaired ventilatory responses to arterial hypoxemia or hypercarbia, hypovolemia, hyponatremia, hypoglycemia, and delayed gastric emptying time (Bennett-Guerrero et al., 1997).

Fluid management must be closely followed in patients with DI. Exogenous replacement of ADH is with either **desmopressin** or aqueous vasopressin. Desmopressin lacks the vasoconstrictor effects of vasopressin. Therefore, desmopressin administration is less likely to cause hypertension or abdominal cramping than vasopressin. Those on baseline therapy may require some degree of fluid restriction, while those manifesting DI acutely intraoperatively will need adequate resuscitation and possible treatment. In the conscious patient with intact thirst mechanism, desmopressin may be administered intranasally on a daily basis and fluid intake monitored closely. Management through fluid restriction and volume contraction alone is also possible (Laxton & Petrozza, 2007).

Management of the unconscious surgical patient is more difficult. For the patient with preexisting DI, desmopressin may be either withheld several days before surgery or continued until the evening before surgery. Intraoperatively, DI is seen most frequently in neurosurgical patients, and osmotic diuresis with mannitol is avoided and urine output monitored closely. If urine output rises abruptly and simultaneously obtained urine and serum osmolalities suggest DI, intravenous vasopressin administration should begin. Postoperative DI most commonly begins the evening following surgery and may resolve in 3 to 5 days if osmoregulatory structures have not been permanently injured. Perioperative glucocorticoid administration may facilitate development of polyuria.

SUMMARY

1. The pituitary gland is instrumental in regulating many hormonal systems. Patients with adrenal insufficiency and hypothyroidism are at greatest risk.
2. The primary risk factor for hypopituitarism is a tumor and its subsequent treatment. In children, one may see empty sella syndrome.
3. Pathology should be identified and treatment initiated prior to elective and nonemergent surgery. One should have a high index of suspicion for adrenal suppression and the need for stress-dose steroids prior to or during surgery and also for the intraoperative manifestations of DI during surgical tumor resection.

ANNOTATED REFERENCES

- Vance ML. Hypopituitarism. *N Engl J Med* 1994; 330: 1651–1662.

  This article is a thorough overview of the etiology, clinical features, diagnosis, and treatment of hypopituitarism.

Further Reading

Bennett-Guerrero E, Kramer DC, Schwinn DA. Effect of chronic and acute thyroid hormone reduction on perioperative outcome. *Anesth Analg* 1997; 85: 30–36.

Bowden SA, Klingele KE. Chronic bilateral slipped capital femoral epiphysis as an unusual presentation of congenital panhypopituitarism due to pituitary hypoplasia in a 17-year-old female. *Int J Pediatr Endocrin* 2009, Article ID 609131.

Laxton MA, Petrozza PH. Pituitary tumors: diabetes insipidus. In Atlee J, ed. *Complications in Anesthesia*, 2nd ed. Philadelphia: Saunders, 2007: 712–713.

Schneider HJ, Aimaretti G, Kreitschmann-Andermahr I, Stalla GK, Ghigo E. Hypopituitarism. *Lancet* 2007; 369(9571): 1461–70.

49

Mitochondrial Disorder for Muscle Biopsy

J. FAY JOU, LORI A. ARONSON, AND
JACQUELINE W. MORILLO-DELERME

INTRODUCTION

Mitochondrial disease (mtD) is a genetically, biochemically, and clinically heterogeneous group of disorders that arise most commonly from defects in the oxidative phosphorylation or electron transport chain involved in energy metabolism. These patients have an increased risk for cardiac, respiratory, neurologic, and metabolic complications from anesthesia. Consequently, there are several anesthetic considerations for patients with mtD.

LEARNING OBJECTIVES

1. **Identify common clinical presentations of a patient with mtD.**
2. **Anticipate anesthetic implications for the disease.**
3. **Discuss anesthetic management for patients with mtD.**

CASE PRESENTATION

A 7-year-old girl with difficulty swallowing, choking, and gagging due to Chiari I malformation is scheduled for posterior fossa decompression with monitoring of evoked potentials. She presents for a pre-anesthesia consultation. The patient's medical history is significant for **complex I mitochondrial disease**, coenzyme Q10 deficiency, and adrenal insufficiency. Her symptoms include myopathy, fatigability, chronic "wet" cough, history of frequent pneumonias, chronic sinusitis, and respiratory muscle weakness. She uses a respiratory vest daily for chest physiotherapy and had a normal sleep study 9 months earlier. She has a history of aspiration, mild gastroparesis, and gastroesophageal reflux disease (**GERD**), for which she had a gastrostomy tube placement. The patient is prone to dehydration and ketotic **hypoglycemia exacerbated by illness**. Her parents have heard that **propofol** should not be used in mtD patients but are concerned that their daughter might be at risk for **malignant hyperthermia (MH)**.

DISCUSSION

1. What is a mitochondrial disease? How does it present?

mtD is a heterogeneous group of disorders that arise as a result of defects in the oxidative phosphorylation or electron transport chain involved in energy metabolism. The disease can be broadly classified into primary disorders and secondary disorders. Primary disorders can be caused by either inherited or spontaneous mutations or deletions of nuclear DNA (nDNA) or mitochondrial DNA (mtDNA). In general, nDNA mutations present in childhood and mtDNA mutations present in late childhood or adult life. Secondary disorders are caused by a broad spectrum of free radicals, drugs, or diseases in which abnormal mitochondrial functions have been postulated or demonstrated. These metabolic diseases, inherited or acquired, include untreated hyper- and hypothyroidism, diabetes mellitus, systemic lupus erythematosus, and certain types of cancer. Drugs such as aspirin, statins, chemotherapy, and agents used to treat human immunodeficiency virus infections have also been implicated (Naviaux, 1997).

A confounding feature of mtD is that identical genetic mutations may not produce identical diseases. Table 49.1 summarizes the protean presentation of mitochondrial disorders. Conversely,

---

Table 49.1

COMMON CLINICAL PRESENTATIONS OF MITOCHONDRIAL DISEASE

Systems	Presentation
Airway/ Breathing	Frequent pulmonary infections, respiratory muscle weakness, central alveolar hypoventilation syndrome, obstructive sleep apnea, macroglossia, stridor, choking episodes
Cardiac	Exercise intolerance, conduction defects (heart blocks) that may require a pacemaker, pre-excitation syndromes (Wolff-Parkinson-White), cardiomyopathy (dilated or hypertrophic)
Neurology	Seizure disorder, encephalopathy, dementia, ataxia, stroke-like episodes, myoclonus, dysphagia, ophthalmoplegia, hearing loss, neuropathy
Endocrine	Diabetes mellitus, exocrine pancreatic dysfunction, hypo/hyperthyroidism
Fluid/ Electrolytes/ Nutrition	Intolerance to fasting, dietary restrictions, failure to thrive, nutritional supplementation, altered glucose level, elevated lactate level, altered renal function
GI	Aspiration risks, swallowing difficulties, GI dysmotility, gastroesophageal reflux disease (GERD), altered hepatic function, cholestasis
Hematology	Anemia, neutropenia
Musculoskeletal	Hypotonia, weakness, myopathy, muscle wasting

different genetic mutations can lead to the same disease. Due to a large overlap, there is no clear correlation between clinical findings and the site of biochemical defect. The prevalence of mtD at birth is 1:5,000. A conservative estimate for the prevalence of all mtD is 11.5/100,000 (~1/8,500).

2. What preoperative testing is necessary?

In addition to baseline vital signs and physical exam, one should consider obtaining a complete blood count, basic metabolic panel, liver function test, thyroid function test, urine analysis, blood gases, chest x-ray, pulmonary flow-volume loops, sleep study, ECG, and echocardiography as indicated by the patient's condition.

3. Is a "clean" anesthetic technique necessary? What is the risk of MH in a patient with mtD?

Susceptibility to **MH** is a recognized complication of neuromuscular disorders and was previously thought to have an association with mitochondrial myopathies. There are currently only two disorders for which a clear link to MH has been established: central core disease and King Denborough syndrome.

Although the association between mtD (including mitochondrial myopathies) and MH has now mostly been dismissed, guidelines for the anesthetic management of these patients remain lacking, especially if patients present with neuromuscular deficits of unknown etiology. Flick et al. (2007) concluded that in a diverse population of children undergoing muscle biopsy for known or suspected neuromuscular disorder, the estimated risk of MH or rhabdomyolysis is 1.09% or less. Each clinician must decide whether this risk justifies the use of a "clean" anesthetic technique to avoid MH.

4. What is the best anesthetic plan for this patient?

Because mtD arises from a variety of molecular changes, patients with mtD will have diverse responses to anesthetics. While there is no clear guidance in the literature as to the best anesthetic technique, the overall aim is to *maintain normoglycemia* and *normovolemia* and *avoid* further *metabolic stresses* that may provoke or worsen lactic acidosis (Wallace et al., 1998).

Sedative premedication should be given judiciously to avoid respiratory depression. Impaired respiratory responses to hypoxemia and hypercarbia have been reported in these patients, along with prolonged somnolence following barbiturates. Impaired upper airway and lower esophageal sphincter tone may predispose mtD patients to reflux and aspiration. In patients with overt signs of **GERD** and/or bulbar muscle dysfunction, the use of reflux prophylaxis, including adequate fasting, cricoid pressure, and rapid-sequence intubation, should be considered (possibly with the avoidance of succinylcholine). Pharmacologic prophylaxis with histamine-2 receptor antagonists, proton pump inhibitors, and nonparticulate antacids may also be indicated.

Induction of anesthesia should be undertaken with several considerations in mind. Sensitivity to intravenous induction agents has been described, although thiopental, propofol, and ketamine have all been used safely. Potent inhalational anesthetic agents appear to be safe in the majority of mtD patients, but patients with **complex I dysfunction** are more sensitive. At concentrations of about 2 MAC (minimal alveolar concentration), the activity of complex I was reduced by about 20% in the presence of halothane or isoflurane and by about 10% in the presence of sevoflurane (Hanley et al., 2002). Though these inhibitory effects are unlikely to compromise cardiac performance, careful titration of these volatile agents is advisable.

Patients with mtD often have underlying **hypoglycemia** and *lactic acidosis*, which may be *exacerbated by the surgical stress response*. The hypoglycemia is due to inability of the diseased mitochondria to sustain their energy requirements from fatty acid oxidation during periods of fasting and stress, thus leading to the depletion of carbohydrate stores. Anaerobic metabolism of glucose can cause serum lactate levels in these patients to rise acutely. Adequate dextrose-containing *lactate-free fluids* should be administered preferably up to 3 hours before induction and maintained throughout perioperative care.

5. Should muscle relaxants be avoided?

There has been one case report of a child with mtD who developed myotonic rigidity and signs of MH after the administration of succinylcholine with induction of general anesthesia. While mtD patients may not be susceptible to MH, risks for rhabdomyolysis and hyperkalemia still exist. Succinylcholine has the potential to cause unexpected cardiac arrest from hyperkalemia due to rhabdomyolysis in children with myopathies. Avoidance of succinylcholine in mtD patients is recommended, given the availability of alternative relaxants.

Nondepolarizing muscle relaxants in children with mtD have varying effects. Given the potential for prolonged neuromuscular blockade, the use of shorter-acting nondepolarizing muscle relaxants and close monitoring with a nerve stimulator are recommended.

6. Is propofol safe for these patients?

Propofol has high plasma clearance and rapid metabolism, making it an ideal agent for total intravenous anesthesia (TIVA) and for sedation. However, because mtD patients may be more susceptible to the effects of an increased lipid load, the safe total dose and duration of propofol infusion are not known. Even in normal children, there have been cases in which short-term high-dose propofol infusions have resulted in propofol infusion syndrome (PRIS).

Propofol's impairment of mitochondrial function may play a role in PRIS. It uncouples oxidative phosphorylation and respiratory chain *in vitro* by inhibition of the mitochondrial enzyme complex I and dose-dependent inhibition of complex II and depolarizes mitochondrial membrane potential by modifying ATPases (Rigoulet et al., 1996). Additionally, the lipid component in the propofol formulation can compound the accumulation of toxic fatty-acid intermediates. Avoidance of propofol in the more symptomatic patients should be considered; its use in these patients has been associated with an increased incidence of metabolic acidosis, prolonged anesthesia recovery, and ICU admission.

Should propofol infusions be necessary, monitor lactate levels, ensure adequate carbohydrate intake (6 mg/kg/min) to suppress fat metabolism, minimize exposure by using it in combination with other anesthetics (e.g., ketamine, opioids, dexmedetomidine), and avoid prolonged use.

7. What are the options for postoperative analgesia?

Pain management in mtD patients is critical because the response to pain may worsen their risk of metabolic acidosis from depleted energy stores and increased oxygen demand. A multimodal analgesic approach should be used involving opioids, nonsteroidal anti-inflammatory drugs, and local and regional anesthesia.

Although opioids have been used without adverse event, cautious titration of sedative-hypnotics and opioids is still advised. Decreased ventilatory response to both hypoxia and hypercarbia (unrelated to muscle weakness) has been described. Regional techniques lessen the potential for lactic acidosis by reducing anesthetic requirement, thus minimizing risks of respiratory depression.

If a regional anesthetic technique is possible, this may be the technique of choice. Assessment of coagulation function should precede any neuraxial technique due to the possibility of hepatic dysfunction in patients with mtD. Long-acting local anesthetics (bupivacaine, levobupivacaine, ropivacaine) have been shown *in vitro* to inhibit complex I and uncouple oxidative phosphorylation, causing mitochondrial membrane depolarization and Ca^{2+} dysregulation (Nouette-Gaulain et al., 2007). Maslow and Lisbon (1993) observed that mtD patients with demyelination of the spinal cord or peripheral nerves may be predisposed to develop seizures, strokes, and possibly aggravation or precipitation of spinal-peripheral nerve pathology. While it is possible that patients without clinically evident neuropathy are at no increased risk of sequelae from regional anesthesia and interactions with local anesthetics, it may be prudent to avoid regional anesthetic techniques if the patient demonstrates any evidence of peripheral nerve or spinal cord abnormalities.

8. What postoperative complications are likely?

Postoperative complications are related to the clinical condition of the patient prior to surgery and the complexity of the surgical procedure. Adverse events reported include respiratory difficulties, cardiac arrhythmias, and new neurologic problems such as stroke, worsening of the overall neurologic status, seizures, prolonged coma, and death. It is important to maintain anticonvulsant therapy up to the time of surgery, and promptly resume therapy (or intravenous or rectal equivalent) postoperatively. Close postoperative monitoring for respiratory compromise and cardiovascular instability is important to help prevent complications.

SUMMARY

1. Patients with mitochondrial disorders display wide variation in their clinical presentation and disease severity. Multiple organ systems are often affected.
2. Mitochondrial disorders have not been linked to an increased incidence of MH.
3. Adequate dextrose-containing, lactate-free intravenous fluids should be administered in the perioperative period.
4. Succinylcholine is probably best avoided. Nondepolarizing muscle relaxants can have a prolonged duration of action.
5. Propofol should be avoided in the more symptomatic mtD patients.
6. Meticulous preoperative assessment, a thoughtful anesthetic plan, and close monitoring of the patient allow for the safe administration of general anesthesia to mtD patients. Metabolic decompensation from general anesthesia is rare.

ANNOTATED REFERENCES

- Driessen J, Willems S, Dercksen S, Giele J, van der Staak F, Smeitink J. Anesthesia-related morbidity and mortality after surgery for muscle biopsy in children with mitochondrial defects. *Pediatr Anesth* 2007; 17: 16–21.

  This is a retrospective case review study of 155 children who underwent diagnostic muscle biopsy for suspected mtD and muscle disorders. With standard preoperative assessment, monitoring, and anesthesia management, there were no serious adverse events attributed to anesthesia in the 122 children who were later diagnosed with mtD.

- Flick RP, Gleich SJ, Herr MMH, Wedel, DJ. The risk of malignant hyperthermia in children undergoing muscle biopsy for suspected neuromuscular disorder. *Pediatr Anesth* 2007; 17: 22–27.

  This is a retrospective case review of 274 children who received a volatile anesthetic agent or succinylcholine while undergoing diagnostic muscle biopsy for suspected neuromuscular disorder. No patient exhibited signs or symptoms of MH or rhabdomyolysis.

- Footitt EJ, Sinha MD, Raiman JA, Dhawan A, Moganasundram S, Champion MP. Mitochondrial disorders and general anaesthesia: a case series and review. *Br J Anaesth* 2008; 100: 436–441.

  This is a retrospective case review study of 38 mtD patients who had undergone 58 episodes of general anesthesia. There were no episodes of MH and no documented intraoperative complications attributable to general anesthesia.

Further Reading

Chinnery PF. Mitochondrial disorders overview. *GeneReviews*. Accessed Feb. 5, 2011. http://www.ncbi.nlm.nih.gov/books/NBK1224/.

Hanley PJ, Ray J, Brandt U, Daut J. Halothane, isoflurane, and sevoflurane inhibit NADH:ubiquinone oxidoreductase (complex I) of cardiac mitochondria. *J Physiol* 2002; 544(3): 687–693.

Maslow A, Lisbon A. Anesthetic considerations in patients with mitochondrial dysfunction. *Anesth Analg* 1993; 76: 884–886.

Naviaux RK. The spectrum of mitochondrial disease. In Weber K, ed. *Mitochondrial and Metabolic Disorders: A Primary Care Physician's Guide*, 1st ed. Oradell, NJ: Psy-Ed Corp., 1997: 3–10.

Nouette-Gaulain K, Sirvent P, Canal-Raffin M, Morau D, Malgat M, Molimard M, Mercier J, Lacampagne A, Sztark F, Capdevila X. Effects of intermittent femoral nerve injections of bupivacaine, levobupivacaine, and ropivacaine on mitochondrial energy metabolism and intracellular calcium homeostasis in rat psoas muscle. *Anesthesiology* 2007; 106: 1026–1034.

Rigoulet M, Devin A, Avéret N, Vandais B, Guérin B. Mechanisms of inhibition and uncoupling of respiration in isolated rat liver mitochondria by the general anesthetic 2,6-diisopropylphenol. *Eur J Biochem* 1996; 241: 280–285.

Wallace JJ, Perndt H, Skinner M. Anaesthesia and mitochondrial disease. *Paediatr Anaesth* 1998; 8: 249–254.

50

Obesity

VIDYA CHIDAMBARAN AND
SENTHILKUMAR SADHASIVAM

INTRODUCTION

Over the past few decades, obesity rates have doubled among adolescents and tripled among children in the United States. The risk for anesthesia-related morbidity is higher in obese children, so anesthesiologists need to have a comprehensive knowledge of the pathophysiology of obesity in children and its unique anesthetic implications.

LEARNING OBJECTIVES

1. Understand the anesthetic implications of obesity and its effects on various body systems.
2. Know the principles of perioperative management of obese children.
3. Gain a working knowledge of pharmacokinetics of common anesthetic drugs in obese children and dosage implications.

CASE PRESENTATION

*A 10-year-old boy who weighs 98 kg and is 140 cm tall (BMI 50) presents for hip pinning of his slipped capital femoral epiphysis. He has a history of **sleep and behavioral disturbances**, and a sleep study* showed a Respiratory Disturbance Index of 36. He has been fitted with **nasal continuous positive airway pressure (CPAP)** of 8 cmH$_2$O but has not tolerated it well. He has a history of mild, controlled **asthma** and is **not very active,** especially due to his hip pain. He takes thyroxine for **hypothyroidism** and is on metformin 500 mg/day for **non-insulin-dependent diabetes mellitus.** An echocardiogram showed left ventricular dilation but adequate cardiac function. He has properly fasted. His physical examination is significant for BP of 130/82, obesity with rolls of fat behind his neck, a double chin, and a pear-shaped appearance. He is nervous and tearful. On **airway** examination, he has adequate mouth opening, restricted neck extension, and a Mallampati class 3 airway. He is given **midazolam** 15 mg orally preoperatively, which makes him very sleepy. On arrival to the OR, his room air oxygen saturation is 94%. Monitors are placed, he is given nitrous oxide and oxygen by mask, and IV access is secured on the second attempt. Sheets are stacked under his head and shoulders. After preoxygenation for 3 minutes, **rapid-sequence induction** is done with propofol and succinylcholine (suxamethonium). The patient **desaturates** to 78% before the airway is intubated and secured. Despite clear bilateral breath sounds, **high airway pressures** are needed to ventilate the patient with a tidal volume of 8 mL/kg. After a few breaths with airway pressures of 35 cmH$_2$O and positive end-expiratory pressure (PEEP) of 5 cmH$_2$O, his saturation normalizes. An orogastric tube is placed and **300 mL of gastric fluid** is suctioned. Maintenance of anesthesia is with oxygen/air, desflurane, cisatracurium, fentanyl, and then morphine towards the end of the operation.

At the end of surgery, he is given **ketorolac** for pain relief and prophylactic ondansetron to prevent nausea/vomiting. Neuromuscular relaxation is reversed and the patient is **extubated awake** in the OR. The patient complains of hip pain and is given 0.5 mcg/kg of fentanyl. As the patient is being transported to the recovery room, his airway becomes obstructed, requiring a vigorous jaw thrust and positive pressure by mask. In the recovery room, a lubricated nasal airway is inserted, but he continues to snore and remain sleepy with an oxygen saturation oxygen of 92%. CPAP is initiated and his saturations improve to 96%. Due to his need for pain medication and his sleep *apnea, he is admitted for overnight observation and monitoring and is discharged uneventfully the next day.*

DISCUSSION

1. How is obesity defined in children?

Obesity refers to an individual who has excess body fatness. Different criteria have been used to describe obesity in children, including a body weight that is 20% or more than the recommended body weight for age and height. In adults, obesity can easily be defined with reference to Body Mass Index (BMI = weight in kilograms/height in meters^2). An adult with a BMI above 25 is considered "overweight," a BMI above 30 is "obesity," a BMI above 35 is "morbid obesity," and a BMI above 50 is "super-morbid obesity." In children, the BMI reference changes with age and sex. On a gender-specific BMI-for-age growth chart (Centers for Disease Control and Prevention), children whose BMI-for-age percentile measurements are between the 85th and 95th percentile are "overweight," and those above the 95th percentile are "obese" (Ogden & Flegal, 2010). Other terms used for calculation of drug doses are: ideal body weight (IBW) = 22 × (height in m)^2 and lean body mass (LBM), which comprises all nonfatty tissues and accounts for 99% of the body's metabolic activity. Obesity is associated with a 20% to 40% increase in LBM.

2. What are the effects of obesity on various organ systems? What are the anesthetic implications?

Airway: Obese children have an increased risk of *difficult mask ventilation* (7.4% vs. 2.2% in non-obese), airway obstruction, bronchospasm, and overall *critical respiratory events*. In adults, morbid obesity and neck thickness are risk factors for difficult intubation. However, in children, few studies predict difficult laryngoscopy (1.3% vs. 0.4%) (Nafui et al., 2007). Others report equivalent rates of difficulty in intubation (10%) in obese and non-obese children. The following factors can contribute to a difficult airway in obese children: diminished mandibular and atlanto-occipital joint mobility, narrowed upper airway and small mouth, short distance from mandible to sternal fat, and redundant oral tissue. Positioning the patient with the head and shoulders elevated, so that the ears and the sternum are at the same level, can improve the laryngoscopic view dramatically in obese patients (Collins et al., 2004). It is important to have help and emergency airway backup available.

Childhood obesity is highly associated with *obstructive sleep apnea* (OSA). Unlike adults, OSA in children is associated more with hyperactivity and learning difficulties than daytime somnolence. Disordered sleep breathing (as in the case scenario) occurs four to five times more frequently in obese children than their normal-weight counterparts. Polysomnography can be used to quantify sleep apnea and to assess the need for **CPAP** during sleep to improve OSA symptoms.

Respiratory: Obese children have reduced lung volumes and forced expiratory volume (FEV)/forced vital capacity (FVC) ratios, in addition to lower functional residual capacity (FRC) and higher oxygen consumption. Rapid oxygen **desaturation** occurs on induction and during periods of apnea. Obese children have reduced chest compliance due to the weight of the fat rolls on the neck and chest as well as an increased risk of developing asthma. Practically, preoxygenation in the upright position helps reduce desaturation episodes, and alveolar recruitment strategies such as elevated peak inspiratory pressures and optimal PEEP may be required for successful ventilation intraoperatively.

Cardiac: Obesity is associated with *hypertension* due to increased cardiac output and increased hemodynamic load. Echocardiogram findings show increased ventricular dimensions and early subclinical findings of ventricular dysfunction, though cardiac reserves are preserved. In patients with OSA, increased oxygen demand, hypoxia, hypercapnia, increased pulmonary blood flow, and polycythemia are common physiologic changes. The extreme example is the patient with Pickwickian syndrome who is hypercapnic and has right ventricular strain/failure and somnolence (obesity hypoventilation syndrome). It is important to assess cardiac function with an echocardiogram in inactive children who fit this picture, or who are coming in for a major operation.

Gastrointestinal: Traditionally, morbid obesity has been associated with an increased incidence of gastroesophageal reflux, hiatal hernia, attenuated gastric emptying, and lower gastric pH, with a predisposition to aspiration during bag-mask ventilation and intubation. Gastric acid pretreatment with proton pump inhibitors, histamine receptor-2 blockers, and sodium bicitrate has been advised preoperatively. Recent evidence refutes this increased risk for aspiration in obese children. The gastric fluid volume in obese children (1 mL/kg IBW) was found to be no different from non-obese children (Cook-Sather et al., 2009).

Endocrine: Obese children are at increased risk for diabetes, which may require treatment, and the metabolic syndrome (obesity, elevated triglycerides, low HDL cholesterol, hypertension, and increased plasma glucose). Hypothyroidism is also frequently associated with obesity.

Mental Health: The social stigma associated with childhood obesity can be profound. Overall, 35% of obese children have a psychiatric diagnosis.

Thromboembolic: Longer hospital stays with immobilization increase the risk of **deep vein thrombosis and pulmonary embolism.** Therefore, compression stockings and other preventive measures are indicated.

3. What are other perioperative considerations in caring for an obese patient?

Preoperative: Preoperative laboratory studies may be indicated based on the planned operation and the patient's medical condition. Arterial blood gas determination may be indicated in patients with Pickwickian syndrome, and preoperative glucose measurement is important for diabetic patients. Premedication must be individualized and given judiciously, especially in the face of OSA, when the patient must be monitored closely with pulse oximetry and direct observation.

Intraoperative: Intravenous access may be difficult due to obesity. Routine noninvasive monitors are acceptable. However, if an appropriate-size blood pressure cuff fails to read due to the thickness or conical shape of the arm or forearm, an arterial line may be necessary for monitoring blood pressure. Careful padding of pressure points is important as these patients are at increased risk for neuropathies. As in adults, regional anesthesia techniques may be more challenging in obese children due to difficult positioning, increased fatty tissue, and increased lordosis. Despite these difficulties, regional anesthesia may significantly decrease the opioid doses needed for postoperative analgesia. Though most data regarding neuraxial blocks and obesity come from obstetrics, it would be prudent to assume that reduced epidural local anesthetic volume is needed for similar levels of anesthesia compared to non-obese patients. Lastly, it appears safer to extubate obese children awake.

Postoperative: It is important to watch for airway obstruction, apnea, and respiratory failure. Preoperative CPAP should be resumed postoperatively. Caution might be warranted while using positive airway pressure by mask after gastric bypass surgery due to the risk for gastric insufflation and anastomotic leak. It is important to remember that patients with sleep apnea are very sensitive to respiratory depressants and opioids. Pain control can be achieved by patient-controlled analgesia or carefully titrated doses of analgesics. Use of regional techniques and non-opioid analgesics like ketorolac are important adjuncts that decrease the risk of respiratory depression. Patients with severe sleep apnea should be **admitted** for **observation** and **monitoring** after general anesthesia.

4. How is medication dosing altered in an obese child like this one?

With a paucity of information specifically on the pharmacokinetics and pharmacodynamics of many common drugs, including anesthetic agents, in obese children, conclusions are largely drawn from adult literature. Generally, volume of distribution

(V_d) determines the loading dose for a drug and clearance determines the maintenance dose. Hence, *highly lipophilic* drugs as propofol, fentanyl, dexmedetomidine, cisatracurium, and benzodiazepines have increased V_d and are dosed to total body weight (TBW). Sodium thiopental (thiopentone) is an exception and is dosed to IBW, as obese patients have increased sensitivity to its effects. Remifentanil has a lower-than-expected V_d for lipid-soluble drugs and, due to its rapid extrahepatic metabolism, is dosed based on IBW, not TBW.

Weakly lipophilic drugs, such as ketamine, vecuronium, rocuronium, and morphine, are dosed by lean body mass (about 20% more than IBW) because their limited volume of distribution is not influenced by fat stores. The V_d of muscle relaxants and other *hydrophilic* drugs is not affected by increased fat stores, and hence they are dosed based on IBW. Table 50.1 summarizes the pharmacological effects of obesity.

For the patient in the case presentation (TBW 98 kg, IBW 22 × 1.4^2 = 41.8 kg, LBM = 120% of IBW = 50.16 kg), the following doses are used:

- **Propofol:** 1 to 2 mg/kg (TBW) = 2 × 98 ∼ 200 mg. Clearance and V_d have been found to correlate with TBW. Rates for infusion have been successfully calculated using an empirical formula "Corrected weight = IBM + [0.4 × excess weight]." Caution needs to be exercised in administering boluses based on TBW, especially for drugs that cause hemodynamic changes; it is best to administer these drugs by *titration to clinical effect*.
- **Fentanyl:** 1 to 2 mcg/kg (TBW) = 100 to 200 mcg, followed by morphine at the end of the case (0.1–0.2 mg/kg) (LBM) = 5 – 10 mg
- **Succinylcholine:** 1 to 2 mg/kg at TBW (not IBW, as would be expected, given that succinylcholine is a hydrophilic drug; this is due to increased plasma cholinesterase activity in the obese population) = 98 to 190 mg. Usually, a dose of 120 to 150 mg is adequate.

Table 50.1

GENERAL PHARMACOKINETIC IMPLICATIONS OF OBESITY

Physiological Factors	Volume of Distribution		Clearance		Dosing Recommendations, Based on Weight	
	LD	HD	LD	HD	LD	HD
Body composition*						
Increased adipose tissue ↑↑	↑	↔	↔	↔	Loading dose—total body weight	Dose based on ideal body weight
Increased lean body mass ↑	↑	↔	↑	↑	Maintenance dose—lean body weight	
Organ function and blood flow						
Increased renal blood flow, increased GFR, increased tubular secretion	↔	↔	↑	↑	Insufficient data for dose recommendations	
Altered hepatic metabolism (fatty degeneration of the liver)	↔	↔	↓	↓	Insufficient data for dose recommendations	

(continued)

Table 50.1 (continued)

Physiological Factors	Volume of Distribution		Clearance		Dosing Recommendations, Based on Weight	
	LD	HD	LD	HD	LD	HD
Protein binding changes	**Effect**				**Recommendations**	
Increased concentrations of free fatty acids, cholesterol, triglycerides, and lipoproteins inhibit protein binding	Increased free drug levels				No dosage changes recommended	
Plasma albumin unchanged, increased α_1-acid glycoprotein	Decreased free drug levels					

LD, lipophilic drugs; HD, hydrophilic drugs.

* 75% excess weight is fat mass generally, but there is high variability in fatness for same BMI.

Sources: (1) Casati A, Putzu M. Anesthesia in the obese patient: Pharmacokinetic considerations. *J Clin Anesth* 2005; 17(2): 134–145 and (2) Mulla H, Johnson TN. Dosing dilemmas in obese children. *Arch Dis Childhood Education Practice* 2010; 95(4): 112–117.

- **Cisatracurium:** 0.1 mg/kg (TBW) = 10 mg. There is some evidence for prolonged duration of action when dosed to TBW.
- **Local anesthetics** should be dosed based on IBW. Doses should be reduced by 25% for epidural and spinal techniques due to engorged epidural veins and reduced volume of the spaces.
- **Desflurane** has been suggested to be the inhaled anesthetic of choice due to its rapid recovery profile and low solubility.

SUMMARY

1. Careful preoperative airway evaluation is fundamental, and intravenous induction may be preferred in an obese child with severe OSA due to prolonged second stage on inhalation induction and risk for airway obstruction. Rapid-sequence intubation may still be advisable for morbidly obese children.
2. Obese children with OSA may be extremely sensitive to narcotics and respiratory depressants.
3. Preoxygenation in the upright position helps reduce desaturation episodes.
4. Alveolar recruitment strategies such as elevated peak inspiratory pressures to ventilate and optimal PEEP to prevent atelectasis are important for successful ventilation intraoperatively.
5. Opioid-sparing analgesics and regional analgesia are important for quicker postoperative recuperation. Use lower incremental doses of local anesthetic when dosing an epidural block in obese patients.

ANNOTATED REFERENCES

- Mulla H, Johnson TN. Dosing dilemmas in obese children. *Arch Dis Child Educ Pract Ed* 2010; 95 (4): 112–117.

  A guide to optimal dosing in children, with discussion of factors affecting pharmacokinetics.

- Nafiu OO, Reynolds PI, Bamgbade OA, Tremper KK, Welch K, Kasa-Vubu JZ. Childhood body mass index and perioperative complications. *Pediatr Anesth* 2007; 17(5): 426–430.

  In this retrospective review of 6,094 children who underwent general anesthesia, difficult airway, upper airway obstruction in the PACU, PACU stay longer than 3 hours, and the need for two or more antiemetics were more common in overweight and obese than normal-weight children.

- Samuels PJ. Anesthesia for adolescent bariatric surgery. *Int Anesthesiol Clin* 2006; 44(1): 17–31.

  A comprehensive review of anesthetic considerations for morbidly obese children undergoing bariatric surgery.

Further Reading

Almarakbi WA, Fawzi HM, Alhashemi JA. Effects of four intraoperative ventilatory strategies on respiratory compliance and gas exchange during laparoscopic gastric banding in obese patients. *Br J Anaesth* 2009; 102(6): 862–868.

Casati A, Putzu M. Anesthesia in the obese patient: Pharmacokinetic considerations. *J Clin Anesth* 2005; 17: 134–135.

Collins JS, Lemmens HJ, Brodsky JB, Brock-Utne JG, Levitan RM. Laryngoscopy and morbid obesity: a comparison of the "sniff" and "ramped" positions. *Obes Surg* 2004; 14(9): 1171–1175.

Cook-Sather SD, Gallagher PR, Kruge LE, Beus JM, Ciampa BP, Welch KC, Shah-Hosseini S, Choi JS, Pachikara R, Minger K, Litman RS, Schreiner MS. Overweight/obesity and gastric fluid characteristics in pediatric day surgery: implications for fasting guidelines and pulmonary aspiration risk. *Anesth Analg* 2009; 109(3): 727–736.

Ogden CL, Flegal KM. Changes in terminology for childhood overweight and obesity. *National Health Statistics Reports*, June 25, 2010. Accessed Feb. 27, 2011. http://cdc.gov/nchs/data/nhsr/nhsr025.pdf.

Rowland TW. Effect of obesity on cardiac function in children and adolescents: A review. *J Sports Sci Med* 2007; 6: 319–326.

Tait AR, Voepel-Lewis T, Burke C, Kostrzewa A, Lewis I. Incidence and risk factors for perioperative adverse respiratory events in children who are obese. *Anesthesiology* 2008; 108(3): 375–380.

PART 11

CHALLENGES IN THE

PERINATAL PERIOD

51

Exploratory Laparotomy for Necrotizing Enterocolitis

DUGALD McADAM

INTRODUCTION

The survival rates of very-low-birth weight (VLBW; birth weight <1,500 g) and extremely-low-birth weight (ELBW; birth weight <1,000 g) infants have increased with improvements in antenatal and postnatal care. These include the use of antenatal steroids, artificial surfactant, and ventilation strategies that have reduced injury to the neonatal lung. As a result, the pediatric anesthesiologist is now more often faced with the task of safely caring for these infants, often in unfamiliar environments, and sometimes during episodes of life-threatening illness. One example is necrotizing enterocolitis (NEC) requiring surgical management.

LEARNING OBJECTIVES

1. Know the comorbidities of the population commonly presenting with NEC.
2. Understand the anesthetic challenges and issues related to operating in the neonatal intensive care unit (NICU).
3. Appreciate the preoperative measures required to ensure safety in NICU.
4. Develop a plan for managing "massive transfusion" in the neonate.

CASE PRESENTATION

*A 17-day-old, 920-g girl requires an urgent laparotomy. She was born at 24 weeks' gestation and was intubated and ventilated at birth for poor respiratory effort. At day 13 she was extubated to nasal CPAP. On day 17 she is re-intubated for signs of **sepsis** (shock, tachypnea, and increased work of breathing). During fluid resuscitation, a radial arterial line, a urinary catheter, and a 4Fr triple-lumen internal jugular central line (CVC) are inserted. X-ray reveals **free intraperitoneal gas**. She is scheduled for an urgent laparotomy. Due to escalating ventilator requirements, she is placed on a **high-frequency oscillating ventilator** (HFOV), with ΔP 30 mmHg, mean airway pressure of 14 cmH_2O, frequency of 8 Hz, and FiO_2 of 0.8. Preoperatively her vital signs are pulse 190/min, blood pressure 42/20 mmHg, SpO_2 89%, and esophageal $T°$ 36.3. Her abdomen is tense and distended. She appears mottled with some generalized edema. She is passing 1 mL/hour urine. The chest x-ray shows no focal changes; the endotracheal and nasogastric tubes are in good position. Her medications are dobutamine and dopamine (both 20 mcg/kg/min), morphine (40 mcg/kg/hour), midazolam (1 mcg/kg/min), antibiotics, and maintenance fluids 1 mL/hr (10% dextrose, 0.225% saline, 20 mmol/L KCl). Cranial and renal ultrasounds are normal. An echocardiogram shows a moderate-sized patent foramen ovale (PFO), a large **patent ductus arteriosus (PDA)** with left-to-right shunt and some evidence of **pulmonary hypertension**. Arterial blood gas results are pH 7.13, pCO_2 64 mmHg, pO_2 51 mmHg, Hb 106 g/L, and lactate 5.3 mmol/L.*

*In the NICU, anesthesia comprises fentanyl (5 mcg initially, then 2.5-mcg boluses dependent on hemodynamcs) and pancuronium 0.2 mg. Surgery reveals extensive peritoneal soiling and a 50-cm segment of necrotic distal small bowel; it is managed with bowel resection, peritoneal lavage, and an ileostomy with distal mucus fistula. Hepatic bleeding is noted; the MAP drops to 18 mmHg. There is no response to a bolus of 15 mL/kg of **fresh packed red blood cells** (PRBCs), 15 mL/kg of fresh frozen plasma (FFP), and 0.4 mL **calcium gluconate** 10%. Norepinephrine (noradrenaline) 0.4 mcg/kg/min is started. MAP increases to 31 mmHg. During wound closure, further **hepatic*** *bleeding occurs; she is given 20 mL/kg fresh PRBC, 10 mL/kg cryo-precipitate, 15 mL/kg platelets, and three doses of 0.4 mL* **calcium gluconate** *10%. The bleeding continues. The abdomen is packed and a bolus of 180 mcg* **recombinant factor VIIa** *is given; bleeding reduces to allow abdominal wall closure. She is discharged from the NICU 4 months later.*

DISCUSSION

1. What is NEC and who gets it?

NEC is a severe *inflammatory disorder* of the intestine that may progress to full-thickness necrosis and perforation. It may involve a localized segment of bowel or be more generalized. The pathogenesis is still not fully understood. It most commonly affects premature neonates, with the incidence decreasing as the gestational age increases. Its diagnosis is associated with significant morbidity and mortality. The typical baby at risk of NEC is one who already has cardiorespiratory *complications of prematurity*. Abdominal distention, bile-stained vomiting, and occult or gross blood in the stool are the usual clinical features. Lethargy, apneic spells, respiratory insufficiency, and poor perfusion may be early, nonspecific signs. Sepsis may be suspected before the diagnosis of NEC is made. Deterioration can be rapid with circulatory compromise, acidosis, coagulopathy, and multiorgan failure. The optimal surgical management of perforated NEC remains unclear (Moss et al., 2006).

2. What are the preoperative cardiorespiratory issues for consideration?

At the time of diagnosis, these neonates are almost always ventilated. The use of pre-delivery maternal steroids, artificial surfactant administration, and early use of noninvasive ventilation to the preterm neonate have reduced morbidity and mortality in this population. Unfortunately, the incidence of bronchopulmonary dysplasia and chronic lung disease in this population has not been reduced, perhaps because many more of these preterm neonates are surviving. A tense, distended abdomen further compromises respiratory function and **HFOV** is frequently required. The specialized nature of such ventilation requires perioperative cooperation between the neonatologist and anesthesiologist. The ex-premature neonate has a cardiovascular system that tolerates deviations from homeostasis poorly. The myocardium is less able to generate force and is more dependent on extracellular **calcium** than in older children. It has limited functional reserve and copes poorly with increases in afterload (Lönnqvist, 2004) or significant changes in preload. There is also a high incidence of structural heart disease in this population, the most common being **PDA**, with an incidence of up to 80% in those weighing less than 1,200 g. The shunt is usually left to right through the PDA, causing excessive pulmonary circulation at the expense of systemic oxygen delivery. This shunt may be reversed where **pulmonary hypertension** is present (precipitated in part by systemic acidosis and hypoxia in the sick neonate). A laparotomy with significant fluid shifts may well worsen already marginal cardiac function. A preoperative cardiology consultation with echocardiography is important; the cardiac function and ventricular filling can be quantified and congenital heart disease can be evaluated.

3. What are the other essential features of the preoperative visit?

After establishing the comorbidity, degree of cardiorespiratory compromise, and level of ventilator and pharmacology support, a certain attention to detail is required before proceeding to surgery. In particular, recent arterial blood gas analysis, complete blood count, coagulation studies, and electrolytes (including Ca^{2+}) are reviewed, as well as a "babygram" x-ray to confirm the position of lines and the endotracheal tube. Treatable lung pathology is excluded (e.g., pneumothorax). Glucose will need to be measured before and during the surgery. Intra-arterial blood pressure monitoring is highly desirable (if not essential) for this surgery, both for continuous measurement and for blood sampling. Central venous access is also considered "essential" for expected inotrope delivery and fluid balance monitoring; however, if invasive monitoring is not in place, time taken to achieve it needs to be weighed against surgical delay. Good peripheral access is mandatory in the absence of a CVC. Finally, parents need to be counseled about transfusion and the high perioperative risk.

4. Should this procedure be performed in the OR or NICU?

Advantages of using the OR are familiarity with equipment for all staff, the ability to deliver volatile anesthesia, and better surgical lighting conditions. Disadvantages of using the OR include the need to disrupt any complex ventilator strategy for transport, the development of hypothermia in transit, and inadequate surgical access and lighting (Frawley et al., 1999). Consequences of changing to hand ventilation for transport include loss of PEEP, atelectasis, hypoxemia, and risks of barotrauma or volutrauma. It is more difficult to manage critical incidents during transport; in addition, movement carries the risk of inadvertent extubation, venous line removal, or endobronchial tube migration. **HFOV** would contraindicate transport to the OR. The decision to operate in the NICU alerts the anesthesiologist to the fact that the neonate is *too critically unwell* to be moved.

5. How should the NICU environment be prepared for surgery?

Having a trained assistant and second anesthesiologist is ideal. To avoid hypothermia, a U-shaped blanket can be placed around the baby and heated with a forced-air warmer; the usual overhead heater may need to be turned off during surgery itself. Waterproof drapes prevent irrigation and preparation fluid from spilling and coming into contact with the rest of the baby. *All fluids should be warmed;* a fluid warmer, with access ports on either side of the warming device, can be connected to the patient using a short, minimum-volume (0.5 mL) extension tube. IV fluids can therefore be aspirated through the warming device before manual injection to the patient with minimal dead space. In addition to standard monitoring, a pre- and post-ductal saturation probe, a transcutaneous CO_2 monitor, and an esophageal temperature probe are useful. Before surgical draping, all IV and arterial lines are reviewed for access points and potential sites of kinking. It is imperative to have *rapid access to the endotracheal tube, and an alternate ventilatory source* (e.g., a Neopuff™ T-piece resuscitator [Fisher & Paykel Healthcare, Auckland, New Zealand]). Appropriately sized suction catheters should be ready. *Emergency drugs, inotropes, and neonatal airway* equipment should be checked. **Bleeding** should be anticipated; blood products need to be ready and checked in the room; an irradiated (to prevent graft-versus-host disease) bag of PRBC containing at least one blood volume (approximately 100 mL in this case), a thawed unit of FFP, and a 50-mL bottle of 4% albumen would be a reasonable reserve available at the bedside.

6. What are the major intraoperative risks?

Sepsis, potentially massive **bleeding** (see Chapter 24), maintaining euthermia, and combating glucose instability, on the background of significant comorbidity are the major challenges (Table 51.1). In the infant presented, the estimated total blood volume is 90 to 100 mL/kg (i.e., 82–92 mL). A preoperative *massive blood loss plan* needs to have been made. Communication with the surgical team is both visual and verbal, with constant surveillance of the operative field, monitors, and surgical suction. There are various formulas for calculating maximal allowable blood loss before blood transfusion should start. However, it is expected that transfusion of blood products would start as soon as bleeding is identified. Warmed PRBCs are administered, guided by ABP, CVP, and [Hb]. Note there will be no hypovolemic arterial waveform "swing" with respiration if the neonate is on **HFOV**. Extrapolating from studies of transfusion in preterm neonates not acutely bleeding (Bell, 2008), a reasonable hemoglobin target is probably 10 g/dL.

Table 51.1

CHECKLIST TO PREVENT AND MANAGE COMMON INTRAOPERATIVE RISKS

Intraoperative Risk	Action
Airway disconnection, tube kinking	Prevention: Check airway and connections before draping. During the case: Always have access to the tube and alternative ventilator source.
Changing ventilatory requirement with opening abdomen, closure, worsening sepsis	Monitor ABG, CO_2, SpO_2 closely and be prepared to change ventilation.
Worsening cardiovascular function due to sepsis, bleeding, coagulopathy, or hypocalcemia	Have inotropes ready, measure IABP. Have a plan and blood products ready (see text). Predict hypocalcemia after blood products; measure and treat.
Hyperkalemic dysrhythmias	Prevent: use new blood (? washed).
Hypothermia	Measure temperature, use plastic drapes and a forced-air warmer.
Loss of IV access (kinking, disconnection, blockage)	Prevention: Check that lines are secure and not kinked before draping. Consider multiple IV access and establish central access. During the case: Check the IV line and connections if the patient is not responding to fluid bolus.
Hypoglycemia	Monitor glucose hourly.

Coagulopathy can develop due to **sepsis**, hypothermia, and dilution of coagulation factors and platelets. Once blood loss exceeds one blood volume it would be expected that clinical clotting factor deficiency would be demonstrated clinically in the surgical field (Barcelona et al., 2005). To prevent impending coagulopathy it is reasonable to begin FFP when blood volume transfused reaches 40 mL/kg (or sooner if there is diffuse microvascular bleeding and abnormal INR/APTT). Platelet numbers have been shown to be reduced to 60%, 40%, and 30% of their initial value after one, two, and three blood volumes have been lost, respectively. The lowest acceptable platelet count during neonatal surgery is unknown. In the setting of ongoing bleeding and a worsening coagulation profile, a platelet count of above 100×10^9/L is an acceptable target, but recommendations vary (Chang, 2008). Platelet transfusion is usually not required until between one and two blood volumes have been lost, depending on the initial platelet count. Fibrinogen as cryoprecipitate should be replaced when the level is less than 1 g/L, or when hemorrhage is uncontrolled, and one blood volume replacement is being approached.

Of particular importance to the neonate is the risk of hyperkalemic arrest; the [K+] is high in stored PRBCs due to irradiation and prolonged storage. Thus, neonates should be given **fresh PRBCs** and the time between irradiation and administration should be minimized. Methods to prevent hyperkalemic arrhythmias include washing and warming packed cells prior to transfusion. Infusing via a peripheral vein will reduce the concentration of potassium being presented to the atria, and thus the risk of nodal dysfunction (Sloan, 2011). Citrate is used as an anticoagulant in stored blood products and binds calcium and magnesium. The highest amount of citrate is found in FFP and platelets. **Hypocalcemia** not only worsens hypokalemia but also has an especially strong negative effect on inotropy in neonates.

7. In addition to coagulopathy, why else may these children bleed?

Fluid overload in the setting of NEC is a significant problem. Preoperative aggressive filling is associated with liver congestion;

surgically entering a tense abdomen may release any tamponade effect on the liver. Rapid hepatic expansion can follow, eventually leading to capsular rupture and **spontaneous hepatic bleeding** (Pumberger et al., 2002). If fluid therapy is too aggressive intraoperatively, spontaneous intraoperative liver hemorrhage may occur. This is a separate issue from iatrogenic injury due to surgical trauma. It is vital to communicate closely with the surgical team about the status of hepatic congestion and enlargement during the operation. Cardiovascular instability in children with NEC needs to be treated with ongoing liberal transfusion of blood products. Low systemic vascular resistance and increased capillary leak seen in these patients may continue to cause unacceptable hypotension despite adequate volume resuscitation. Increasing doses of inotropes in such cases may be protective for hepatic hemorrhage. There are many case reports of **recombinant factor VIIa** being used successfully for liver hemorrhage in this situation (Matthew & Young, 2006), and this could be considered for resuscitation of a baby *in extremis from hemorrhage*.

SUMMARY

1. NEC most commonly affects the smallest and sickest preterm neonates, with coexistent conditions of prematurity.
2. Communication and planning between the neonatologist, surgeon, and anesthesiologist is vital. This will optimize decisions such as where to operate, how to ventilate, and how to respond early to bleeding.
3. Massive transfusion in the neonate with NEC should be expected, and this should be communicated to the blood bank prior to the start of the case.
4. Judicious use of increasing inotropes as well as ongoing transfusion should be considered to support a "septic" circulation.

ANNOTATED REFERENCES

- Barcelona SL, Thompson AA, Cote CJ. Intraoperative pediatric blood transfusion therapy: a review of common issues. Part II: transfusion therapy, special considerations, and reduction of allogenic blood transfusions. *Pediatr Anesth* 2005; 15: 814–830.
  This second of two articles gives comprehensive coverage of transfusion and massive transfusion in the pediatric patient, including complications and methods to reduce allogenic administration.
- Lönnqvist PA. Major abdominal surgery of the neonate: anaesthetic considerations. *Best Pract Res Clin Anaesthesiol* 2004; 18(2): 321–342.
  A very good summary of neonatal physiology and pathophysiology and general principles of caring for babies with specific abdominal conditions.
- Royal Children's Hospital (Melbourne). *Massive Transfusion Clinical Practice Guidelines, 2005.* Accessed Dec. 2, 2010. http://www.rch.org.au/clinicalguide/cpg.cfm?doc_ id=11225.
  Practical guidelines and a flowchart for management of massive transfusion, and suggested triggers for red cell and component administration.

Further Reading

Bell EF. When to transfuse premature babies. *Arch Dis Child Fetal Neonatal* 2008; 93: F469–473.

Chang T-T. Transfusion therapy in critically ill children. *Pediatr Neonatol* 2008; 49(2): 5–12.

Frawley G, Bayley G, Chondros P. Laparotomy for necrotizing enterocolitis: Intensive care nursery compared with operating theatre. *J Paediatr Child Health* 1999; 35: 291–295.

Mathew P, Young G. Recombinant factor VIIa in paediatric bleeding disorders: a 2006 review. *Haemophilia* 2006; 12: 457–472.

Moss RL, Dimmitt RA, Barnhart DC. Laparotomy versus peritoneal drainage for necrotizing enterocolitis and perforation. *N Engl J Med* 2006; 354: 2225–2234.

Pumberger W, Kohlhauser C, Mayr M, Pomberger G. Severe liver hemor-rhage during laparotomy in very low birthweight infants. *Acta Pædiatr* 2002; 91: 1260–1262.

Sloan RS. Neonatal transfusion review. *Pediatr Anesth* 2011; 21: 25–30.

52

Former Premature Infant for Hernia Repair

GEOFF FRAWLEY

INTRODUCTION

There has been a marked improvement in the survival rates of premature infants. Coincident with the increase in survival has been an increase in ex-premature infants presenting for surgery. Hernia repair is the most common surgery in ex-premature infants, with the incidence of inguinal hernias being inversely proportional to gestational age at birth (13% incidence in infants born <32 weeks' gestation and 30% in those born with a birth weight <1,000 g). Postoperative apnea is a significant complication in this age group. Both awake regional and general anesthetic techniques are widely used for infant hernia repair; the choice often is based more on anesthetic preference than on evidence from prospective randomized controlled trials.

LEARNING OBJECTIVES

1. **Know the risk of apnea and/or bradycardia in the postoperative period and contributing factors that increase the risk.**
2. **Understand the risks and benefits of different anesthetic techniques for infant hernia repair.**
3. **Understand the basic principles in avoiding and managing apnea in this group.**

CASE PRESENTATION

A 5-month-old, former 28-week estimated gestational age **premature infant** *presents with an incarcerated inguinal hernia that needs urgent repair. The infant had been intubated at birth due to respiratory distress syndrome and remained intubated for 2 weeks, followed by a further 3 weeks of nasopharyngeal continuous positive airway pressure (nCPAP). Episodes of* **apnea** *were treated with intravenous and then oral caffeine. Echocardiography had revealed a patent ductus arteriosus, which closed with indomethacin treatment. He went home about 1 month ago with an apnea and bradycardia monitor. The current medications are iron and vitamin supplements, and he weighs 5 kg.*

An awake **spinal anesthetic** *is given with* **1 mL of 0.5% bupivacaine** *without epinephrine (adrenaline). The block is rapidly effective. The surgery starts well but the inguinal hernia is larger than expected and surgical repair is long and difficult. After taking* **60 minutes** *to repair the first side, the surgeon starts the contralateral side. Twenty minutes later the infant becomes unsettled and his leg movement becomes troublesome to the surgeon. A general anesthetic is now given. Induction is with sevoflurane and a size 1 laryngeal mask (LMA) is used for the airway. Upon removal of the LMA in the operating room, there is occasional apnea with oxygen desaturation to 88%. The infant requires intermittent stimulation and positive-pressure ventilation via an anesthetic circuit. The infant is transferred to the PACU once respiration is regular.*

In the PACU, the infant again has bradycardia to 80 bpm with **apneas** *requiring intermittent stimulation to maintain saturations above 85%.* **Caffeine** *(10 mg/kg) is given. The surgeon asks if the baby can be* **discharged to home**.

DISCUSSION

1. What factors increase the risk of postoperative apnea?

Ex-premature infants have been identified as a group at risk of postoperative apnea and oxygen desaturation. In the most comprehensive review, Coté et al. combined data from eight prospective studies (255 patients) and found that gestational age at birth (GA), postmenstrual age (PMA), and anemia were independent risk factors for postoperative apneas. They concluded that the risk of **apnea** in an infant born at 35 weeks is at least 5% until a PMA of 48 weeks and at least 1% until a PMA of 54 weeks. The risk of apnea in an infant born at 32 weeks is at least 5% until a PMA of 50 weeks and at least 1% until a PMA of 56 weeks (Coté et al., 1995). Major changes in neonatal and anesthetic care make it difficult to interpret this paper in the setting of modern anesthetic practice. Coté et al. analyzed studies where halothane and enflurane were used, and the new volatile anesthetic agents have a markedly different postoperative complication profile. Additionally, the use of opioids, ketamine, and benzodiazepines increases the risk for postoperative apnea. In a more recent but smaller study, Murphy et al. (2008) found a lower overall incidence of apnea, and the following were identified as risk factors: a past history of apnea, lower birth weight, lower GA at birth, and a complicated medical history.

Although it is difficult to exactly identify those at risk, prematurity and low PMA are still generally regarded as the most significant risk factors for postoperative apnea. PMA is the time elapsed between the first day of the last menstrual period and birth (gestational age) plus the time elapsed after birth (chronological age).

2. Which anesthetic is best?

The goal of anesthesia for the ex-premature infant having hernia repair is to provide acceptable operating conditions, a safe anesthetic, and an anesthetic that will minimize intra- and postoperative cardiorespiratory complications. General anesthesia (GA) with regional nerve blockade, awake spinal anesthesia (SA), and awake caudal anesthesia (CA) are options well described in the anesthesia literature. The choice of anesthetic for these patients is often based on a practitioner's passion toward a technique and level of experience rather than scientific evidence.

GA: The greatest concern with GA is the increased risk of postoperative apnea. It is usually assumed that GA increases the risk compared to awake regional techniques, but the evidence is far from clear. Some of the older studies used older anesthetic agents, and in the GA arm regional blockade was not used to reduce anesthetic requirements. Studies using newer anesthetic agents (sevoflurane or desflurane) combined with presurgical regional anesthesia find less evidence for an increase in ventilatory impairment postoperatively. While the incidence may be less compared to older agents, postoperative apnea can still occur following sevoflurane and desflurane anesthesia. Sale et al. (2006) compared respiratory events in ex-premature infants receiving sevoflurane or desflurane using nasal thermistry and impedance for 12 hours before and after surgery. The incidence of *preoperative* apnea was 27% in the sevoflurane group and 40% in the desflurane group and increased postoperatively to 33% and 60% respectively. Others have reported apnea occurring far less frequently. One reason why the incidence varies between studies is that the definition of apnea and how it is detected both vary from study to study. The actual clinical significance of a short self-limiting apnea is also unknown.

Apart from increased risk of apnea, there are several other reasons that make GA a less appealing option. Awake regional anesthesia avoids the requirement for tracheal intubation and the potential for further airway trauma in infants who have been previously intubated and are at risk for subglottic stenosis or cysts. There is also an unknown effect of GA on the developing brain.

Awake spinal: This technique has been demonstrated to reduce the risk of postoperative apnea in at-risk neonates. The largest series published describing SA is the Vermont Infant Spinal Registry's 1,554 infants (Williams et al., 2006). Successful spinal anesthesia was achieved in 97.4% of infants. This contrasts with smaller series that have reported a significantly higher incidence of failed access to the subarachnoid space, bloody taps, and blocks requiring supplementation. In the Vermont Infant

Registry study, over 75% of infants required no more than comforting the child with stroking and a pacifier. Other studies titrate small doses of midazolam 20 to 50 mcg/kg or propofol 0.25 to 0.5 mg/kg to calm fussy babies. However, adding *supplemental sedation or converting to GA significantly increases the risk of postoperative apnea.*

SA is best performed in the lateral decubitus position using the intercristal line as the anatomical landmark. Not all infants are suitable for SA for hernia repair. SA requires cooperation between the anesthetist and the surgeon to produce optimal conditions. Some surgeons feel that large or technically challenging repairs cannot be performed within the time constraints imposed by SA.

Table 52.1 lists cases where SA could have significant advantages over GA. Finally, it should be noted that SA is also associated with a small but finite risk of aseptic meningitis after subarachnoid block. Strict asepsis is essential.

Awake Caudal: Successful CA in awake infants has been reported. Bupivacaine 0.25% is commonly used at doses ranging

---

Table 52.1

INFANTS IN WHOM SPINAL ANESTHESIA MAY OFFER SIGNIFICANT ADVANTAGES

Ex-premature infants born at <35 weeks' gestational age

Infants with a PMA <45 weeks

Past or current apnea of prematurity requiring caffeine or methylxanthines

Chronic lung disease requiring home oxygen

Significant neonatal history, including IVH, NEC, retinopathy of prematurity

High-risk infants with congenital heart disease and airway anomalies

Any infant without absolute contraindications

Infants booked as day-case surgery

---

from 0.8 to 1.2 mL/kg (2.0–3.0 mg/kg). Epinephrine is essential to slow absorption, lower peak plasma levels, and permit early recognition of intravascular injection despite a negative aspiration test. Drawbacks to caudal block are the slow onset, inconsistent motor block, short duration, increased risk of local anesthetic toxicity from the larger dose used, and the risk of inadvertent intravascular injection. A recent study comparing awake spinal to awake caudal anesthesia in premature and ex-premature infants failed to demonstrate any advantage to awake caudal over SA. The rate of postoperative apneas in the CA group was 8.9% compared to 5.6% in the SA group (Hoelzle et al., 2010).

3. What is the role of prophylactic caffeine?

There is limited evidence that **caffeine** and theophylline can reduce the rate of postoperative apnea after GA. A Cochrane Review stated that caffeine can be used for this indication but emphasized the small number of patients studied. It is not clear whether there is a benefit in giving caffeine prophylactically to all patients receiving GA with newer insoluble agents such as sevoflurane or desflurane (Henderson-Smart & Steer, 2005).

4. How should postoperative apnea be handled?

In any case of irregular breathing after GA, **caffeine** or aminophylline should be given without delay. Of the methylxanthines, theophylline is the most extensively used, but caffeine is at least as effective as theophylline, has a longer half-life, is associated with fewer adverse events, and is easier to administer. Any postoperative bradycardia or apnea is predictive of both early and late cardiorespiratory events and mandates admission until a 12-hour event-free interval has elapsed.

5. Where should this patient go after recovery? When can the child go home?

The best **time to discharge** these patients is controversial. The most widely practiced and conservative measure is to admit all ex-premature infants less than 60 weeks PMA for overnight

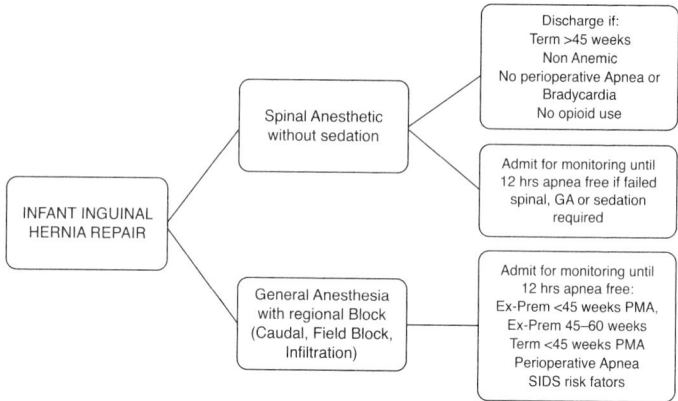

FIGURE 52.1 Decision tree algorithm for management of infants presenting for inguinal hernia repair.

apnea monitoring, regardless of the anesthetic. Certainly this needs to be the case for infants on apnea monitors or methylxanthine drugs, or those who have received any form of a perioperative CNS-depressing medication. Babies at risk for sudden infant death syndrome (e.g., parental smoking, single-parent families, low socioeconomic status) should be considered for admission as well. Some units consider "early" discharge for uncomplicated infants who do not have any risk factors and who have demonstrated no apnea, bradycardia, or desaturations during the surgery and for 8 hours postoperatively. Figure 52.1 summarizes an algorithm to consider for the management of the former premature infant.

SUMMARY

1. **Premature infants less than 60 weeks PMA are at increased risk for postoperative apnea. Other factors**

that may increase this risk include anemia, previous history of apnea, and a complicated neonatal course.

2. There is some evidence that awake regional anesthesia reduces the risk of apnea compared to GA. However, the use of sedative drugs during regional anesthesia is associated with an increased risk of apnea.

3. The use of awake regional techniques is largely determined by the experience of the anesthetist involved and the speed and skill of the surgeon.

ANNOTATED REFERENCES

- Coté CJ, Zaslavsky A, Downes JJ, Kurth CD, Welborn LG, Warner LO, Malviya SV. Postoperative apnea in former preterm infants after inguinal herniorrhaphy. A combined analysis. *Anesthesiology* 1995; 82: 809–822.

  This classic article used meta-analysis of risk factors to identify infants at risk of postoperative apnea and remains the most quoted article on this topic.

- Henderson-Smart DJ, Steer P. Prophylactic caffeine to prevent postoperative apnea following general anesthesia in preterm infants (Cochrane Review). *The Cochrane Library*, Issue 1, 2005.

  A short Cochrane meta-analysis that recommends caffeine prophylaxis in newborns at risk of apnea but warns about the small numbers in the series examined.

- Williams RK, Adams DC, Aladjem EV, Kreutz JM, Sartorelli KH, Vane DW, Abajian JC. The safety and efficacy of spinal anesthesia for surgery in infants: the Vermont Infant Spinal Registry. *Anesth Analg* 2006; 102: 67–71.

  The combined data from 30 years of spinal anesthesia at a single institution.

Further Reading

Abajian JC, Mellish RW, Browne AF, Perkins FM, Lambert DH, Mazuzan JE. Spinal anesthesia for surgery in the high-risk infant. *Anesth Analg* 1984; 63: 359–362.

Breschen C, Hellstrand E, Likar R, Lonnqvist PA. Bupivacaine plasma concentrations associated with clinical and electroencephalographic signs of early central nervous system toxicity in infants during awake caudal anaesthesia. *Anaesthetist* 1988; 47: 290–294.

Frawley G, Ingelmo P, Smith K. Relative potencies of bupivacaine, levobupivacaine and ropivacaine for neonatal spinal anaesthesia. *Br J Anaesth* 2009; 103(5): 731–738.

Hoelzle M, Weiss M, Dillier C, Gerber A. Comparison of awake spinal with awake caudal anesthesia in preterm and ex-preterm infants for herniotomy. *Paediatr Anaesth* 2010; 20(7): 620–624.

Murphy J, Swanson T, Ansermino M, Milner R. The frequency of apneas in premature infants after inguinal hernia repair: do they need overnight monitoring in the intensive care unit? *J Pediatr Surg* 2008; 43: 865–868.

Sale SM, Read JA, Stoddart PA, Wolf AR. Prospective comparison of sevoflurane and desflurane in formerly premature infants undergoing inguinal herniotomy. *Br J Anaesth* 2006; 96: 774–778.

Welborn LG, Rice LJ, Hannallah RS, Broadman LM, Ryttimann UE, Fink R. Postoperative apnea in former preterm infants: prospective comparison of spinal and general anesthesia. *Anesthesiology* 1990: 72; 838–842.

Williams JM, Stoddart PA, Williams SAR, Wolf AR. Postoperative recovery after inguinal herniotomy in ex-premature infants: comparison between sevoflurane and spinal anaesthesia. *Br J Anaesth* 2001; 86: 366–371.

53

Tracheoesophageal Fistula Repair

LORNA RANKIN

INTRODUCTION

Tracheoesophageal fistula (TEF) and esophageal atresia (EA) is a congenital malformation occurring in 1:3,000 to 4,500 births. The condition presents specific challenges to the anesthesiologist in the perioperative period. The presence of a fistula means that infants born with TEF/EA are at risk of aspiration and positive-pressure ventilation may be hazardous. These babies often have coexistent problems associated with prematurity and low birth weight, and 50% have associated abnormalities, most commonly congenital cardiac malformations.

LEARNING OBJECTIVES

1. Know the anatomy of the various abnormalities of the trachea and esophagus and the commonly associated conditions.
2. Identify how TEF/EA presents and what investigations are required during the preoperative assessment.
3. Assess the potential problems associated with anesthetizing an infant with TEF/EA.
4. Construct an appropriate postoperative management plan.

CASE PRESENTATION

*A 1.6-kg girl is born at 32 weeks' gestation. No polyhydramnios or other antenatal problems were present. Apgar scores were 8 at 1 minute and 10 at 5 minutes. She is now spontaneously ventilating with normal saturations in air and no increased work of breathing. The baby is transferred to the NICU for feeding. On arrival, placement of a nasogastric tube (NGT) was unsuccessful; the whole body x-ray ("babygram") demonstrates the **NGT** is **coiled in the upper esophagus,** and **gas is noted in the stomach** (see Fig. 53.2 below). Based on this, a diagnosis of TEF/EA is made with surgical consultation. On examination she is well perfused with no dysmorphic features. Cardiorespiratory examination is normal. She has passed urine and meconium. Maintenance IV fluid of 10% dextrose is continued at 60 mL/kg/day. The baby is kept 30 degrees head up to prevent aspiration and the NG tube is suctioned regularly. An **echocardiogram** excludes cardiac disease and confirms a left-sided aortic arch. Complete blood count, urea, electrolytes, and renal and cranial ultrasounds are normal. A type and screen is taken and she is booked on the emergency surgical list.*

*In the warmed OR, the baby is placed on a blanket connected to a forced-air warmer. IV dextrose is continued. Anesthesia is induced using sevoflurane/oxygen. **Gentle positive-pressure ventilation** is applied with no significant expansion of the stomach. She is nasally intubated with a size 3 uncuffed endotracheal tube (ETT) after muscle relaxant; the tube is passed into the bronchus and gently pulled back until bilateral air entry is heard. Hand ventilation using an Ayres T-piece is possible without stomach expansion, so fentanyl 2 mcg/kg, atracurium, and antibiotics are given. A 24G radial arterial line and nasopharyngeal temperature probe are inserted. Anesthesia is maintained with sevoflurane at end-tidal 2.8% in an oxygen/air mix with FiO_2 0.4. Rigid esophagoscopy shows a blind-ended upper esophageal pouch; no upper pouch fistula is seen. She is positioned in the left lateral position and tube position and ventilation are rechecked. A right thoracotomy and extrapleural dissection allows the fistula to be* *ligated. The FiO$_2$ is increased to 0.8 to compensate for the SpO$_2$ fall due to lung retraction. There is a short gap, so the upper and lower esophageal segments are anastomosed over a size 10 nasogastric feeding tube; during this, the mean blood pressure (MAP) drops 20 mmHg. This is instantly corrected with release of the surgical traction.* **Hand ventilation** *is required throughout the procedure; this allows instant recognition of two episodes of* **large airway obstruction** *due to surgical retractors. A total of 30 mL/kg of albumin is given for the 150-minute procedure. A* **morphine infusion** *is started at 10 mcg/kg/ hr. The baby is transferred ventilated to the NICU to allow controlled extubation the following morning.*

DISCUSSION

1. What are the anatomical variants of TEF/EA, and what are the common associations?

In the majority of patients (80–85%) the lesion consists of EA with a distal esophageal pouch and a proximal TEF (Holder et al., 1987). The remaining 15% to 20% of patients have variations on this (Fig. 53.1).

Urgent diagnosis and treatment is important to avoid aspiration of saliva, feeds, and possibly gastric contents. TEF/EA is linked with other clinical defects in more than 50% of babies; the most common is cardiac (30%). The most frequent cardiac anomalies are ventriculoseptal defects and tetralogy of Fallot (Greenwood & Rosenthal, 1976). **Echocardiogram** is also used to exclude a right-sided aortic arch, which would influence the surgical approach. This anomaly occurs in 2.5% of cases. There is a link with malformation associations such as VACTERL (vertebral, anorectal, cardiac, tracheoesophageal, renal, and limb defects), CHARGE (coloboma, heart defects, anal atresia, retarded growth, genital hypoplasia, ear anomalies) and trisomy 18. Isolated abnormalities also occur, such as renal abnormalities, imperforate anus, duodenal atresia, and cleft lip and palate.

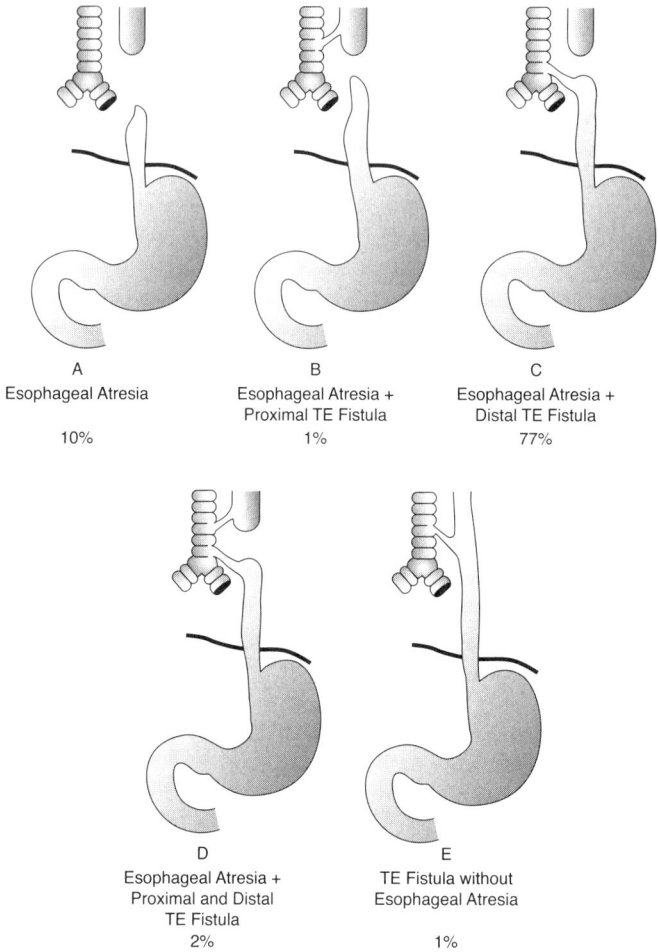

A	B	C
Esophageal Atresia	Esophageal Atresia + Proximal TE Fistula	Esophageal Atresia + Distal TE Fistula
10%	1%	77%

D	E
Esophageal Atresia + Proximal and Distal TE Fistula	TE Fistula without Esophageal Atresia
2%	1%

FIGURE 53.1 Anatomic variants of tracheoesophageal fistula.

2. How does TEF/EA present and how is it diagnosed?

TEF/EA can present *in utero* with the absence of stomach bubble on ultrasound, or it may be suspected in the presence of polyhydramnios. The majority of TEF/EAs are diagnosed postnatally. The baby may be "mucousy," and EA is confirmed with the inability to pass a NG tube. However, it may be that TEF/EA is not discovered until the baby chokes or aspirates on feeding. An isolated TEF can present at an older age with recurrent pneumonia. A "babygram" x-ray is the initial investigation used to diagnose EA. Typically the **NG tube is coiled in the upper mediastinum** and **air in the stomach** confirms the presence of a TEF (Fig. 53.2). The x-rays are also useful to examine the vertebrae for bony abnormalities, check the positions of umbilical lines (and ETT), and look for signs of aspiration or congenital heart disease. Electrolytes should be checked as they may become deranged with large amounts of suctioned secretions and subsequent replacement.

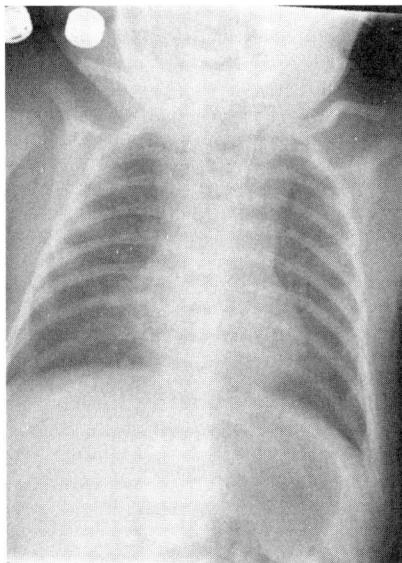

FIGURE 53.2 Typical radiograph of a baby with a TEF. Note nasogastric tube coiled in esophagus and air bubble in stomach.

3. What are the key problems associated with anesthetizing an infant with TEF/EA?

Comorbidities: Infants with extreme prematurity or severe lung disease can be difficult to ventilate; the ventilatory gasses can easily flow down the low-resistance fistula, and this is worsened if lung compliance is poor. The result is inadequate ventilation and gastric distention; the latter can further impede ventilation or even cause gastric rupture and pneumoperitoneum. In the past, a gastrostomy would have been performed in these high-risk neonates and thoracotomy postponed until respiratory function improved (Ulma et al., 2001). However, in these cases it is now generally accepted that emergency transpleural ligation of the TEF is the procedure of choice, with the aim to reoperate in 8 to 10 days to divide the fistula and repair the atresia. Very-low-birth weight (<1,500 g) premature infants have a higher rate of anastomotic complications and overall morbidity; a staged repair is often considered. This involves ligation and division of the TEF with gastrostomy placement followed by a delayed primary repair when the child is clinically stable or has reached a weight of 2,000 g (Greenwood & Rosenthal, 1976). Premature or low-birth weight babies can also have hypoglycemia and hypocalcemia, which need to be evaluated and treated pre- and intraoperatively. Particular care needs to be taken with temperature control, and checking ETT placement with any position change.

Location and Size of Fistula: In an otherwise well infant the majority of anesthetic problems are due to the location and size of the fistula. Carinal and multiple fistulas make it difficult to exclusively ventilate the lungs. Rigid bronchoscopy performed before intubation and thoracotomy has been used to assess the presence, type, size, and location of the fistula. It may also aid in the diagnosis of tracheomalacia or bronchial abnormalities, which can alter the surgical plan and influence the timing of extubation. Flexible bronchoscopy through the ETT could be used during initial intubation and following changes in the patient position, to confirm placement below the TEF and above the carina. However, in premature infants the airway may be too small to accommodate the endoscope. The main disadvantage to presurgical bronchoscopy is that preterm infants with severe respiratory compromise may not tolerate spontaneous ventilation. Complications such as desaturation, airway trauma, or laryngo- or bronchospasm can occur. Controversy still exists as to how to induce and intubate while minimizing ventilatory difficulties. In theory, maintaining spontaneous ventilation seems to be the optimal technique, as the negative intrathoracic pressure causes the gas to preferentially enter the lungs rather than the TEF. However, in an already compromised neonate with poor lung compliance, adequate gas exchange may not be possible without **positive-pressure ventilation**. Inadequate depth of anesthesia can lead to coughing, splinting, or inadequate ventilating conditions. Some authors choose to use succinylcholine (suxamethonium) before intubation (McEwan, 2004).

Surgical Retraction: Lung retraction can be tolerated poorly, requiring high FiO_2 and altering ventilation settings. Direct **large airway compression** can also occur; for these reasons many anesthetists prefer to **hand ventilate** throughout these periods for immediate recognition of altered respiratory physiology. Surgical compression of the great vessels and right atrium can cause rapid loss in preload and hence a rapid fall in MAP. This is one reason an arterial line is useful (although some would argue not "absolutely essential"). Continued open dialog with the surgeon throughout the case is essential.

4. How can positive-pressure ventilation difficulties after intubation be managed?

After intubation, it is usually difficult to maintain spontaneous ventilation until the time of fistula ligation; the combination of lung retraction, opioids, and comorbid lung insufficiency requires positive-pressure ventilation. Ventilation problems occur due to gas preferentially flowing into the fistula rather than the lungs. Various anesthetic and surgical maneuvers are possible; the choice depends on the clinical urgency and the *predetermined plan* made between the anesthesiologist and the surgical team (Table 53.1).

Table 53.1

ANESTHETIC AND SURGICAL TECHNIQUES TO MANAGE PROBLEMS WITH POSITIVE-PRESSURE VENTILATION.

Anesthetic Technique	Advantage	Disadvantage
Maintain spontaneous ventilation	Avoid positive-pressure ventilation down fistula	Inadequate ventilation or apnea during thoracotomy
"Blind" placement of ETT below fistula	Simple if anatomy allows	May not be possible if fistula is at or below level of carina
Bronchoscopic ETT placement	Accuracy ensured	ETT may be too small for bronchoscope; time-consuming in an emergency
Occlusion of fistula with embolectomy balloon catheter via trachea (with or without bronchoscope)	Can be effective	Difficult in practice if unfamiliar with technique; time-consuming in emergency
Deliberately intubate the bronchus	Can be effective	Difficult to intubate the correct (left) bronchus; right bronchial intubation is not sustainable intraoperatively with right thoracotomy
Surgical Technique	Advantage	Disadvantage
Emergency ligation of fistula	Effective; probably *most preferable technique* unless the baby is in extremis. Surgeon familiar with technique.	Requires lateral positioning

Table 53.1 (*continued*)

Surgical Technique	Advantage	Disadvantage
Needle decompression of stomach	Rapid; used if gastric distention is causing cardiorespiratory depression or imminent gastric rupture	Temporary measure, invasive
Gastrostomy to decompress stomach	Can keep patient supine. An underwater seal may reduce ventilation "egress" into the decompressed stomach (Domajnko et al., 2007).	More time-consuming than needle decompression. Invasive. Inevitable gastropexy caused may make long-gap esophageal anastomosis more difficult. May reduce fistula resistance and worsen ventilation.
Occlude fistula with embolectomy catheter via gastroscopy	Effective	Can be difficult, time-consuming
Occlude gastroesophageal junction	Effective; performed supine; some may reserve this for those in extremis	Invasive, time-consuming

Reprinted from Knottenbelt G, Skinner A, Seefelder C. Tracheo-oesophageal fistula and oesophageal atresia. *Best Pract Res Clin Anaesthesiol* 2010; 24: 387–401, with permission from Elsevier.

5. What are the postoperative respiratory complications?

Generally, infants return to the NICU for postoperative management of pain and ventilation. The timing of extubation depends on many factors, including preoperative lung disease, prematurity, congenital abnormalities, and surgical preference. Airway edema and postoperative stridor may occur. The most common early postoperative complication is pneumonitis or atelectasis from secretions in the bronchial tree. Severe tracheomalacia and bronchomalacia occur in 10% to 20% of infants. It can result in apnea, cyanotic spells, and reintubation. Rare life-threatening tracheomalacia may require urgent aortopexy.

6. What are the potential analgesic modalities?

Intravenous opioid infusion, regional techniques, epidural catheters, extrapleural catheters, or a combination have all been used. The choice depends on several factors, including the timing of extubation, the type of ventilation being used, and the operator's familiarity with a technique and ability to care for a modality on the ward or NICU.

Continuous **infusions of morphine** or fentanyl have been used safely and with good effect. Some institutions prefer the use of fentanyl due to concerns over accumulation of morphine and its metabolites in neonates. Epidural catheters can be inserted via the caudal, lumbar, or thoracic spaces and advanced to the mid-thoracic level; verification of the tip is recommended, and this can be achieved by electrical stimulation, ultrasound, or x-ray screening (see chapter 58). Local anesthetic clearance is reduced in the neonate, so both maximum dose and duration should be reduced; most limit infusions to 48 hours. Regional techniques can reduce opioid requirement and ventilator days; the evidence for improved outcome is lacking.

SUMMARY

1. TEF/EA represents a perioperative challenge; up to 30% of patients are preterm,

2. Many patients have respiratory compromise, and up to 50% have other congenital comorbidities.
3. The surgery involves the lateral position and thoracotomy with the inherent potential hemodynamic, ventilatory, and analgesic problems.
4. Communication with cardiologists, surgeons, and neonatologists is essential to optimize the preoperative assessment, intraoperative emergency planning, and postoperative analgesia and ventilation.

ANNOTATED REFERENCES

- Knottenbelt G, Skinner A, Seefelder C. Tracheo-oesophageal fistula and oesophageal atresia. *Best Pract Res Clin Anaesthesiol* 2010; 24: 387–401.

   An excellent recent article. A good overview of anesthetic management of TEF/EA, including recent evidence for the use of preoperative bronchoscopy.
- McEwan A. Anaesthesia for repair of oesophageal atresia and trachea-oesophageal fistula. In Stoddart PA, Lauder GR, eds. *Problems in Anaesthesia: Paediatric Anaesthesia*. London: Taylor and Francis, 2004: 7–11.

   A nice summary chapter of the anesthetic management of TEF/EA.

Further Reading

Domajnko B, Drugas GT, Pegoli W Jr. Temporary occlusion of the gastroesophageal junction: a modified technique for stabilisation of the neonate with esophageal atresia and tracheoesophageal fistula requiring mechanical ventilation. *Pediatr Surg Intern* 2007; 23: 1127–1129.

Greenwood RD, Rosenthal A. Cardiovascular malformations associated with tracheoesophageal fistula and oesophageal atresia. *Pediatrics* 1976; 57: 87–91.

Holder TM, Ashcraft KW, Sharp RJ. Care of infants with oesophageal atresia, tracheoesophageal fistula and associated abnormalities. *J Thorac Cardiovasc Surg* 1987; 94: 828–835.

Orenstein S, Peters J, Khan S Youssef N, Hussain SZ. The digestive system. Congenital abnormalities: esophageal atresia and trachesophageal fistula. In Behrman RE, Kliegman RM, Jenson HB, Stanton BF, eds. *Nelson Textbook of Paediatrics*, 18th ed. Philadelphia: Saunders Elsevier, 2007: 1219–1220.

Petrosyan M, Estrada J, Hunter C, Russell W, Stein J, Ford H, Anselmo DM. Esophageal atresia/tracheoesophageal fistula in very low birth-weight neonates: improved outcomes with staged repair. *J Pediatr Surg* 2009; 44: 2278–228.

Ulma G, Geiduschek J, Zimmerman A, Morray J. Esophageal atresia and tracheosophageal fistula: anesthesia for thoracic surgery. In Gregory GA, ed. *Pediatric Anesthesia*, 4th ed. Philadelphia: Churchill Livingstone, 2001: 440–443.

54

Omphalocele/Gastroschisis Repair

PETER STODDART

INTRODUCTION

Congenital abdominal wall defects (AWD) comprise gastroschisis and omphalocele (exomphalos). Nearly all AWDs require urgent intervention within a few hours of birth. The current incidence of omphalocele (3 per 10,000) and gastroschisis (4–5 per 10,000) has been increasing over the past few decades; however, improved management of these congenital defects has resulted in a fall in mortality to less than 5%. The anesthetic management of both conditions is essentially the same.

LEARNING OBJECTIVES

1. To be able to compare and contrast the AWDs: gastroschisis and omphalocele.
2. To develop a plan for the perioperative management of AWD.
3. To review the complications and outcomes of AWD.

CASE PRESENTATION

A 2.25-kg boy is vaginally born at a district hospital at 36+4 weeks to a 15-year-old primigravida mother. There is meconium-stained amniotic fluid and the Apgar scores are 7 at 1 minute and 9 at 5 minutes. The neonate has a "matted" gastroschisis that is wrapped in **plastic wrap** *(Fig. 54.1) by the midwife prior to transfer to the Special Care Baby Unit. The infant has a size 8FG* **orogastric** *tube inserted and is started on 80 mL/kg/24 hr IV 10% dextrose. The infant needs IV 2x 22.5 mL 4.5%* **human albumin (HAS)** *in response to an increasing heart rate and an increase in capillary filling time to 5 seconds.* **Prophylactic antibiotics** *and IM vitamin K are also administered. Due to the distance and delays in road transport, it took 8 hours from delivery until the baby arrived in the surgical neonatal intensive care unit (NICU).*

The pediatric surgeon decides to reduce the viscera in the OR under general anesthesia. The OR is **warmed** *to 26°C (humidity 50%), and the infant is laid on an air mattress attached to a forced-air warmer. An overhead heater is used while monitoring is applied (including pre- and post-ductal SpO_2). The stomach is emptied by aspirating the orogastric tube while turning the infant prone, then supine. Anesthesia is induced with O_2/air/sevoflurane and the infant is intubated following 1 mg atracurium and 5 micrograms fentanyl. He is ventilated to normocapnea using pressure-controlled ventilation. On the table the surgeons remove the plastic wrap (Fig. 54.2) and find prolapsed thickened distended bowel, mainly midgut and ascending colon, with a possible ileocecal atresia. During a dilute Gastrografin enema to empty the bowel of meconium, the nasopharyngeal temperature falls to 35°C. When the bowel is reduced into the peritoneal cavity, the* **tidal volume falls** *despite raising the ventilation pressures from 12/4 to 26/4 cmH_2O. The* **$ETCO_2$ drops** *to 22 mmHg, heart rate rises from 130 to 166, and the* **post-ductal saturations drop** *compared to the measured SpO_2 in the right hand. The mean BP falls from 38 to 30 mmHg despite two further doses of 25 mL 4.5% HAS. Primary closure is abandoned and a spring-loaded silo (Fig. 54.3) is inserted; cardiovascular stability returns and ventilation pressures normalize. A peripherally inserted central catheter (PICC) is inserted for* **parenteral nutrition** *before returning to the NICU. The baby is extubated 12 hours later and nursed supine with the silo suspended above. Over 72 hours the remaining bowel returns*

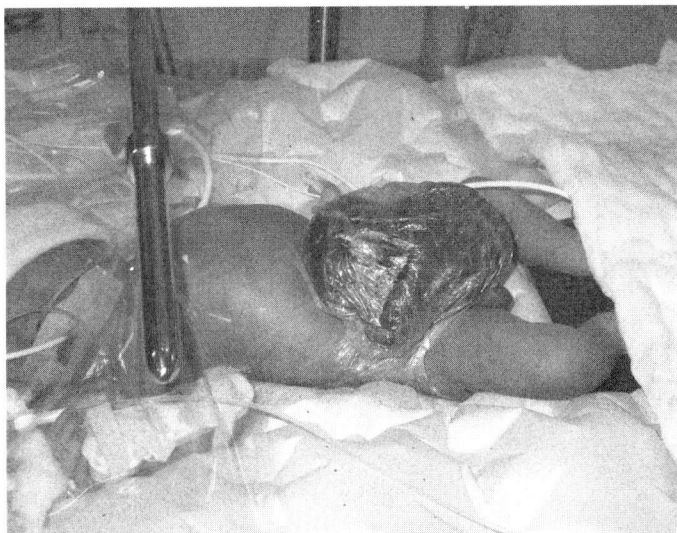

FIGURE 54.1 On arrival to the OR, the baby's intestines were covered by plastic wrap to prevent evaporative losses.

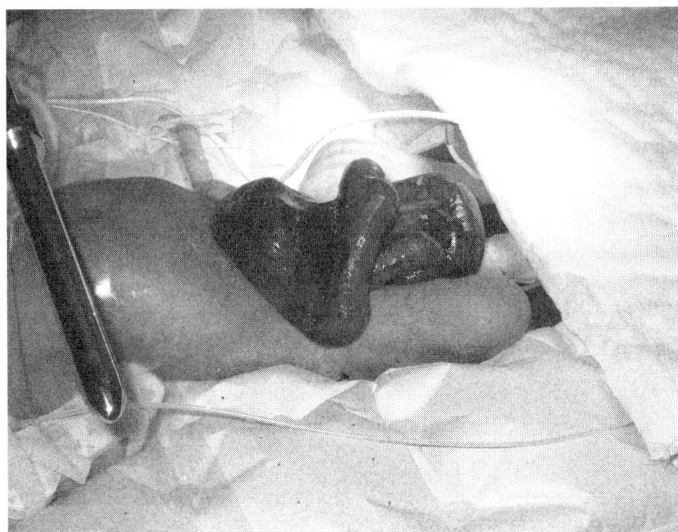

FIGURE 54.2 Gastroschisis unwrapped intraoperatively.

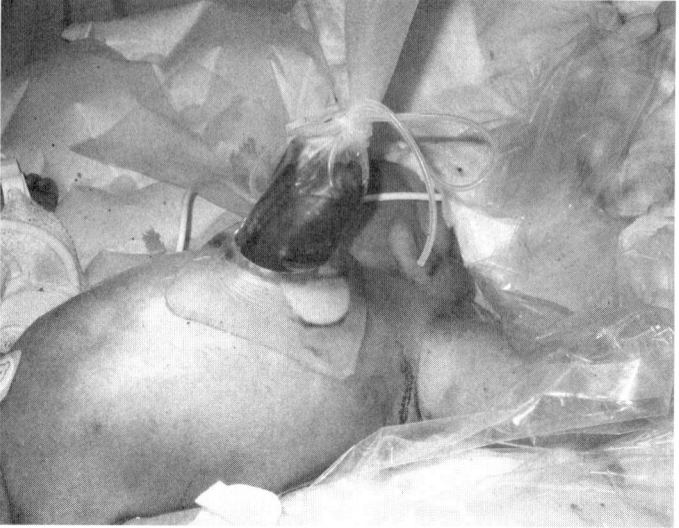

FIGURE 54.3 Silo reduction of gastroschisis.

into the abdominal cavity. The silo is removed and the abdomen is closed by pulling the umbilical cord over the deficit, and a dressing is applied. Over the ensuing weeks, the suspected atresia is excluded and enteral feedings are gradually started with success.

DISCUSSION

1. What are the similarities and differences between gastroschisis and omphalocele?

There are two major causes of congenital AWD: omphalocele and gastroschisis. Their surgical and anesthetic management is similar; however, they have different etiologies and comorbidities, so their overall prognoses differ (Table 54.1).

Gastroschisis can be classified into simple or complex; the latter is associated with bowel atresia (sometimes multiple) or other congenital abnormalities. Complex gastroschisis therefore has a

---

Table 54.1

COMPARISON OF OMPHALOCELE WITH GASTROSCHISIS

Omphalocele	*Gastroschisis*
• Herniation of viscera into base of umbilical cord through a central defect; a membranous sac covers and protects the viscera, but this may rupture, especially at birth.	• Evisceration of gut and potentially other organs through 2- to 5-cm defect lateral to umbilicus (nearly always right-sided); no sac: viscera exposed to chemical burn from amniotic fluid and environment
• Failure of gut to migrate back into abdominal cavity between 6th and 10th week after conception	• Abnormality; lateral ventral wall folds fail to close during 4th week after conception, a similar mechanism to neural tube defects
• Incidence 3:10,000	• Incidence 4 to 5:10,000: associated with young maternal age and deprivation, geographic clusters; higher in Northern European compared with Mediterranean countries
• Lower risk of prematurity	
• 75% have associated congenital abnormalities, including chromosomal, cardiac, GU, craniofacial	• 60% associated with prematurity and intrauterine growth retardation
	• Lower risk for congenital abnormalities, 10% to 30%

---

poorer prognosis. Omphalocele is classified into minor (defects <5 cm) or major (defects >5 cm). The major defect may or may not include the liver in the sac. Omphalocele is associated with chromosomal abnormalities (e.g., trisomy 13, 18, 21, Turner, Klinefelter's), syndromes including Beckwith-Wiedemann, cardiac defects (e.g., ASD/VSD, tetralogy of Fallot, and transposition of the great vessels), and lung hypoplasia.

2. What are the management priorities for AWD?

The primary goal for a neonate with gastroschisis is to reduce the evisceration. The ideal way to minimize the delay before reduction of the viscera is to make an antenatal diagnosis with ultrasound and deliver the baby in an obstetric unit with an attached neonatal surgical unit. However, premature delivery may prevent *in utero* transfer. If there is no significant viscero-abdominal cavity disproportion, a simple gastroschisis may be reduced at the bedside. However, in the case presentation, reduction was not immediately possible and the neonate needed to be transferred to the regional NICU. In these situations fluid and heat loss must be minimized by covering the bowel with simple **plastic wrap**, or placing the viscera and abdominal defect (including the lower extremities) in a "bowel bag." It is vital to maintain the vascular integrity of the bowel by *avoiding accidental volvulus*; therefore, the color and perfusion should be monitored. Prior to definitive treatment the baby should be positioned supine in a thermoneutral neonatal cot/incubator with *ongoing fluid resuscitation*; in the United Kingdom this normally includes bolus infusions of **human albumin** 4.5%. To aid reduction of the viscera an **orogastric tube** is required to decompress the bowel and is preferable to a nasogastric tube in potentially obligate nasal-breathing premature infants. Many surgeons also use a Gastrografin lavage, as in the scenario. However, there is no evidence that it increases primary closure rates, and it does risk a significant acute core temperature drop.

Wound infection/sepsis is a particular risk following surgical reduction, especially if a silo or a patch is used, so **antibiotics** are started prior to surgery. Unruptured omphalocele sacs do not require additional cover but may need physical support to avoid rupture in major omphalocele defects. Associated abnormalities are common, so all infants with omphalocele routinely require an *echocardiogram* before surgery. Cardiac defects may also occur in 10% of infants with gastroschisis, so preoperative echocardiography should also be strongly considered for these infants too. Enteral **nutrition** is frequently delayed because of raised intra-abdominal pressure and/or additional gastrointestinal anomalies such as atresias, necrotizing enterocolitis (NEC), and intra-abdominal sepsis. Nutrition should therefore be initiated parenterally with early minimal enteral trophic feeding if possible.

3. What is the physiological effect of reducing the viscera, and what is abdominal compartment syndrome (ACS)?

Returning the viscera into the abdominal cavity causes a rise in intra-abdominal pressure depending on the disparity between the volume of viscera reduced and the volume of the abdominal cavity. This can result in respiratory and cardiovascular compromise. Lung expansion is limited by splinting of the diaphragm, which will cause a fall in tidal volume and atelectasis. Cardiac output will fall (and right atrial pressure will rise) due to a reduction in venous return from the lower body and an increase in afterload. A rise in intra-abdominal pressure above 15 mmHg reduces renal perfusion with disruption of fluid and salt homeostasis. Above 20 mmHg, ACS develops due to compromised splanchnic blood flow. Visceral ischemia (particularly bowel and liver) leads to prolonged ileus, metabolic acidosis, NEC, and sepsis (Marven & Owen, 2008). Therefore, ACS must be avoided by individualizing the visceral reduction depending on the degree of abdominal cavity disproportion.

Intra-abdominal pressure may be measured via a nasogastric tube or bladder catheter. If the pressure does not rise above 20 mmHg during the reduction of a gastroschisis under general anesthesia, primary closure of the abdomen can be achieved. However, in the United Kingdom, intra-abdominal pressure is not routinely measured directly. Instead, surrogate measures are used, such as an acute **fall in ETCO$_2$** (reflecting falls in tidal volume or cardiac output), a significant **fall in measured tidal volume**, a rise in inspiratory plateau pressure above 25 cmH$_2$O, or a significant **fall in lower limb SpO$_2$** compared to post-ductal upper limb SpO$_2$. If any of these occur, primary closure should be abandoned, as in the scenario presented. In most units a silo would be used to achieve a staged abdominal closure, or occasionally a prosthetic patch is used (particularly in omphalocele major defects).

4. What are the complications of AWD?

Preoperative and intraoperative fluid losses from exposed bowel and "third spacing" are large, so infants need up to 200 mL/kg/24 hr of crystalloid, with colloid supplement as indicated by heart rate, blood pressure, and capillary refill. Postoperatively babies often become edematous and hyponatremic due to renal dysfunction, so urine output, serum electrolytes, and fluid input need to be carefully monitored. Some infants may need inotropic support to improve renal and splanchnic perfusion pressure. Temperature control can be difficult, with extensive heat loss due to evaporation from exposed viscera, especially in small premature infants. This is minimized with early coverage of viscera by reduction into the abdominal cavity or into a silo. Other warming techniques include maintaining ambient OR temperatures above 27°C and using heat and moisture exchange (HME) filters, warm air blowers, overhead heaters, warmed IV fluid, and occlusive surgical drapes to keep the rest of the baby dry.

Postoperative intestinal dysfunction and failure is common due to a combination of inflammation, intestinal anomalies, atresias, dilatations, raised intra-abdominal pressure, and NEC. In view of the frequent prematurity of these infants and prolonged gastrointestinal dysfunction, nutritional support is required. **Parenteral nutrition** should be instituted via a peripherally placed intravenous Silastic feeding catheter or, if there is prolonged gut failure, a cuffed Hickmann/Broviac central line. Early trophic feeding with expressed human milk is of benefit to premature infants and potentially those with gastroschisis. Sepsis is a significant problem, particularly in very small neonates at high risk of NEC and wound and line infection. Signs of sepsis need to be actively sought if there is any deterioration in the baby's condition.

5. What is the long-term outcome of AWD?

The mortality of AWD is dependent on coexisting genetic or congenital abnormalities and the prematurity or growth retardation of the neonate. In a recent American study on gastroschisis in low-risk neonates mortality was 2.9%, compared with 24.4% in high-risk neonates (Chang et al., 2010). High risk was associated with NEC, complex cardiac anomalies, or lung hypoplasia/bronchopulmonary dysplasia. A rare but significant problem is intestinal failure secondary to short bowel syndrome caused by intrauterine or post-delivery volvulus, atresia, or NEC. This results in prolonged parenteral nutrition dependency and a need for small bowel with or without liver transplantation.

Usually a good cosmetic result is achieved if multiple surgeries are not required and the umbilical cord is preserved (ultimately in the correct position). Initially many neonates are growth-retarded, but following successful treatment most will attain a normal IQ and exercise tolerance.

SUMMARY

1. Gastroschisis and omphalocele are associated with different comorbidities and therefore different prognoses.
2. The aim of management is to reduce the eviscerated organs back into the abdominal cavity; primary closure of the abdomen is ideal, but abdominal compartment syndrome must be avoided.
3. Nutritional support is universally required until full enteral feeding is established.
4. Long-term prognosis is good except in the presence of significant prematurity, growth retardation, or associated genetic or congenital anomalies.

ANNOTATED REFERENCES

- Holland AJ, Walker K, Badawi N. Gastroschisis: an update. *Pediatr Surg Internat* 2010; 26: 871–878.

The most recent review of gastroschisis, including antenatal care and overall prognosis.

• **Marven S, Owen A. Contemporary postnatal surgical management strategies for congenital abdominal wall defects** *Seminar Pediatr Surg* **2008; 17: 222–235.**

This is an excellent review of the various options for the surgical management of AWD. It discusses the risks of ACS and outcomes of treatment.

Further Reading

Chang DC, Salazar-Osuna JH, Choo SS, Arnold MA, Colombani PM, Abdullah F. Benchmarking the quality of care of infants with low-risk gastroschisis using a novel risk stratification index. *Surgery* 2010; 147: 766–771.

Sadler T. Embryological origin of ventral body wall defects. *Sem Pediatr Surg* 2010; 19: 209–214.

Vachharajani AJ, Rao R, Keswani S, Mathur AM. Outcomes of exomphalos: an institutional experience. *Pediatr Surg Internat* 2009; 25: 139–144.

55

Congenital Diaphragmatic Hernia Repair

ANNE C. BOAT AND
SENTHILKUMAR SADHASIVAM

INTRODUCTION

Congenital diaphragmatic hernia (CDH) affects approximately 1 in 2,500 live births and results from an embryologic defect in diaphragm formation allowing abdominal contents to enter the fetal pleural cavity. Prognosis and treatment options vary depending on the extent and location of the diaphragmatic hernia, but CDH remains a significant cause of neonatal morbidity and mortality. Anesthesia for neonatal repair of CDH can be involved, as patients often have many organ systems affected by their disease process.

LEARNING OBJECTIVES

1. Understand the pathogenesis of CDH.
2. Know the prognostic indicators and treatment options for CDH.
3. Review the anesthetic considerations of a neonate for CDH repair.

CASE PRESENTATION

*An 11-day-old 3.5-kg boy was born at 38 weeks with a prenatal diagnosis of left-sided CDH and is now scheduled for CDH repair. The prenatal predictors of CDH severity include a **lung-to-head ratio** (LHR) of **1.6**, a **McGoon Index** of 1.49, and a percent predicted lung volume at 34 weeks of 26%. The patient was born via spontaneous vaginal delivery and was intubated immediately after birth. Currently, the patient is ventilated with pressure control/pressure support ventilation at a rate of 40 bpm, with peak inspiratory pressures of 23 cmH$_2$O and a FiO$_2$ of 0.30. He is also on inhaled **nitric oxide** at 20 ppm for pulmonary hypertension estimated to be at systemic level. **Echocardiography** shows a small patent ductus arteriosus with bidirectional shunting and normal right and left systolic ventricular performance. Head ultrasound reveals a grade 1 intraventricular hemorrhage. He is sedated with a midazolam infusion and intravenous morphine as needed.*

DISCUSSION

1. What is the embryologic defect causing CDH formation?

A common pleuroperitoneal cavity exists in the fetus during the first 4 weeks of human gestation. Subsequently, a pleuroperitoneal membrane forms and becomes the diaphragm at about 8 weeks' gestation, dividing this common cavity into the chest and abdomen. The left posterolateral section of this membrane is the last to develop. When incomplete closure of the pleuroperitoneal membrane occurs, abdominal contents such as small and large intestine, stomach, spleen, and liver can herniate and migrate into the chest cavity (Fig. 55.1). CDHs are classified by their location in the diaphragm, with left posterolateral positioning (foramen of Bochdalek) occurring most frequently. Other possible diaphragmatic sites for visceral herniation include right posterolateral, anterior through the foramen of Morgagni, and through the esophageal hiatus.

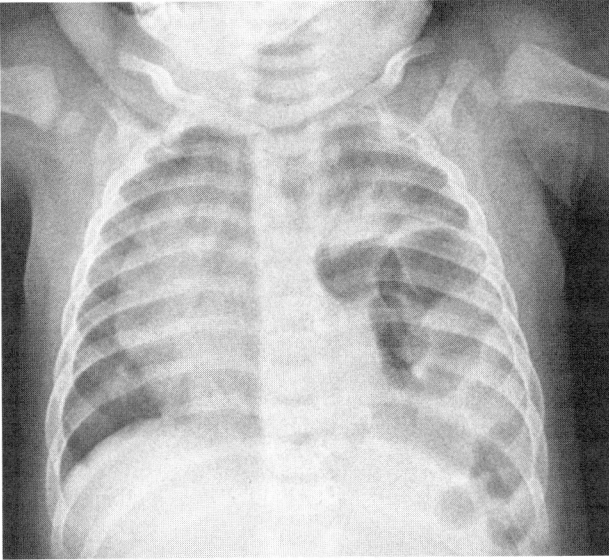

FIGURE 55.1 Typical radiograph of baby with CDH. Note bowel in left hemithorax with displacement of thoracic contents to the right.

2. What is the pathophysiology of CDH?

The presence of abdominal organs in the pleural cavity produces a mass effect resulting in lung compression, pulmonary hypoplasia, pulmonary vascular changes, and cardiac malposition. Pulmonary hypoplasia is more pronounced in the ipsilateral lung, but lung development in the contralateral lung can also be affected. Visceral herniation occurs during a critical time in lung development when the bronchi and pulmonary arteries are undergoing branching. Subsequently, CDH patients have abnormal pulmonary vasculature due to lung hypoplasia-associated reduction in the vascular cross-sectional area and abnormal thickening of the walls of the pulmonary arteries (Chinoy, 2002). The decreased functional lung volume and the increase in pulmonary vascular resistance lead to postnatal hypoxemia, acidosis, and, in severe cases, right heart failure. The hypoxemia and acidosis then further worsens the pulmonary vasoconstriction; this in turn exacerbates the cyanosis and respiratory distress. Cardiac malposition (mesocardia or dextroversion) is frequently found with left-sided CDH. Vascular compression of the inferior vena cava can occur and produce shock-like clinical conditions. Finally, congenital heart diseases have been found in association with CDH in up to 23% of patients (Greenwood et al., 1976).

3. How is CDH diagnosed?

With the detailed level of prenatal care performed today, CDH is often diagnosed prenatally with ultrasonography or fetal MRI. The diagnosis of CDH should be considered in any newborn with signs of respiratory failure shortly after birth. On physical examination of a patient with left-sided CDH, a scaphoid abdomen is often noted with a barrel-shaped chest and decreased or absent breath sounds over the left part of the chest. A chest radiograph shows dilated loops of bowel in the chest and a shifting of the mediastinum to the right (Fig. 55.1).

4. What prognostic indicators are used to determine the severity of CDH?

Commonly used prognostic predictors of CDH severity are liver position and **lung-to-head ratio** (LHR) on fetal ultrasound. Presence of liver in the chest or a LHR of less than 1.0 is associated with severe CDH and increased mortality. Several other predictors of CDH severity have been proposed, including the **Modified McGoon Index (MMI)**. Echocardiography determines the MMI, which is a ratio of the combined diameter of the pulmonary arteries to the aorta at the level of the diaphragm. Studies have shown that a MMI below 1.3 is associated with higher mortality (Suda et al., 2000). Other factors that have been used as predictors of outcome include birth weight, low Apgar scores, and size of the diaphragm defect (CDH Study Group, 2007). An important determination to make in a fetus/neonate diagnosed with CDH is the presence of chromosomal abnormalities and/or other congenital anomalies. Congenital anomalies most commonly associated with CDH involve the central nervous, gastrointestinal, genitourinary, and cardiovascular systems. Severe or lethal congenital anomalies may preclude aggressive CDH treatment.

5. What are the available treatment options?

The focus of treatment in patients with CDH is medical management followed by surgical repair of the diaphragm. Respiratory and cardiovascular compromise is not solely caused by the mass effect of the abdominal contents in the thorax; it is *primarily* due to pulmonary hypoplasia and pulmonary hypertension causing right-to-left cardiac shunting, hypoxemia, and right heart failure. With CDH patients, medical stabilization often means sedation and positive-pressure ventilation to prevent hypoventilation, acidosis, and worsening of pulmonary hypertension. However, ventilator-associated lung injury due to barotrauma caused by overdistention of the lungs and oxygen toxicity can worsen pulmonary status. The ventilation strategy should achieve preductal oxygen saturation of greater than 85% while maintaining a $PaCO_2$ of 45 to 55 mmHg and a pH greater than 7.3, with peak inspiratory pressures 25 cmH_2O or less. Neonates who require more than 25 cmH_2O peak pressures for adequate oxygenation may benefit from high-frequency oscillatory ventilation (HFOV) with decreased risk of barotrauma. In theory, a higher oxygen tension will improve pulmonary blood flow by decreasing pulmonary hypertension, while lower peak inspiratory pressures reduce the possibility of further mechanical lung injury.

Other strategies for improving pulmonary blood flow include **inhaled nitric oxide** (iNO) and HFOV. Nitric oxide is an endogenous regulator of vascular tone, and iNO can act as a selective vasodilator of the pulmonary vasculature. Although the use of iNO has shown benefit in other causes of neonatal pulmonary hypertension, the abnormal pulmonary vessels in some CDH patients with hypoplastic lungs may not respond appropriately to vasodilators, and vasodilators may even worsen the condition (Finer & Barrington, 2006). The effectiveness of iNO in patients with CDH remains controversial. HFOV uses an oscillator to produce high respiratory rates at low tidal volumes. This method is thought to evenly inflate the lungs and decrease overdistention and the subsequent release of inflammatory mediators from the lungs (Van den Hout et al., 2009).

When medical stabilization fails, extracorporeal membrane oxygenation (ECMO) is often used to support cardiopulmonary status. ECMO will temporarily stabilize the patient's condition, allowing for time or medications to improve the pulmonary hypertension and respiratory failure. Exclusion criteria for ECMO include preterm birth before 34 weeks, weight less than 2 kg, presence of a grade II or greater intracranial hemorrhage, and the presence of an irreversible disease process. A CDH infant can undergo diaphragm repair either on ECMO or after ECMO decannulation.

More recent techniques for CDH treatment involve fetal interventions. These include fetal endoscopic tracheal occlusion and ex-uterine intrapartum treatment (EXIT)-to-ECMO procedures. Fetal tracheal occlusion is thought to promote fetal lung growth by preventing the outward movement of fluid from the lungs and increasing lung volumes. However, improvement in survival rates or morbidity with fetal tracheal occlusion has not been proven (Harrison et al., 2003). EXIT-to-ECMO procedures are performed in fetuses with severe CDH needing ECMO support at birth. To avoid the unstable period after delivery but before ECMO initiation, the fetus undergoes ECMO cannulation while still on uteroplacental circulation. Once ECMO and invasive monitoring are established, the umbilical cord is cut and the fetus is delivered.

6. What are the anesthetic considerations for a neonate with CDH?

Depending on the status of a patient for CDH repair, the surgery may occur in the operating room or in the intensive care setting if the patient is on ECMO. In either situation, extensive knowledge of the patient's hospital course, medications, and ventilatory status is essential prior to providing an anesthetic for CDH repair. This includes understanding of coexisting congenital anomalies, results of **echocardiograms**, blood gases, need for pulmonary vasodilators, need for inotropes, and sedation requirements. The patient is usually placed in the supine position for a transabdominal approach to the CDH repair. The diaphragmatic defect is typically closed primarily, and if the defect is large, a prosthetic patch is often used. Vascular access for a CDH repair includes peripheral intravenous lines and an arterial line (preferably right radial to measure the pre-ductal oxygen saturation). Central venous access may be necessary, but care must be taken not to damage neck veins that may be used for ECMO cannulation at a later time.

During the CDH repair, close attention must be paid to ventilatory parameters such as tidal volume, peak inspiratory pressure, and blood gas measurements. Before surgery, a nasogastric tube should be placed to prevent gaseous distention of the bowel in the chest, which could further decrease functional lung volume. Similarly, prolonged mask ventilation and nitrous oxide should be avoided as they may contribute to bowel distention. High ventilatory pressures should be avoided and "gentle ventilation" should be considered (Van den Hout et al., 2009). Sudden elevations in peak inspiratory pressures, a decrease in lung compliance, or sudden hypotension should alert the anesthetist to the possibility of pneumothorax. Pneumothorax usually occurs in the ipsilateral side but can also occur in the contralateral lung. If pneumothorax occurs, surgeons should be prepared for immediate chest tube placement.

Myocardial function and cardiac output must also be closely monitored. Treatment of hypotension and fluid management is paramount in maintaining adequate cardiac output. If hypotension and poor perfusion are not responsive to crystalloid/colloid administration, then the addition of inotropic support (such as dopamine, epinephrine, or dobutamine) may be necessary. Hypocalcemia may occur following transfusion of blood products and must be corrected to maintain optimal cardiac function. Although the use of iNO in CDH patients is controversial, if the patient is already on iNO, it may be prudent to continue with it during the procedure as there is the potential for rebound pulmonary hypertension and right ventricular dysfunction if the iNO is discontinued abruptly.

As with all newborns brought to the operating room, it is important to avoid hypothermia, which can increase oxygen consumption and alter platelet function. Warming the operative room, fluid warmers, warming blankets, and radiant warmers are important means to maintain normal body temperature in the newborn.

The type of anesthetic agent used during CDH repair depends on the cardiovascular status of the patient, type of ventilator, and preference of the anesthesiologist. Halogenated inhalational anesthetics may be used but can cause hemodynamic instability even at lower doses. The hemodynamic stability afforded by intravenous fentanyl is often preferred. If the conventional ventilator on the anesthesia machine does not allow for adequate ventilation with varying modes of ventilation or for the use of iNO, it may be prudent to use the ICU ventilator. The addition of a neuromuscular blocking agent is recommended to decrease the amount of anesthetic used. Since CDH patients are sedated throughout the period of medical stabilization prior to surgical repair, they have often developed a tolerance to narcotic agents and benzodiazepines and may require higher doses.

SUMMARY

1. CDH is a failure of the closure of the diaphragm during the early stages of fetal life, allowing abdominal contents to herniate into the chest cavity and causing lung hypoplasia and other morbidities. The most common site of a CDH is in the posterolateral aspect of the diaphragm.

2. The presence of abdominal viscera in the chest cavity results in pulmonary hypoplasia and an alteration

in the structure of pulmonary vessels, leading to pulmonary hypertension. Pulmonary hypertension and right heart failure is a major source of morbidity and mortality in neonates with CDH.

3. Treatment now consists of delayed closure of the diaphragm after medical stabilization of the patient. Treatment options range from conventional ventilation to ECMO to fetal surgery.

4. Anesthesia for CDH repair requires close attention to the ventilatory status of the patient. Pneumothorax is a risk in both the ipsilateral and contralateral lungs and should be considered if there is a sudden increase in peak inspiratory pressure, decrease in lung compliance, or hypotension. A "gentle ventilation" strategy may decrease the likelihood of pneumothorax and barotrauma to the hypoplastic lungs.

5. Preexisting pulmonary hypertension treated with inhaled NO may need to be continued intraoperatively to avoid sudden rebound pulmonary hypertension.

6. Cardiovascular status must also be monitored closely with invasive lines and aggressive treatment of hypotension.

ANNOTATED REFERENCES

- Finer N, Barrington KJ. Nitric oxide for respiratory failure in infant born at or near term. *Cochrane Database of Systematic Reviews* 2006; 4. Art. No.: CD000399.

A review of the use of iNO for respiratory failure in term or near-term infants. The review found the outcome of infants with CDH was not improved and may have been slightly worsened with iNO.

- Suda K, Bigras J-L, Bohn D, Hornberger LK, McCrindle B. Echocardiographic predictors of outcome in newborns with congenital diaphragmatic hernia. *Pediatrics* 2000; 105: 1106–1109.

    A study aimed at identifying echocardiographic predictors of outcome for infants with isolated CDH. Measurement of the hilar pulmonary arteries may be an indicator of the adequacy of the pulmonary vascular bed, which may help guide treatment.

- Van den Hout L, Sluiter I, Gischler S, De Klein A, Rottier R, Ijsselstijn H, Reiss I, Tibboel D. Can we improve outcome of congenital diaphragmatic hernia? *Pediatr Surg Internat* 2009; 25: 733–743.

    A nice review of CDH discussing etiology, prenatal predictors of survival, treatment strategies, and long-term outcomes.

Further Reading

Chinoy MR. Pulmonary hypoplasia and congenital diaphragmatic hernia: advances in the pathogenetics and regulation of lung development. *J Surg Res* 2002; 106: 209–223.

Congenital Diaphragmatic Hernia Study Group. Defect size determines survival in infants with congenital diaphragmatic hernia. *Pediatrics* 2007; 120; 651–657.

Greenwood RD, Rosenthal A, Nadas AS. Cardiovascular abnormalities associated with congenital diaphragmatic hernia. *Pediatrics* 1976; 57(1): 92–97.

Harrison M, Keller R, Hawgood S, Kitterman J, Sandberg P, Farmer D, Lee H, Filly R, Farrell J, Albanese C. A randomized trial of fetal endoscopic tracheal occlusion for severe fetal congenital diaphragmatic hernia. *N Engl J Med* 2003; 349: 1916–1924.

Langham MR Jr, Kays DW, Ledbetter DJ, Frentzen B, Sanford LL, Richards DS. Congenital diaphragmatic hernias: epidemiology and outcome. *Clin Perinatol* 1996; 23: 671–688.

56

Myelomeningocele Repair

ANNE C. BOAT AND
SENTHILKUMAR SADHASIVAM

INTRODUCTION

Myelomeningocele (MMC) is a spinal birth defect that occurs due to failure in the closure of the embryologic neural tube. The meninges and/or neural structures are exposed, resulting in nerve damage. MMCs are associated with significant direct morbidity as well as with Chiari II malformations and hydrocephalus. The degree of sensory and motor deficits depends on the level of the defect, with bowel and bladder function often affected. Due to the risk of infection with an exposed spinal cord, surgical repair is usually performed in the first 24 to 48 hours of life. Anesthesia for MMC repair presents a unique challenge since positioning of these patients must prevent direct pressure on the exposed neural tissue.

LEARNING OBJECTIVES

1. Understand the pathogenesis and potential causes of MMC.
2. Review the treatment options for MMC, including postnatal and fetal repair.
3. Review the anesthetic considerations for MMC repair.

CASE PRESENTATION

*A full-term baby girl with known **MMC**, **Chiari II malformation**, and **hydrocephalus** was born via cesarean section. Apgar scores were 7 and 8 at 1 minute and 5 minutes. Birth weight was 4,070g. The MMC was noted to be ruptured at birth and was covered with **saline-soaked gauze**. She was transferred to the NICU. Prenatal studies included a fetal MRI showing a low lumbar, upper sacral open neural tube defect, severe hydrocephalus, and a Chiari II malformation with **herniation of the posterior fossa and brain stem** contents into the low cervical spinal canal. Fetal echocardiography showed normal cardiac anatomy. On physical exam, the infant is pink and active with no apparent distress. Macrocephaly is noted, with a head circumference of 46 cm with full and bulging anterior and posterior fontanels. Examination of the back shows a 6 × 3-cm sacral lesion covered by a thin membrane. Spontaneous movement is present in all four extremities. The patient is positioned prone, on room air, with a saline drip over the MMC to keep the membrane and neural tissue moist. The neurosurgeon wants to proceed to the operating room immediately for MMC repair and possible ventriculoperitoneal (VP) shunt placement.*

DISCUSSION

1. What is a MMC, and at what point in embryologic development does it occur?

MMC, also known as spina bifida, is a birth defect that occurs during the third to fourth week of embryologic development, causing an abnormality in the spinal column and spinal cord. Incomplete closure of the neural tube causes a cleft in the vertebral column through which meninges, neural tissue, and cerebrospinal fluid can herniate. When only meninges protrude through the defect, the term "meningocele" is used. However, when meninges and neural elements are involved, it is called a **myelomeningocele**. The opening may occur anywhere along the spinal column, but low thoracic, lumbar, and sacral regions are most commonly affected (Fig. 56.1). Typically, the exposed neural tissue develops abnormally, forming a flat neural placode. The neural placode is then thought to be further damaged by *in utero* exposure to amniotic fluid. This is the "two-hit" hypothesis of the development of neurologic damage in MMC. The first insult occurs with initial exposure and abnormal formation of the cord, the second with the chronic irritation of the exposed cord to amniotic fluid, leading to further damage.

Although most patients with MMC are born alive and are relatively healthy, there are significant lifelong morbidities associated with this congenital defect. Depending on the location of the lesion, sensory and motor function and bowel, bladder, and sexual function are affected.

2. Why are hydrocephalus and Chari II malformations strongly associated with MMC?

A majority of infants with MMC develop **hydrocephalus**. Of the infants who develop hydrocephalus, up to 81% will require

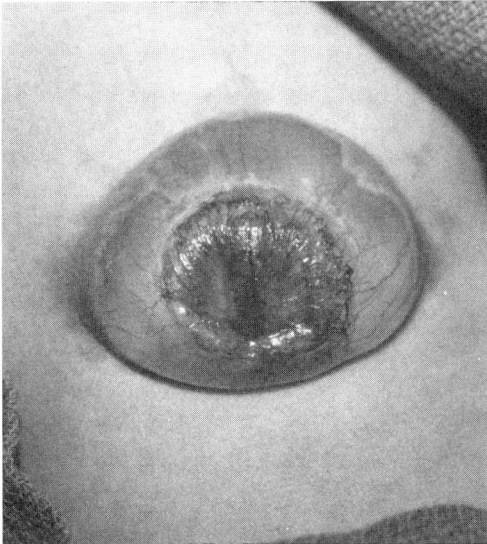

FIGURE 56.1 Lumbar myelomeningocele.

cerebrospinal fluid shunt placement. Evidence of hydrocephalus may occur within the first week of life, as repair of the MMC often worsens the degree of hydrocephalus. While some argue that placement of a cerebrospinal fluid shunt at the time of the MMC repair will decrease the hospital stay, others feel that MMC repair and shunt placement performed together will prolong surgery and increase the risk of shunt infection. Delaying VP shunt placement to allow for a period of observation for meningitis or ventriculitis after MMC repair has been shown to decrease morbidity and mortality, especially in cases with a ruptured MMC. Prolonged antibiotic therapy is often necessary for treatment of shunt infection. In addition, not all infants with MMC require a VP shunt.

Hydrocephalus is likely secondary to the **Chiari II malformation**, which is seen universally in patients with MMC. Chiari II malformations involve **herniation of the cerebellum and brain stem** tissue through the foramen magnum into the cervical spine. Symptoms associated with a Chiari II malformation include difficulty swallowing, inspiratory stridor, apnea, impaired cough/gag reflex, weakness or spasticity of the upper extremities, and difficulties with balance and coordination. One in three patients with MMC will be symptomatic from their Chiari II malformation, so one must handle airway management and neck positioning with care. It is important that the signs and symptoms of a Chiari II malformation are recognized early and followed with a decompressive procedure; otherwise, respiratory failure and loss of neurologic function can occur. 15% of MMC patients with a symptomatic Chiari II malformation will die by 3 years of age and one third will have permanent neurologic damage (Stephenson, 2004). Elevated intracranial pressure can mimic symptoms of Chiari II malformation. Therefore, it is important to rule out increased intracranial pressure as the cause of a patient's symptoms, often by radiologic or surgical evaluation of the ventriculoperitoneal shunt.

3. What are potential causes of MMC?

MMC affects approximately 1 in 2,000 live births and is thought to be caused by genetic as well as non-genetic factors (Mitchell et al., 2004). A family history of a sibling with MMC significantly increases the risk. MMC is a multifactorial polygenetic trait. Non-genetic factors associated with neural tube defects include folate deficiency, use of folate antagonists such as carbamazepine, valproic acid, and trimethoprim, and maternal pregestational diabetes mellitus. The incidence of neural tube defects decreases with maternal folic acid supplementation before and during early pregnancy, and MMC is becoming increasingly rare in communities that have adopted routine folate supplementation. Folate plays an important role in nucleic acid synthesis and methylation reactions, but the exact method by which low folate levels contribute to neural tube defects has yet to be fully understood.

4. What are the treatment options for MMC?

The treatment options for MMC include postnatal surgical repair in the first 24 to 48 hours of life or *in utero* repair of the lesion. Advances in prenatal diagnostic testing and imaging permit prenatal diagnosis of MMC. This allows for a planned cesarean section prior to the onset of labor, reducing the risk of rupture of membranes, and allows delivery in a medical center with pediatric neurosurgery services.

After birth and initial physical examination of the infant, the patient is placed prone or lateral to prevent pressure on the neural placode. The defect is covered with **sterile saline-soaked gauze** to prevent drying out of the neural tissue and further trauma. Postnatal MMC repair involves reconstruction of the neural placode, with care taken to prevent future tethering of the spinal cord with closure of the dura, the muscular layer, and the skin (Gaskill, 2004). The cerebrospinal fluid is cultured at the time of surgery and the infant often remains on antibiotic therapy until cultures are negative.

Fetal surgery for MMC is undergoing investigation. The rationale behind *in utero* repair of MMC is the fact that additional trauma to the neural placode is believed to occur during its prolonged exposure to amniotic fluid and subsequent direct trauma or pressure on the neural tissue. This theory has been supported by both human and animal data (Bouchard et al., 2003; Meuli et al., 1996). With the routine use of ultrasonography for fetal screening and the ability to confirm the diagnosis of MMC with a fetal MRI, the diagnosis is often made by 18 weeks of gestation. This allows for fetal surgery to occur in the window of 19 to 25 weeks' gestation, when the integrity of the fetal tissue is amenable to repair but before extensive damage to the neural placode occurs.

A multicenter prospective randomized clinical trial called the Management of Myelomeningocele Study (MOMS) compared such midgestation surgery with standard postpartum repair. The authors found much lower rates of demise (fetal or neonatal) and need for and placement of a VP shunt by 1 year of age. There was also significant improvement in the composite score for mental development and motor function at 30 months. Improvements were seen in **hindbrain herniation** at 12 months and percentage of patients who were ambulatory at 30 months of age. Potential benefits of prenatal surgery must be balanced against associated higher rates of preterm birth, intraoperative complications, and uterine-scar defects apparent at delivery, along with a higher rate of maternal transfusion at delivery (Adzick et al., 2011).

5. What are the anesthetic considerations for MMC repair?

Preoperatively, it is important to establish if there is coexisting disease. Many infants with MMC have been found to have a shortened trachea, and a chest x-ray may help assess that. The anesthesia provider should perform a thorough cardiac exam and review results of echocardiography. Screening echocardiograms have been suggested for all neonates with MMC, as over one third of patients have congenital heart disease. Most commonly seen cardiac anomalies are secundum atrial septal defects and ventricular septal defects, with girls affected more than boys. Most patients with MMC develop hydrocephalus, and some may have an enlarged head, making airway management difficult. However, the increase in intracranial pressure often happens after the MMC defect is closed. All neonates with MMC have a

Chiari II malformation, but not all are symptomatic. Symptomatic patients may present with inspiratory stridor due to dysfunction of cranial nerve X (vagus nerve), apnea or disordered breathing due to disruption of the medullary respiratory center, or diminished gag reflex and dysphagia due to dysfunction of cranial nerve IX (glossopharyngeal nerve). Other signs and symptoms may include hypotonia, opisthotonos, nystagmus, and a weak cry.

Patients for MMC repair should have peripheral intravenous access established prior to surgery. Volume status needs to be assessed preoperatively as there is the potential for significant fluid loss from the MMC. IV fluid replacement with crystalloid should cover maintenance requirements plus these losses. Glucose may be added to the IV fluids to prevent hypoglycemia, and glucose levels should be monitored at regular intervals. It is usually not necessary to establish central venous access or place an arterial line for open MMC repair. Blood loss is not usually significant unless a large rotation flap is required to cover the defect. However, two well-functioning peripheral IVs are recommended.

Positioning of patients for induction of anesthesia and intubation can be a challenge. Care must be taken not to place pressure on or traumatize the MMC sac. This can be achieved by intubating the patient in the lateral position or placing the patient supine with the MMC sac supported in the hollowed portion of a cushioned ring. The approach to the airway should account for the fact that Chiari II malformations may cause significant cervical cord and brain stem compression, which is accentuated by cervical flexion during laryngoscopy and intubation. MRI images are helpful in understanding the extent of cord and brain stem compression.

After intubation, the patient is turned prone and supported on hip and chest rolls. It is important that the rolls are placed to minimize an increase in intra-abdominal pressure, which could compromise ventilation and cause increased surgical bleeding through engorged epidural veins. Anesthesia can be maintained with a combination of IV opioids and inhalational anesthetic agent.

Use of neuromuscular blocking agents should be discussed with the neurosurgeon prior to surgery; they may be undesirable if the surgeon plans to use nerve stimulation during surgery. Attention should be paid to maintaining the patient's body temperature. This may be achieved by preventing preoperative hypothermia, warming the room temperature, and using a forced-air warming blanket.

If comorbid conditions affect the airway or respiratory center, patients may need to remain intubated in the postoperative period to protect the airway and to ensure adequate ventilation. Otherwise, extubation can often be achieved with close monitoring for postoperative apnea. Some centers have used spinal anesthesia for MMC repair with direct injection of hyperbaric local anesthetic into the caudal aspect of the MMC sac (Viscomi et al., 1995). This approach prevents the need for intubation and general anesthesia but is limited by the duration of the block and the risk of a "high spinal." At this time, spinal anesthesia is not a widely accepted anesthetic technique for MMC repair.

SUMMARY

1. MMC occurs due to a failure in the closure of the neural tube in the third to fourth week of gestation in 1:2,000 live births. Loss of sensory and motor function at and below the level of the lesion and bowel and bladder dysfunction are often seen.
2. Chiari II malformation is seen in conjunction with MMC and contributes to the hydrocephalus seen in the majority of patients with MMC.
3. Anesthetic considerations for MMC repair (performed in the first 24–48 hours of life) include comorbidities (congenital heart disease and symptomatic Chiari II malformations), careful positioning, and evaluation

and treatment of patient's volume status. MMC patients are at risk for hypoventilation in the postoperative period.
4. MMC patients return to the operating room frequently through their lifetime and are at risk for developing latex allergies.

ANNOTATED REFERENCES

- Gaskill A. Primary closure of open myelomeningocele. *Neurosug Focus 2004;* 16: 1–4.

  A nice review of the neurosurgical technique for postnatal MMC repair. It is helpful for anesthesia providers to understand the phases of surgical care and the postoperative course.
- Mitchell L, Adzick NS, Melchionne J, Pasquariello P, Sutton L, Whitehead A. Spina bifida. *Lancet* 2004; 364, 1885–1895.

  A thorough review of MMC, including epidemiology, diagnosis, treatment, and prevention. If the reader were to pick one review article to read on MMC, this should be it.
- Stevenson KL. Chiari II malformation: past, present and future. *Neurosurg Focus* 2004; 16(2): E5.

  This is an informative review of Chiari II malformations, including an extensive explanation of the clinical complexity of presenting signs and symptoms. Multiple images illustrate the anatomic derangement found with Chiari II malformations.

Further Reading

Adzick NS, Thom EA, Spong CY, et al.; the MOMS Investigators. A randomized trial of prenatal versus postnatal repair of myelomeningocele. *N Engl J Med* 2011; 364: 993–1004.

Bouchard S, Davey MG, Rintoul NE, Walsh DS, Rorke LB, Adzick NS. Correction of hindbrain herniation and anatomy of the vermis after in utero of myelomeningocele in sheep. *J Pediatr Surg* 2003; 38: 451–458.

Hirose S, Farmer D. Fetal surgery for myelomeningocele. *Clin Perinatol* 2009; 6(2): 431–438.

Meuli M, Meuli-Simmen C, Hutchins GM, Yingling CD, Timmel GB, Harrison MR, Adzick NS. In utero repair of experimental myelomeningocele saves neurologic function at birth. *J Pediatr Surg* 1996; 31: 397–402.

Rintoul NE, Sutton LN, Hubbard AM, Cohen B, Melchionno J, Pasquariello P, Adzick NS. A new look at myelomeningoceles: functional level, shunting, and the implications for fetal intervention. *Pediatrics* 2002; 109, (3): 409–413.

Ritter S, Lloyd YT, Shaddy, RE, Minich LL. Are screening echocardiograms warranted for neonates with meningomyelocele? *Arch Pediatr Adolesc Med* 1999; 153: 1264–1266.

Sival DA, Begeer JH, Staal-Schreinemachers AL, Vos-Niel JM, Beekhuis JR, Prechtl HF. Perinatal motor behavior and neurological outcome in spina bifida aperta. *Early Hum Dev* 1997; 50: 27–37.

Viscomi CM, Abajian JC, Wald SL, Rathmell JP, Wilson JT. Spinal anesthesia for repair of meningomyelocele in neonates. *Anesth Analg* 1995; 81: 492–495.

PART 12

CHALLENGES IN REGIONAL

ANESTHESIA AND PAIN

57

Caudal vs. Penile Block

CHARLES B. EASTWOOD AND
KENNETH R. GOLDSCHNEIDER

INTRODUCTION

Circumcision is a commonly performed operation. Although the medical necessity of routine circumcision is debated, common indications for the procedure include religious beliefs, parental preference, hygienic concerns, phimosis, and paraphimosis. As with any surgical procedure, adequate postoperative pain control is an important consideration. A variety of analgesic options for circumcision exist, each with potential risks and benefits.

LEARNING OBJECTIVES

1. Discuss post-circumcision analgesia.
2. Understand basic anatomy and technique pertaining to caudal and penile blocks.
3. Identify potential risks and benefits of caudal versus penile blockade.

CASE PRESENTATION

A 2.5-year-old boy presents for circumcision. His parents report that providing adequate hygiene for their son has been difficult due to increasing difficulty with and pain during foreskin retraction. He has no allergies, has had no surgeries, and is otherwise healthy. He walks and runs but is not yet toilet-trained. Physical examination reveals **numerous skin bruises** *on the shins, knees, and forehead. Exam of the spine reveals a* **dimple** *that can be probed to an end point. No further dermatologic anomalies are seen. His parents express a desire to "not use strong pain medications" after the operation. During the discussion of* **caudal blockade**, *they express concern because a neighbor's child was diagnosed with a tethered cord after the pediatrician found a dimple on routine exam. After induction, an ultrasound-guided* **penile block** *is performed. The child requires acetaminophen and a small dose of fentanyl in the recovery room and is discharged home with acetaminophen for further analgesia.*

DISCUSSION

1. What is the significance of a sacral dimple?

Physical examination of this patient shows a "sacral **dimple**." Although this variant may occur in up to 4% of normal children, it is a finding that is also associated with tethered cord syndrome (spinal dysraphism). Additional skin findings in patients with spinal dysraphism include overlying pigmentation changes, hypertrophic growths, lipomas, dermal sinuses, skin appendages, and hemangiomas (Zywicke & Rozzelle, 2011). Significant medical history findings that point to underlying spinal cord and/or vertebral disease include progressive motor or sensory deficits, difficulty playing sports due to poor coordination of the lower extremities, frequent falls, and urologic or bowel control problems causing delayed or renewed problems with toilet training. History or physical examination that is significant for one or more of these issues should lead the anesthesiologist to consider non-neuraxial approaches to postoperative pain. As a tethered cord can lead to delayed but progressive neurologic problems, the placement of a caudal injection in that context might confound the causality of such changes, and it is a relative contraindication to performing the block. **Penile block**s and systemic analgesics provide viable, safe alternatives. If there is a suggestion that the child may have a tethered cord, then further workup, in coordination with the pediatrician, should be discussed with the parents. In this boy, the **dimple** has an easily seen end point and no associated stigmata. Such shallow dimples are not associated with spinal dysraphism, and reassurance is the only intervention required.

2. What is the innervation of the penis?

The pudendal nerve (S2–S4) and the pelvic plexus give rise to penile innervation. The majority of penile sensation is carried by the pudendal nerve, which divides deep to Buck's fascia to form the dorsal nerves to the penis. The dorsal nerves travel lateral to the superficial and deep dorsal veins and dorsal arteries on the dorsal aspect of the penis.

3. How are caudal and penile nerve blocks performed?

Caudal blocks are essentially a variety of epidural analgesia. They generally involve a single injection of local anesthetic, with or without additives, into the epidural space. The space is accessed by inserting a needle through the sacrococcygeal ligament, which overlies the sacral hiatus. The landmarks for this block are the posterior superior iliac spines (PSIS), which form the base of an equilateral triangle projecting downward, with the apex approximating the sacral hiatus. Just prior to the inferior tip of the triangle are the sacral cornua, which can be palpated as two small prominences between 0.3 and 1 cm apart. These form the base of a smaller triangle with the coccyx, which is covered by the sacrococcygeal membrane. To perform a **caudal block**, the child is placed in a lateral decubitus position with knees drawn towards the chest. After confirmation of landmarks and location of the sacral hiatus, the area is prepared with a sterilizing solution such as povidone–iodine or chlorhexidine. As for any neuraxial procedure, strict attention to sterile technique is necessary during this block.

Different practitioners may select different needles for the **caudal block**. Short-bevel needles are advocated by some for their improved tactile sensation as tissue layers are penetrated. Others prefer intravenous catheters because they would be difficult to advance into the intraosseous space, thereby reducing the potential for intraosseous injection of large volumes of local anesthetic, with subsequent systemic toxicity. Advantages of the catheter technique include being able to leave it in place, under sterile dressing, for reinjection at the end of a longer case, sparing the need for another needle stick.

After the needle pierces the skin just inferiorly to the sacral cornua, the needle is advanced at a 45-degree angle with the bevel facing anteriorly. This orientation of the bevel theoretically reduces the likelihood of puncturing the sacral cortex. Following puncture of the sacrococcygeal membrane, felt as a distinct "pop," the needle's angle is dropped to approximate the angle of the sacral canal. After advancing a further 1 to 2 mm, the needle or catheter is advanced. At all points in the procedure needle and catheter advancement should not meet resistance; otherwise, misplacement of the needle should be suspected, equipment withdrawn, landmarks reconfirmed, and the procedure started again.

A short length of sterile IV extension tubing, connected to and flushed with the syringe containing the caudal block solution, is attached to the needle or catheter hub. It is common practice to connect the syringe directly to the needle; however, the tubing prevents motion in the injecting hand from altering the depth or angle of the needle. Aspiration is performed to check for the presence of blood or cerebrospinal fluid (CSF). Following negative aspiration the block solution is injected in a slow, fractionated fashion, with repeated checks for blood or CSF. Dosing for caudal blocks has traditionally been cited as up to 1 mL/kg (depending on the concentration of local anesthetic and the size of the child). As the dermatomes involved in circumcision are limited (see above), 0.5 mL/kg will generally suffice and will reduce the potential for toxicity. Epinephrine (adrenaline) is often added to allow for monitoring of electrocardiographic (ECG) changes suggestive of intravascular injection. Some choose to avoid it because ECG changes are not entirely reliable under anesthesia, and the vasoconstrictive effects of larger doses of caudal dosing may affect blood flow to the distal cord. This in theory might cause ischemic damage to the spinal cord or nerve roots. A test dose followed by the balance of the dosing with plain local anesthetic is a reasonable compromise.

A number of different approaches to **penile nerve blocks** have been described. A dorsal penile nerve block (DPNB) is performed by inserting the needle at the inferior edge of the pubic ramus at the midline to a depth (0.5–1 cm, depending on the size of the child) where one feels the needle "pop" through the superficial fascia (Scarpa's fascia). The needle should be angled first to one side of midline, then the other. After negative aspiration, injection of local anesthetic without epinephrine commences. Any resistance to injection should prompt one to reposition the needle to avoid damaging the neurovascular bundle, which is located in the midline. Although this block covers the majority of penile innervation, it may miss lateral and ventral regions of sensation. Ultrasound seems to have a role in improving the success rate of the **penile block**, but experience with ultrasound is still growing. A ring block is performed by subcutaneous infiltration of local anesthetic around the base of the penis. Combining DPNBs with deposition of local anesthetics at different points around the base of the penis has also been described. Whichever penile nerve block is selected, care must be taken to use epinephrine-free solutions to avoid the risk of vasoconstriction-induced penile ischemia.

4. What are the potential risks of caudal anesthesia versus penile nerve blockade?

Any procedure that involves a needle puncture risks bleeding or infection. All perineural injections carry the risk of injury to nerves, although these appear to be more theoretical than actual. Large retrospective studies suggest that the risks of permanent nerve injury after caudal injection are very small (e.g., Giaufré et al., 1996; Llewellyn & Moriarty, 2007). Risks specific to caudal anesthesia include epidural hematoma or abscess, dural puncture with "high" or "complete" spinal anesthesia, post-dural puncture headache, and intravascular or intraosseous injection of large volumes of local anesthetic with subsequent systemic toxicity. Regarding risk assessment for bleeding, the physical examination and history must account for the child's developmental stage. In this child, the **numerous bruises** are compatible with an active toddler whose frequent falls will result in bruising that suggests a pattern consistent with forward (if unsteady) motion. Bruising in areas not expected to bear the brunt of falls, such as the buttocks, back, or abdomen, along with bleeding with dental hygiene, would warrant more concern.

Risks of the penile nerve block include hematoma, intravascular injection, penile ischemia (if epinephrine is used), infection, and incomplete block. Despite the wide range of variety and severity of complications possible with these techniques, major adverse events are rare.

Due to the rarity of complications and paucity of good data, it is difficult to clearly say which block has higher risk, but a few issues may sway one's decision towards one block versus the other. If there is reason to suspect spinal deformity, then the **penile block** becomes more appealing. A caudal block might be favored if greater coverage is needed for other procedures (e.g., hernia repair) that may accompany the circumcision. Skin infections at the site of intended needle puncture should prompt consideration of alternative regional anesthetic approaches; if they involve the base of the penis or the penis proper, cancellation of the surgery itself may be in order. A medical history significant for bleeding disorders or ongoing use of anticoagulants is a contraindication to epidural analgesia.

5. Is there a clear benefit to one regional blockade versus another?

A number of studies have been done comparing different regional anesthetic approaches to post-circumcision analgesia. Most have involved a small number (~50) of patients. The most consistent finding of these studies was similar analgesic efficacy (need for additional analgesia in the immediate postoperative period), with durations of analgesic block lasting 2 to 8 hours for both **caudal** and **penile block**s. Technical failures were reported more frequently with penile nerve blocks, while caudals were associated with a higher incidence of nausea and vomiting, delayed micturition (resolving within 8–9 hours), and motor blockade, which delayed ambulation. For small children, ambulation may not be a practical issue, but for larger children, the need for the parents to carry the child may sway the decision toward a penile block.

One study comparing DPNB, ring block, and topical local anesthetics in newborns undergoing circumcision suggested more complete blockade of penile sensation with ring blocks (Irwin & Cheng, 1996). This study also found, not surprisingly,

---

Table 57.1

PROS AND CONS OF CAUDAL VERSUS PENILE NERVE BLOCKS FOR POST-CIRCUMCISION ANALGESIA

Caudal Block		Penile Nerve Block (PNB)	
Pros	*Cons*	*Pros*	*Cons*
- Decreased opioid use - Improved patient/ parent satisfaction -Option to perform procedure without general anesthetic	- Limited duration - Increased risk profile vs. PNB - Increased nausea/ vomiting vs. PNB - Delayed ambulation & micturition	- Decreased opioid use - Improved patient/parent satisfaction - Decreased nausea/ vomiting - Earlier ambulation & micturition	- Limited duration - Increased failure rate vs. caudal - Risk of hematoma

that any attempt to provide local anesthesia was more effective than placebo at reducing signs of infant pain. A consideration of the analgesic options available, as well as the pros and cons of the two classes of regional analgesics, favors the use of penile nerve block combined with oral acetaminophen and NSAIDs with additional oral opioids as needed.

One particular advantage of caudal anesthesia is the option to run a continuous infusion of 3% chloroprocaine (Henderson et al., 1993) or provide a dense, single-dose block with ropivacaine or bupivacaine. This technique allows a procedure such as circumcision to be performed without general anesthesia, should that be desired. A dextrose pacifier along with the continuous block may provide a comfortable experience for a young infant, although is not effective for older infants and toddlers.

Table 57.1 summarizes the pros and cons of caudal versus penile nerve blocks for post-circumcision analgesia.

SUMMARY

1. Penile and caudal blocks are effective for circumcision pain, with overall data favoring penile blocks.
2. Sacral dimples merit careful examination, but superficial dimples are not contraindications to caudal blocks.
3. When circumcision is combined with another procedure, a caudal block poses advantages over a penile block.

ANNOTATED REFERENCES

· Cyna AM, Middleton P. Caudal epidural block versus other methods of postoperative pain relief for circumcision in boys [review]. *Cochrane Library* 2009; Issue 4.

A comprehensive, up-to-date review of the literature comparing caudal blockade to a variety of analgesic approaches for patients undergoing circumcision.

· **Lander J, Brady-Fryer B, Metcalfe J B, Nazarali S, Muttitt S. Comparison of ring block, dorsal penile nerve block, and topical anesthesia for neonatal circumcision: a randomized controlled trial.** *JAMA* **1997; 278(24): 2157–2162.**

A well-designed study comparing multiple approaches to anesthetizing the penis. An interesting (and controversial) aspect of this study is the inclusion of a placebo control group of patients.

Further Reading

Giaufré E, Dalens B, Gombert A. Epidemiology and morbidity of regional anesthesia in children: a one-year prospective survey of the French-Language Society of Pediatric Anesthesiologists. *Anesth Analg* 1996; 83(5): 904–12.

Irwin MG, Cheng W. Comparison of subcutaneous ring block of the penis with caudal epidural block for post-circumcision analgesia in children. *Anaesth Intens Care* 1996; 24: 365–367.

Llewellyn N, Moriarty A. The national pediatric epidural audit. *Pediatr Anesth* 2007; 17(6): 520–533.

Margetts L, Carr A, McFadyen G, Lambert A. A comparison of caudal bupivacaine and ketamine with penile block for paediatric circumcision. *Eur J Anaesthesiol* 2008; 25: 1009–1013.

Sandeman DJ, Reiner D, Dilley AV, Bennett MH, Kelly KJ. A retrospective audit of three different regional anaesthesia techniques for circumcision in infants. *Anaesth Intens Care* 2010; 38: 519–524.

Weksler N, Atias I, Klein M, Rosenztsveig V, Ovadia L, Gurman GM. Is penile block better than caudal epidural block for postcircumcision analgesia? *J Anesth* 2005; 19: 36–39.

White J, Harrison B, Richmond P, Procter A, Curran J. Postoperative analgesia for circumcision. *Br Med J* 1983; 286: 1934.

Zywicke HA, Rozzelle CJ. Sacral dimples. *Pediatr Rev* 2011; 32:109–114.

58

Neonatal Epidural

DAVID L. MOORE AND
KENNETH R. GOLDSCHNEIDER

INTRODUCTION

Over the past couple of decades there has been increased awareness that opioid use for postoperative pain in neonates may not result in the best outcomes for these patients. Concurrently, there has been an increased use of regional techniques for postoperative pain in the neonate, in particular epidural anesthesia. The most common technique has been an epidural block via a caudal catheter. Caudal catheters can be used for lumbar and thoracic epidural blocks. The caudal catheter technique allows for a theoretically safer means of placement than the classic, at-level, loss-of-resistance technique.

LEARNING OBJECTIVES

1. Know the risks and benefits of regional techniques versus IV opioids for postoperative pain relief in infants.
2. Understand the technique of placing epidural catheters by caudal and lumbar routes.
3. Learn the methods of confirmation for correct positioning of caudal catheters in babies.

CASE PRESENTATION

*A 7-day-old girl, diagnosed antenatally at 20 weeks' gestation with a congenital pulmonary adenomatoid malformation, presents to the operating room for excision of the malformation via a right-sided thoracotomy at T6-7. After smooth induction and intubation, a **hold point (time out)** for epidural placement is observed. The baby is placed in the lateral decubitus position, and her back is prepared in sterile fashion for placement of a thoracic epidural catheter via the caudal space. The distance from the **caudal insertion** site to desired dermatome (T5-6) is measured. An **18-gauge IV catheter** is introduced into the epidural space via the sacrococcygeal ligament. After negative aspiration for blood and CSF, a 1-mL bolus of preservative-free 0.9% saline is used to confirm the minimal resistance associated with the epidural space. A styletted 20-gauge catheter is threaded via the IV catheter to the length measured previously. Once placed, the **position of the catheter tip is confirmed** with fluoroscopy. After removing the IV catheter, the insertion site is dressed and a 0.5-mL/kg bolus of 0.1% bupivacaine is given. An **infusion of 0.2 mg/kg/hr of bupivacaine** is begun and continued into the postoperative period, after an uneventful surgery. The baby is extubated at the end of the procedure and her postoperative course is uneventful and comfortable. The catheter is removed on postoperative day 2.*

DISCUSSION

1. What are the advantages of epidural analgesia in infants?

It is thought that patients undergoing thoracic surgery have better pain control, improved postsurgical ventilation, and less morbidity with epidural analgesia than with opioid analgesia. As newborns and infants have smaller respiratory reserves than older patients and a decreased ability to metabolize morphine, opioid analgesia tends to cause sedation and respiratory depression in infants, often requiring postoperative ventilation. Prolonged intubation and mechanical ventilation can lead to iatrogenic disorders such as subglottic stenosis, ventilator-acquired pneumonia, and pulmonary barotrauma. In addition, reducing exposure to opioids reduces the chances for urinary retention, shortens postoperative ileus, and allows the baby to be awake enough to interact more with the parents. In an otherwise healthy neonate, epidural analgesia allows extubation soon after surgery (Tobias et al., 1996). With careful handling, babies with epidurals can be held by their parents, taking full advantage of their wakefulness.

2. Are there risks specific to epidurals in infants?

The caudal and low lumbar approaches to insertion of thoracic catheters are used to minimize the risk of needle trauma to the spinal cord by using an insertion point below the conus medullaris (usually around L3 in newborns). The dural sac terminates around S3 in neonates, so both such techniques do have the risk of dural puncture. While there have been no known reports of nerve root injury with this technique, the catheter must still be advanced carefully to avoid injury.

For the first 6 months of life the clearance of local anesthetics is lower than in older children. Further, infants have lower blood levels of albumin and alpha-1 acid-glycoprotein, the two proteins that account for the majority of local anesthetic binding in the blood. Therefore, total dosing of local anesthetics for patients under 6 months of age must be lower than that for older patients. **Bupivacaine infusion** rates up to 0.25 mg/kg/hr appear to be safe, although data on exact dosing are lacking. Of note, blood levels of bupivacaine have been found to be still increasing 24 hours into infusion, so cardiopulmonary monitoring is crucial, even if the patient looks otherwise stable in the immediate postoperative period. While there have been no reports of IV lipid use for resuscitation and treatment of local anesthetic toxicity in infants, one would predict that it would be worth using in the event of seizures or cardiovascular signs of toxicity.

2-chloroprocaine is an interesting alternative local anesthetic that may have a role for infants. As an ester, it has a very short half-life, even in fetal blood (Kuhnert et al., 1988), and can be run for long periods without accumulation. The tip of the catheter has to be accurately placed at the desired dermatome, as this anesthetic is usually run alone without opioid additives, and so it does not have the benefit of opioid coverage beyond the immediately affected dermatomes.

The risk of infection is theoretically higher when the caudal approach is used because a higher percentage of colonization has been found in caudal catheters than in lumbar ones. This is due in part to proximity to the anus, but also potentially due to the difficulty in maintaining sterile dressings. Contamination of the insertion site by stool is not uncommon and is an indication to remove that catheter.

3. What are the alternative techniques for placing catheters in the thoracic epidural space in infants?

The caudal approach to thoracic catheters is presented in the scenario. It takes advantage of well-known landmarks and is truly just an extension of a very common block (Bösenberg et al., 1988). An **18-gauge IV catheter** is inserted as an introducer for the catheter, though a Crawford needle may also be used. The epidural catheter is then threaded through it, preceded by a roughly 1-mL bolus of preservative-free 0.9% saline to open the epidural space and facilitate catheter passage. The disadvantage of this technique is that the insertion site is in proximity to the anus, and the ability to maintain sterility postoperatively is limited by proximity to the intergluteal fold. The fold tends to force the center of the dressing off the skin, allowing urine or feces to get underneath. This logistical problem can limit how long the catheter remains in place.

A second technique is less familiar to many but resolves these issues. The modified Taylor technique uses the L5-S1 interspace as the access point (Gunter, 2000). This interspace is the largest in the spinal column and easily allows insertion of an 18-gauge Crawford needle with loss of resistance to preservative-free 0.9% saline. The operator should be aware that the depth is usually around 1 cm, and the ligaments are much softer that those of older children, necessitating a careful technique for loss of resistance. The angle of insertion should be approximately 45 degrees, angled cephalad, to allow passage of the catheter. Once loss of resistance is felt, approximately 1 mL of saline is injected to distend the epidural space, and the catheter can be threaded. Advancement of the catheter should be very easy, as for the caudal approach. Any resistance should result in the catheter being withdrawn and re-advanced after catheter or patient is repositioned (see below). While less familiar, this technique is easily learned and allows the dressing to be placed above the intergluteal fold and away from the anus.

As with any procedure, a **hold point** (also known as a **time out**) should be observed prior to starting to confirm that the correct procedure is being done with the proper equipment on the correct patient, who is in optimal position. This process is relatively new to anesthesiologists but has become common practice to avoid wrong-site procedures and to ensure that the needed equipment is available and preparations have been made prior to starting the procedure.

4. If the catheter will not advance, what are techniques to correct this situation?

It is important that the catheter advances easily through the epidural space to avoid traumatic injury to the structures within the spinal canal. Table 58.1 lists approaches to the catheter that is difficult to advance. Of the radiographic techniques used (see below), fluoroscopy is best for identifying positioning and trajectory of catheters as they are being placed. Withdrawing catheters through a Tuohy needle is often discouraged due to the risk of shearing off a portion of catheter; however, this risk must be weighed against the risks of reinserting the needle.

5. What are the options for confirming placement of the catheter tip?

Correct positioning of a caudal catheter is not guaranteed (Valairucha et al., 2002). Real-time techniques include ultrasound,

Table 58.1

SOLUTIONS FOR INABILITY TO THREAD CATHETER

Lumbar Approach

Immediate resistance
Carefully withdraw catheter; inject ~1 mL saline to recheck loss of resistance and to distend space; lower needle to make angle more acute, and align catheter trajectory with spine.

Delayed resistance
Withdraw catheter ~1 cm and gently twist catheter to change angle slightly while advancing; reduce flexion of spine by repositioning child; consider fluoroscopy to confirm trajectory and rule out coiling.

Caudal Approach

Immediate resistance
Use a stylet, if not used initially; remove catheter and inject with ~1 mL saline to confirm low resistance and to feel for subcutaneous placement as well as to distend the epidural space.

Delayed resistance
Use a stylet, if not used initially; withdraw catheter 1 to 2 cm and twirl catheter 90 to 180 degrees, and re-advance; consider fluoroscopic guidance to look for coiling; gently flex or extend the patient's spine.

fluoroscopy, and stimulation. Ultrasound is a rapid confirmation technique that does not expose the child to radiation. It is limited to infants under 6 months of age due to the technical difficulty in visualization as the spinous processes begin to ossify. **Fluoroscopy** can identify the catheter as it is placed, assuming the catheter is radiopaque or has a stylet. A small amount of neuro-compatible radiocontrast can be used to confirm placement after the stylet is removed. Patient exposure to radiation and availability of a portable image intensifier are limitations to this approach. Lastly, stimulating catheters can be used to create somatic movement corresponding to the dermatomal level traversed by the catheter as it is threaded. Extremely low-current requirements suggest intrathecal placement as a secondary safety monitor.

Radiographs can confirm placement, but one has to use neuro-safe radiocontrast to confirm placement. Also, a radiopaque catheter or a stylet can help with confirmation without the use of dye. Radiographs can lead to delays, especially if placement is incorrect and requires readjustment and repeat confirmation.

SUMMARY

1. Both lumbar (modified Taylor approach) and caudal approaches are viable routes for placing epidural catheters at the thoracic level in babies.
2. Monitoring of epidural infusions in infants differs in the need to watch for delayed local anesthetic toxicity.
3. Confirmation of catheter placement is best done in real time, using either fluoroscopy, stimulation, or ultrasound.

ANNOTATED REFERENCES

- Bösenberg AT, Bland BA, Schulte-Steinberg O, Downing JW. Thoracic epidural anesthesia via caudal route in infants. *Anesthesiology* 1988; 69: 265–269.

  This is a landmark article in which the author demonstrates this technique.

- Bösenberg AT. Epidural analgesia for major neonatal surgery. *Paediatric Anaesthesia* 1998; 8:479–483.

  Bösenberg demonstrates that better postoperative respiratory function by way of epidurals leads to better surgical outcomes. His impetus for providing neuraxial analgesia was the lack of ventilators for his patients.

- Valairucha S, Seefelder C, Houck C. Thoracic epidural catheters placed by the caudal route in infants: the importance of radiographic confirmation. *Paediatr Anaesth* 2002; 12: 424–428.

This report shows the large error rate in placement of these catheters, explaining the need to confirm the position of the catheter.

Further Reading

Anand K. Pharmacological approaches to the management of pain in the neonatal intensive care unit. *J Perinatol* 2007; 27: S4–S11.

Flandin-Blety C, Barrier G. Accidents following extradural analgesia in children. The results of a retrospective study. *Paediatr Anaesth* 1995; 5(1): 41–46.

Gunter JB. Thoracic epidural anesthesia via the modified Taylor approach in infants. *Reg Anesth Pain Med* 2000; 25(6): 561–565.

Guruswamy V, Roberts S, Arnold P, Potter F. Anaesthetic management of a neonate with congenital cyst adenoid malformation. *Br J Anaesth* 2005; 95(2): 240–242.

Kuhnert BR, Kuhnert PM, Philipson EH, Syracuse CD, Kaine CJ, Yun CH. The half-life of 2-chloroprocaine. *Anesth Analg* 1986; 65(3): 273–278.

Tobias JD, Rasmussen GE, Holcomb GW 3rd, Brock JW 3rd, Morgan WM 3rd. Continuous caudal anaesthesia with chloroprocaine as an adjunct to general anaesthesia in neonates. *Can J Anaesth* 1996; 43(1): 69–72.

Tsui BC, Wagner A, Cave D, Kearney R. Thoracic and lumbar epidural analgesia via the caudal approach using electrical stimulation guidance in pediatric patients: a review of 289 patients. *Anesthesiology* 2004; 100(3): 683–689.

Willschke H, Bosenberg A, Marhofer P, Willschke J, Schwindt J, Weintraud M, Kapral S, Kettner S. Epidural catheter placement in neonates: Sonoanatomy and feasibility of ultrasonographic guidance in term and preterm neonates. *Reg Anesth Pain Med* 2007; 32(1): 34–40.

Acute Pain Management

JASON CHOU AND GEORGE CHALKIADIS

INTRODUCTION

Age-appropriate pain assessment and management is vital in the care of children with acute pain. Assessment should happen regularly and should be documented clearly; pain should be treated and routinely reassessed. There are both short- and long-term consequences if pain is poorly treated in the acute and postoperative setting. The most effective analgesia plans are multimodal. This chapter focuses on systemic treatments of pain in the acute setting.

LEARNING OBJECTIVES

1. **Know some age-appropriate pain assessment tools for children.**
2. **Know the basics of age-appropriate pain management in children.**
3. **Understand the role of opioids, nonsteroidal anti-inflammatory drugs, and patient-controlled analgesia in acute and postoperative pain management in children.**

CASE PRESENTATION

A healthy 7-year-old boy weighing 25 kg fell off the top bunk while wrestling with his brother in the bedroom. He sustained a right-sided tibial injury. He is brought to the emergency department by his anxious parents in a distraught state. He is complaining of severe pain in his leg. Acutely, his pain is managed in the triage area with 35 μg **intranasal fentanyl** *while local anesthetic cream is applied to the dorsum of his hand. An x-ray confirms the diagnosis of a comminuted tibial fracture and need for operative treatment. After 10 minutes his* **pain is assessed** *again and a further dose of fentanyl is given.*

During the open reduction and internal fixation of the fracture, the surgeon asks about the postoperative analgesia plan and frowns at the mention of using a patient-controlled analgesia pump **(PCA)** *postoperatively. He is worried that opioids will mask any* **compartment syndrome***. He also asks that no nonsteroidal anti-inflammatory drugs* **(NSAIDs)** *be given or prescribed.*

DISCUSSION

1. **How can one assess the child's pain in the emergency department, in the post-anesthesia care unit, and on the ward?**

Good **pain assessment** allows the early recognition of pain and its effective treatment. It should involve the use of an age- and context-appropriate pain intensity measurement tool in the setting of a clinical interview with the child and/or parent/guardian as well as a physical examination. Three fundamental approaches exist in pain assessment in children: self-report, observational/behavioral, and physiological. Verbal self-report is the "gold standard" in pain measurement and should be used whenever possible. Children's understanding of pain and their ability to describe it changes with age and cognitive ability and is affected by a range of social and cultural factors and other biases. Scales for self-report of pain must therefore be appropriate for the child's age and developmental stage. Assessment should be both regularly and uniformly performed by all staff involved in the child's care.

Self-report of pain is usually possible by the age of 4, and beyond this age children can begin to differentiate "more," "less," or "the same" and can use an image-based, self-report tool such as the OUCHER or Faces Pain Scale (Fig. 59.1). For patients unable to self-report, tools such as the Faces Legs Arms Cry and Consolability (FLACC) scale or Children's Hospital of Eastern Ontario Pain Scale (CHEOPS) can be used. Over 8 years of age, a 0-to-100 visual analog scale or 0-to-10 numeric rating scale may be used.

2. What are effective ways to manage pain acutely in the emergency department?

In children with suspected fractures, opioids are increasingly being given at triage in order to provide timely administration of analgesia. Having an x-ray, rather than examination or casting, is often identified as the most painful period. To avoid the slower onset of the oral route and the distress associated with obtaining IV access or IM injections, intranasal (IN) opioid delivery is increasingly popular. **IN administration of fentanyl** provides comparable analgesia to parenteral morphine with a similar side-effect profile (Borland et al., 2007). Higher doses are required due to the lower bioavailability of the IN route. IN **fentanyl** can be used as an initial analgesic in children in moderate to severe pain

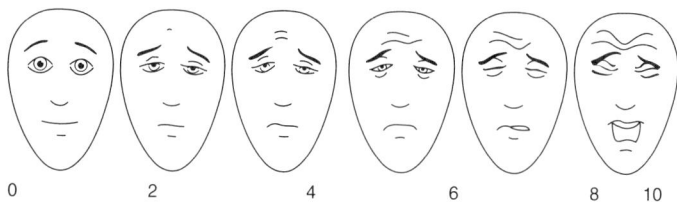

FIGURE 59.1 Faces Pain Scale-Revised (numbers are not shown to the child).
HICKS CL, von Baeyer CL, Spafford P, et al. Faces Pain Scale-Revised: toward a common metric in pediatric pain measurement. *Pain* 2001; 93: 173–183. This Faces Pain Scale-Revised has been reproduced with permission of the International Association for the Study of Pain® (IASP®). The figure may not be reproduced for any other purpose without permission.

or during painful procedures prior to the establishment of IV access. Contraindications include bilateral occluded nasal passages or epistaxis. **Fentanyl** is delivered via a mucosal atomization device (although it can be dripped in, if no such device is available); the dose is divided between each nostril. IN **fentanyl** has a time to onset of action of between 3 and 15 minutes. Therefore, a second dose can be given 10 minutes later. Thereafter, if further analgesia is required, an alternative form and/or route of analgesia needs to be considered. In some countries methoxyflurane 0.2% to 0.7% can also be used and is available as a self-administered inhaler. It reduces pain in children with extremity injuries, but side effects are common and include sedation and vomiting.

IV cannulation can cause significant distress in children. Topical local anesthetic (LA) reduces the pain and anxiety associated with IV cannulation, and amethocaine is more effective than a eutectic mixture of local anesthetics (EMLA®), with a more rapid onset. Even more rapid onset can be attained using lidocaine (lignocaine) iontophoresis or delivery devices that use compressed helium to drive lyophilized lidocaine subcutaneously. Similarly, nitrous oxide (N_2O) also reduces pain and anxiety but has an associated risk of nausea and vomiting. Combining topical LA and N_2O is more effective than either method alone (Hee et al., 2003).

Important nonpharmacological strategies such as distraction, careful positioning, and holding by a parent can reduce pain and anxiety in older children and lower parental perception of distress in younger children.

3. What are options for postoperative analgesia?
IV opioid infusions are safe and effective in the management of postoperative pain in children of all ages. **PCA** can be used in children as young as 5 but requires careful patient selection, patient and parent education, and the availability of suitable equipment and trained staff (including monitoring and acute pain service support). Compared with continuous IV opioid infusions, **PCA**

provides similar efficacy and greater dosing flexibility but is associated with higher opioid consumption and a higher incidence of pruritus (but no difference in other opioid-related side effects). Morphine is the **PCA** opioid of choice. Hydromorphone is an effective alternative when side effects limit the use of morphine, and fentanyl is the alternative opioid of choice in those with renal impairment (or morphine-related side effects). Nausea and vomiting is common (30–45%) and prophylactic antiemetics (e.g., ondansetron or promethazine) should be prescribed. Pruritus is best treated with low-dose IV naloxone, a change of opioid, or addition of a mixed agonist–antagonist, such as butorphanol or nalbuphine.

Acetaminophen (paracetamol) is an effective analgesic that is well tolerated and should therefore be prescribed routinely and regularly postoperatively. Another advantage is that it is available in the IV formulation, which is helpful for patients who are not yet ready for oral medications or who are vomiting postoperatively.

Tramadol is another effective analgesic for postoperative pain. Side effects are similar to opioids (e.g., nausea and vomiting, sedation, and dizziness) with less constipation and pruritus and a low risk of respiratory depression.

4. Does PCA mask the diagnosis of the development of compartment syndrome?

There has been sporadic concern that the use of **PCA** to treat increasing pain can mask the diagnosis of compartment syndrome. Pain is the most reliable (and earliest) symptom of compartment syndrome and should be assessed at rest and with passive movement of the muscles in the affected compartment. The diagnosis can be made more difficult if the child lacks the cognitive or verbal ability to provide meaningful information or localize symptoms.

The current consensus is that it is fortunately very rare for surgical complications to be masked by analgesia. Providing effective analgesia should not increase the risk of missing compartment syndrome as long as regular monitoring and clinical examination with a high vigilance for compartment syndrome is carried out to detect the changes in pain scores and analgesic requirements that are early and sensitive indicators of this condition (Yang & Cooper, 2010). In children at risk of developing compartment syndrome, inadequate analgesia or escalating opioid consumption should immediately trigger orthopedic review to exclude this potentially devastating complication.

5. What is the role of NSAIDs in postoperative analgesia? Do NSAIDs impair bone fusion?

As a component of multimodal analgesia, **NSAIDs** improve analgesia and decrease opioid consumption, especially when combined with acetaminophen. Side effects following short-term use are similar to that of acetaminophen, but **NSAIDs** should be avoided in children with severe asthma and in infants less than 3 months of age.

Evidence for an effect on bone fusion is conflicting, and its clinical significance is unknown. There is animal-model evidence of unknown relevance in humans. The evidence comes from retrospective studies looking at high-dose ketorolac following spinal fusion that have reached different conclusions, and so far there is no evidence from randomized controlled trials or prospective trials. One retrospective study in children found no effect on postoperative complications after fracture repair (Kay et al., 2010). Ketorolac is often seen as the culprit, but it is hardly representative of **NSAIDs** as a class, especially at the high doses given parenterally. **NSAIDs** are, however, effective in reducing the complication of postoperative heterotopic bone formation. They do not affect the risk of refracture in any significant way.

SUMMARY

1. **Age- and context-appropriate pain assessment and measurement, performed regularly, are important components of pain management in children.**

2. Opioids are important analgesics in acute, procedural, and postoperative pain. Multimodal analgesia leads to reduced opioid requirements, better analgesia, and fewer side effects. Nonpharmacological methods should also be incorporated.

3. PCAs provide effective postoperative analgesia. Regular monitoring and clinical examination with a high vigilance for compartment syndrome will allow early identification of this serious complication.

4. There is no good-quality evidence that NSAIDs impair bone fusion in humans, and the analgesic benefits of short-term NSAIDs outweigh this hypothetical risk.

ANNOTATED REFERENCES

- Howard R, Carter B, Curry J, Morton N, Rivett K, Rose M, Tyrrell J, Walker S, Williams G; Association of Paediatric Anaesthetists of Great Britain and Ireland. Special issue: good practice in postoperative and procedural pain management. *Pediatr Anesth* 2008; 18 Suppl 1: 1–81.

  Evidence-based article with recommendations on what constitutes good practice. Section 3, "Pain Assessment," and Section 5, "Postoperative Pain," are particularly pertinent.

- Macintyre PE, Schug SA, Scott DA, Visser EJ, Walker SM; APM: SE Working Group of the Australian and New Zealand College of Anaesthetists and Faculty of Pain Medicine. *Acute Pain Management: Scientific Evidence,* 3rd ed. Melbourne: ANZCA & FPM, 2010.

  Definitive evidence-based book on acute pain management. Chapter 10 is dedicated to the assessment and management of acute pain in all settings in the pediatric patient.

Further Reading

Babl FE, Jamison SR, Spicer M, Bernard S. Inhaled methoxyflurane as a prehospital analgesic in children. *Emerg Med Austral* 2006; 18(4): 404–410.

Borland M, Jacobs I, King B, O'Brien, D. A randomized controlled trial comparing intranasal fentanyl to intravenous morphine for managing acute pain in children in the emergency department. *Ann Emerg Med* 2007; 49(3): 335–340.

Bozkurt P. Use of tramadol in children. *Pediatr Anesth* 2005; 15(12): 1041–1047.

Hee HI, Goy RW, Ng AS. Effective reduction of anxiety and pain during venous cannulation in children: a comparison of analgesic efficacy conferred by nitrous oxide, EMLA and combination. *Paediatr Anaesth* 2003; 13(3): 210–216.

Hicks CL, von Baeyer CL, Spafford PA, van Korlaar I, Goodenough B. The Faces Pain Scale-Revised: toward a common metric in pediatric pain measurement. *Pain* 2001; 93(2): 173–183.

Kay RM, Directo MP, Leathers M, Myung K, Skaggs DL. Complications of ketorolac use in children undergoing operative fracture care. *J Pediatr Orthop* 2010; 30(7): 655–658.

Lejus C. What does analgesia mask? *Pediatr Anesth* 2004; 14: 622–624.

Yang J, Cooper MG. Compartment syndrome and patient-controlled analgesia in children: analgesic complication or early warning system? *Anaesth Intens Care* 2010; 38: 359–363.

60

Peripheral Nerve Block Catheter for Extremity Surgery

ELIZABETH PRENTICE

INTRODUCTION

Continuous peripheral nerve blockade (CPNB) can provide excellent postoperative analgesia. Many adult studies report the effectiveness of CPNB. Although not as widely adopted in pediatrics, several studies support its use. Its niche lies in provision of analgesia after major unilateral limb surgery with severe postoperative pain expected for 48 to 72 hours. Lower limb surgery of this type is more common than upper limb in the pediatric population. Examples include club foot repair, osteotomy, or resection of sarcoma. This chapter presents two cases where CPNB is a good option for postoperative analgesia.

> ## LEARNING OBJECTIVES
>
> 1. Recall the anatomy and techniques for sciatic and infraclavicular blocks.
> 2. Evaluate the indications and contraindications for sciatic and infraclavicular blocks.
> 3. Review the safe management of peripheral nerve catheters in a child.

CASE PRESENTATION 1: LOWER LIMB CPNB

*A 28-kg, 5-year-old boy presents for a **re-do unilateral club foot repair**. He has a history of **obstructive sleep apnea (OSA)**, which only partially improved after a previous adenotonsillectomy; his sleep study still indicates mild to moderate desaturations to the mid 80s. He uses a nocturnal CPAP machine at 5 cmH$_2$O. After his previous operations, he had delayed emergence. He seemed to be very **sensitive to the sedative effects of morphine**. The planned surgery will involve bilateral incisions on the foot with significant bony work. On examination, he is clinically obese (height 114 cm, BMI 21.5) but is otherwise normal. His mother requests that an epidural be avoided, as she had a complicated labor epidural. After induction of general anesthesia, a sciatic nerve block catheter is inserted at the mid-thigh level under ultrasound guidance. A bolus of 10 mL of 0.5% ropivacaine is given and **an infusion of 0.2% ropivacaine** is started and continued at 4 mL/hr for 2 days postoperatively. The block provides excellent analgesia apart from mild pain on day 1 on the medial side of the foot. Oral acetaminophen and tramadol are continued after cessation of the CPNB.*

CASE PRESENTATION 2: UPPER LIMB CPNB

*A 54-kg, 15-year-old boy presents with a painful mass in the left arm. A destructive **osteosarcoma** has been diagnosed in the **proximal humerus**. A staging workup and a biopsy have been performed. He has started adjuvant chemotherapy. A wide surgical resection and reconstruction with a metallic prosthesis is planned as a single-stage procedure. He was nauseated for 12 hours after his previous biopsy. His father had a femoral CPNB for a total knee reconstruction and wonders if a similar technique is possible for his son. The incision will extend from below the deltoid to just proximal to the elbow. After an IV induction, an arterial line is inserted and an **ultrasound-guided infraclavicular brachial plexus block** is performed using 0.2 mL/kg*

*(11 mL) of 0.5% ropivacaine. A brachial plexus catheter is left in situ and a **0.2% ropivacaine** infusion is started intraoperatively and continued postoperatively at 7 mL/hr. The result was excellent analgesia. A trial of cessation of the infusion after 48 hours brings severe pain, uncontrolled by oral acetaminophen (paracetamol) and oxycodone. A bolus of ropivacaine is given and the infusion is continued for another 48 hours.*

DISCUSSION

1. What are the options for postoperative pain relief for Case 1?
The mainstay of analgesia will be either intravenous opioid or a regional technique for the first few postoperative days. Supplemental analgesia such as acetaminophen and tramadol would also be appropriate. NSAIDs are often avoided due to concern regarding effects on delayed bone healing.

Opioid infusion: Opioid side effects include postoperative nausea and vomiting, drowsiness, and respiratory depression, which increase patient morbidity and nursing care and can delay physiotherapy. This patient is at higher risk of experiencing the respiratory depressant effects given his significant **OSA** history, and he may require care in a high-acuity observation unit. If a morphine infusion is used, a reduced dose may be necessary; a ketamine infusion may also be used as an opioid-sparing agent. A patient above the age of 7 is often able to use patient-controlled analgesia (PCA).

Epidural catheter: Although bilateral multilevel lower limb surgery involving osteotomies often warrants continuous epidural blockade (CEB), the risk–benefit analysis can be less clear for unilateral surgery. In addition to the potential neuraxial complications, bilateral block is unnecessary and the associated urinary retention (20% incidence) will require a urinary catheter. The mother wished to avoid an epidural in this case.

Single-shot peripheral nerve block (SIPNB): Given the limited duration of analgesia (8–12 hours), abrupt offset of the SIPNB during the first postoperative night may precipitate uncontrolled pain unless alternative opioid-based analgesia (infusion or PCA) has already been established. It therefore will not avoid opioid side effects. SIPNB is a reasonable choice if the pain is expected to be of shorter duration.

CPNB: Peripheral catheters may be indicated as the operation is associated with severe pain lasting for many days. A postoperative compartment syndrome is less likely in this case than in femoral or tibial procedures, but precautions need to be taken to ensure early diagnosis (see Question 2). In addition to the avoidance of opioids, peripheral nerve catheters provide targeted unilateral blockade, which can improve mobilization. CPNB catheters can be connected to a simple, portable, lightweight plastic automated dosage device.

2. What are the surgical concerns to address before choosing CPNB or CEB?

Limb surgery may predispose to compartment syndrome; the concern often cited is that the diagnosis may be delayed in the presence of anesthetic nerve blockade. This is a difficult issue; the importance of pain in the diagnosis of compartment syndrome is controversial. Virtually all analgesic modalities have been linked to a delayed diagnosis of compartment syndrome; however, reports commonly misattribute analgesia as the *cause* rather than *an association* with a delayed diagnosis. Most practitioners would accept that there is no substitute for regular postoperative vigilance. Trained personnel must be in place to look after the catheter on the ward (see Question 8). Communication with the surgeon about the operative details will allow a sensible risk–benefit analysis discussion. Avoiding dense motor block with dilute local anesthetic solution allows for early detection of a problem (Mar et al., 2009).

3. What are the major nerves that ultimately supply sensation to the foot?

Branches of the sciatic and femoral nerves ultimately supply the foot. The femoral nerve has a small medial cutaneous distribution and the majority of the operative territory is covered in Case Presentation 1 by the sciatic nerve.

4. What is the course of the sciatic nerve?

It originates from the lumbosacral plexus (L4-S3) and comprises the tibial and common peroneal nerves enclosed in a common fibrous sheath. It leaves the posterior pelvic wall through the greater sciatic foramen and enters the region of the buttock slightly medial to the halfway point between the ischial tuberosity and the greater trochanter. It then descends vertically down the midline of the back of the leg; the sciatic nerve can divide into its two components at any stage here, but it is more common to divide at the apex of the popliteal fossa. Tibial nerve branches supply the sole of the foot and common peroneal branches supply the dorsum of the foot.

5. What are the three sites to perform an ultrasound-guided sciatic nerve block?

The anesthetized patient is placed in the semiprone "Sims" position with the leg to be blocked uppermost.

Popliteal level: Place a high frequency (>7 MHz) probe transversely just above the midpoint of the popliteal fossa and locate the popliteal artery. At the popliteal level, the nerve will usually have divided into the common peroneal and tibial components. Moving the probe cephalad, the junction of two nerves identifies the sciatic nerve. The nerves lie lateral and posterior (superficial) to the artery. It will be a hyperechoic (white) structure, and fascicles are often visible. *Practical tip:* Use color flow to locate the artery. If the artery is not clearly visible, move the probe laterally or medially to reduce artifact from the tendons around the knee joint.

Mid-thigh level: The sciatic nerve is located between and deep to the muscle bellies of the biceps femoris (laterally) and the semitendinosis and semimembranosis (medially). *Practical tip:* To confirm the structures, rotate the probe 90 degrees to long axis (LAX); the sciatic nerve is seen as a "band" with a tubular appearance.

Subgluteal level: Position the probe transversely at the subgluteal crease between the ischial tuberosity and the greater trochanter. The sciatic nerve is seen as a flat oval or triangular hyperechoic structure lying lateral to the long head of biceps (Figs. 60.1 and 60.2).

6. How should the needle be oriented in relation to the ultrasound probe?

The ultrasound probe is placed with the long axis in the transverse plane, giving a short axis (SAX) view of the sciatic nerve. The needle is advanced in-plane (IP) from the lateral side of the ultrasound probe and advanced medially towards the nerve. For anesthesiologists used to the landmark technique, a "needle out of plane" (OOP) approach would potentially seem more intuitive,

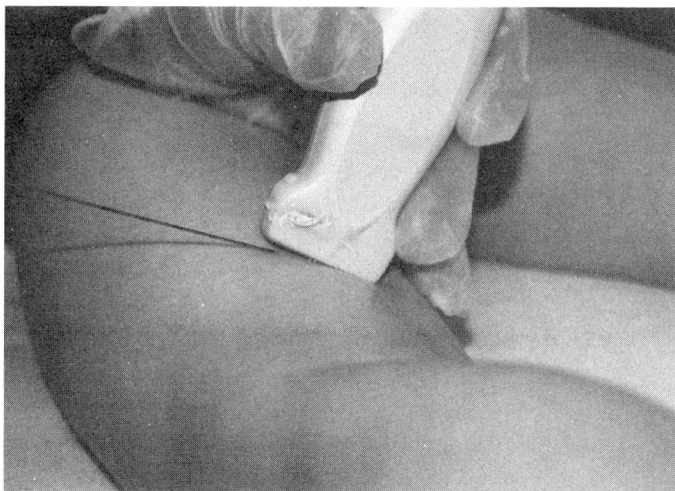

FIGURE 60.1 Needle and ultrasound probe position for mid-thigh approach to sciatic nerve blockade.

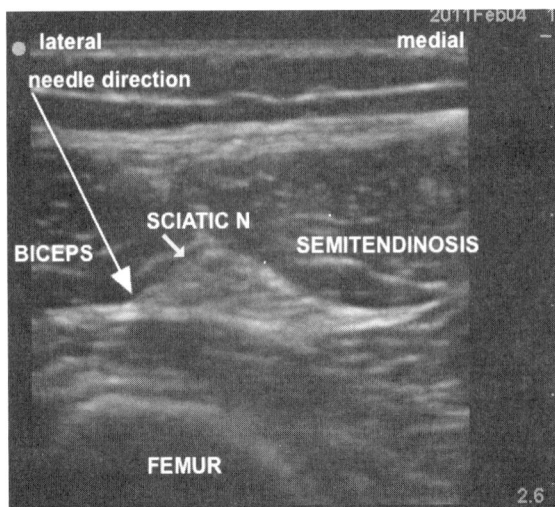

FIGURE 60.2 Ultrasound image of mid-thigh approach to sciatic nerve blockade.

but the IP approach with ultrasound allows continuous observation of the needle. It also allows easier visualization of the catheter tip and provides a longer subcutaneous tract to anchor the catheter.

7. What are the practicalities of inserting a nerve catheter with an ultrasound?

Three hands are needed: one for the needle, one for the probe, and one for the catheter. The procedure is much easier with an assistant, although it is possible to achieve with one operator, by putting the probe to the side while the catheter is advanced. With a SAX IP approach, the introducer needle is positioned at 90 degrees to the long axis of the nerve, so the catheter should be advanced no more than about 1 cm past the needle tip to avoid migration away from the nerve. If a SAX OOP approach is used, the catheter can be advanced further along the line of the nerve. Commercially available CPNB kits usually contain a 18- or

19-gauge Tuohy-tip needle; these needles are unlikely to pierce a nerve and are highly visible on ultrasound. A standard epidural kit can also be used, although the CPNB catheters have multiperforated ends for better local anesthetic distribution.

8. What local anesthetic and what volumes are you going to use?

Levobupivacaine and ropivacaine are commonly used. The **initial bolus** volume should be around 0.3 mL/kg to ensure good spread around the nerves. For example, for a 28-kg child having a single-shot block, 0.3 mL/kg of 0.5% (total 0.3 × 5 = 39 mg = 1.5 mg/kg) levobupivacaine could be given. If direct visualization of spread with ultrasound is possible, the volume may be reduced if desired. The usual bolus maximum safe dose for levobupivacaine and ropivacaine is 2.5 mg/kg. For **infusions**, 0.1 to 0.2 mL/kg/hr of a 0.125% levobupivacaine or 0.2% ropivacaine solution produces good analgesia while avoiding a dense motor block; voluntary limb movement is important to avoid pressure areas and for postoperative assessment.

9. Why was an infraclavicular block chosen for Case 2? How is it performed?

The infraclavicular site is anatomically a good location for a catheter; it provides reliable blockade of the surgical site, and the deeper location of the plexus means the catheter is securely buried before exiting comfortably on the chest wall below the clavicle. In contrast to the interscalene block, phrenic nerve blockade is avoided.

Infraclavicular block is performed with the child in a supine position with the affected arm alongside the body using full barrier precautions. A 10-MHz linear probe is placed just medial to the coracoid and below the clavicle in a sagittal plane. This point is approximately halfway between the shoulder tip and the suprasternal notch. The three cords of the brachial plexus appear as hyperechoic round structures; they are located around the **subclavian artery**: posterior cord deep, lateral cord to the clavicular side, and medial cord between the artery and vein. Posterior and caudal to the vessels the pleura can be seen. An 18-gauge 80-mm Tuohy-tip needle is inserted and positioned posterior to the subclavian artery, avoiding the posterior cord. After negative aspiration, 0.2 mL/kg of 0.5% ropivacaine is injected. A horseshoe-like pattern of local anesthetic is seen. A 20-gauge catheter is threaded approximately 15 mm past the end of the needle. A further 0.1 mL/kg of 0.5% ropivacaine is injected through the catheter to confirm location. The needle is removed and the catheter is taped into position.

10. How should any nerve catheter be monitored on the ward?

Nursing staff need to be trained in looking after patients with a CPNC. *Regular assessment* and documentation of analgesic *efficacy*, degree of *motor blockade*, and local anesthetic side effects (vital signs) is imperative. The infusion needs to be checked for incorrect administration and drug errors. The catheter site is *inspected* for signs of *catheter dislodgement, leakage,* or *infection.* The limb needs to be regularly assessed for *swelling* and *neurovascular compromise.* Clear guidance is required for adverse event management and triggers for medical review.

SUMMARY

1. Many consider CPNB to be the gold standard in providing postoperative analgesia for painful unilateral limb surgery; however, a careful risk–benefit analysis is required before insertion.
2. Nursing staff need to be properly trained in assessing children with CPNB.
3. Ultrasound improves the reliability of successful blockade. It also reduces the volume of local anesthetic required.

ANNOTATED REFERENCES

- Lonnqvist PA. Is ultrasound guidance mandatory when performing pediatric regional anesthesia? *Curr Opin Anesthesiol* 2010; 23(3): 337–341.
  Very good review appraising the use of ultrasound for regional blocks in children.
- Rochette A, Dadure C, Raux O, Capdevila X. Changing trends in pediatric regional anesthetic practice in recent years. *Curr Opin Anesthesiol* 2009; 22(3): 374–377.
  Good overview of this rapidly changing subspecialty.
- Rochette A, Dadure C, Raux O, Capdevila X. Continuous epidural block versus continuous popliteal nerve block for postoperative pain relief after major podiatric surgery in children: a prospective, comparative randomized study. *Anesth Analg* 2006; 102: 744–749.
  Good practical descriptions of the blocks covered in this chapter.

Further Reading

Dadure CS, Bringuier S, Raux O, Rochette A, Troncin R, Canaud N, Lubrano-Lavadera JF, Capdevila X. Continuous peripheral nerve blocks for postoperative analgesia in children: feasibility and side effects in a cohort study of 339 catheters. *Can J Anesth* 2009; 56(11): 843–850.

Gonano C, Kettner SC, Ernstbrunner M, Schebesta K, Chiari A, Marhofer P. Comparison of economical aspects of interscalene brachial plexus blockade and general anaesthesia for arthroscopic shoulder surgery. *Br J Anaesth* 2009; 103(3): 428–433.

Mar GJ, Barrington MJ, McGuirk BR. Acute compartment syndrome of the lower limb and the effect of postoperative analgesia on diagnosis. *Br J Anaesth* 2009; 102(1): 3–11.

Oberndorfer UP, Marhofer P, Bosenberg A, Willschke H, Felfernig M, Weintraud M, Kapral S, Kettner SC. Ultrasonographic guidance for sciatic and femoral nerve blocks in children. *Br J Anaesth* 2007; 98(6): 797–801.

van Geffen GJ, Gielen M. Ultrasound-guided subgluteal sciatic nerve blocks with stimulating catheters in children: a descriptive study. *Anesth Analg* 2006; 103(2): 328–333.

Complex Regional Pain Syndrome in the Emergency Department

GILLIAN R. LAUDER

INTRODUCTION

Acute exacerbation of an ongoing chronic pain can be a diagnostic and clinical dilemma. Chronic pain in children requires an interdisciplinary approach to assessment and treatment. Further, the child must commit to taking an active role in therapy. When this approach is not working, or there is an acute trauma to the affected region, children with chronic pain may present to the emergency department with extreme pain. Acute care health professionals may find themselves unable to modify the pain intensity with standard analgesic medications. The analgesic approach requires careful clinical management and liaison with the chronic pain team supervising the ongoing management of pain.

LEARNING OBJECTIVES

1. Understand that chronic pain is a biopsychosocial problem and needs to be managed with an interdisciplinary approach.
2. Identify key features from the history and examination that determine the nature of the acute exacerbation of pain.

3. **To understand therapeutic options for the ED setting while awaiting follow-up with the chronic pain team.**

CASE PRESENTATION

*Samantha is a 12-year-old, 35-kg girl with a history of left foot **complex regional pain syndrome (CRPS)**. She presents to the emergency department with excruciating (9/10) pain in her left foot. Samantha reports hitting her foot on the dining-room table this evening, which caused an immediate and intense increase in her left foot pain. Her CRPS began 3 months previously: after a minor twist of her ankle during gymnastic practice, she suddenly developed pain in the heel of her left foot. The pain progressed over 2 days to the point she was unable to bear weight; her foot developed purple mottling and felt cold. No inflammatory, orthopedic, thrombotic, or neurologic etiology was found. The bone scan demonstrated delayed uptake in her left foot and the MRI showed increased fluid content of the marrow of the left hind foot. Her physician prescribed gabapentin 100 mg TID, which was increased over 3 days to 200 mg TID. She has used crutches to ambulate since, and had only simple analgesics at home to use. Samantha has been unable to bear weight, undergo the prescribed physiotherapy, or attend school due to tiredness and pain. Simple analgesics have been ineffective, while codeine and tramadol caused nausea and retching. Gabapentin improved the pain initially, but this effect diminished. She is on no other medication and has no past medical history.*

The current heel pain is a constant burning sensation, associated with shooting pains up to her knee; these are variable in intensity and associated with color and temperature changes. The pain is aggravated with light touch (such as putting on a sock), weight bearing, and leaving the foot in a dependent position. There are no other relieving factors. Her pain is worse at night and sleep is difficult due to pain from the touch of blankets and the recurrent shooting pains.

Samantha's appetite, drive, energy, affect, and eating behavior are normal. On examination, Samantha is pleasant and interactive. She is afebrile, with normal vital signs. There is no bruising, laceration, or swelling; however, her foot becomes mottled when hanging in a dependent position. Her distal left leg is slightly cooler than her right, and there is intense pain to light touch on the heel of the left foot, which limits examination. When ambulating, she is able to put pressure on the anterior half of her left foot but not her heel. X-ray of her foot is normal. Samantha is given IV ketorolac 18 mg, oral acetaminophen (paracetamol) (500 mg), and oral clonidine (40 mcg) with moderate effect after 30 minutes. Following a discussion with the chronic pain management team (**CPMT**), she is given an outpatient pain clinic appointment in 1 week, where she will see an **interdisciplinary team** comprising a **physical therapist**, a **psychologist**, and a pain physician and nurse. Her discharge medications are gabapentin 300 mg TID (TDS), amitriptyline 10 mg at bedtime, melatonin 3 mg at bedtime, and once-daily topical 5% lidocaine patches.

DISCUSSION

1. What is CRPS?

CRPS is an unusual condition where pathophysiological changes within the peripheral and central nervous system result in severe pain. The pain is often associated with allodynia (pain from a stimulus that is not normally painful), hyperalgesia (greater-than-normal sensitivity to a painful stimulus or a lowered pain threshold), abnormal sudomotor activity, and changes in the nails, bones, and hair of the affected painful part. However, between patients signs vary, and in individual patients signs vary with time. Specific diagnostic criteria are now well established (Harden et al., 2007). In children **CRPS** may occur as the result of injury, but often there is no predisposing event. The pain of **CRPS** is of neuropathic nature (shooting/burning character) and often does not respond to medications targeted to nociceptive or inflammatory types of pain. The pain is out of proportion to the inciting event. **CRPS** is a diagnosis that should be made only when other conditions that could account for the degree of pain and dysfunction have been excluded.

2. What is the long-term management strategy for CRPS?

Ideally, CRPS, and chronic pain, should be treated by an **interdisciplinary team** that should include the child and family, the family physician, a physiotherapist, a psychologist, a pain physician, a pain nurse, a pharmacist, and an occupational therapist. The interdisciplinary team promotes a self-management approach, allowing children to take control of their symptoms and improve day-to-day biopsychosocial functioning (i.e., a functional rehabilitation approach that focuses on sleep, eating, physical activity, mood, and social and school function). The pain and the consequences of pain, such as poor sleep or anxiety, are managed using a combination of concurrent therapies (Fig. 61.1). These include paced physical activity, psychological support, and psychological therapies used in conjunction with medical interventions (medications or interventional blocks). The principal modality that will improve pain and function in children with CRPS is physical therapies. Key to success is early appropriate intervention, education for the child and family (Lauder & Massey, 2010), and good communication between team members. The interdisciplinary approach has been shown to be effective for pediatric chronic pain (Eccleston et al., 2003; Lee et al., 2002; Maynard et al., 2010; Sherry et al., 1999).

What is appropriate for individual children will depend on findings from the history and examination as well as the expertise of the pain team (Berde & Lebel, 2005). It is important to keep things as simple as possible and to change any treatment modalities in a step-by-step fashion. Improvement may take weeks or months; some children will make a full recovery; others will achieve return to function with ongoing pain; others will progress to adult life with ongoing complex pain problems. The ED is

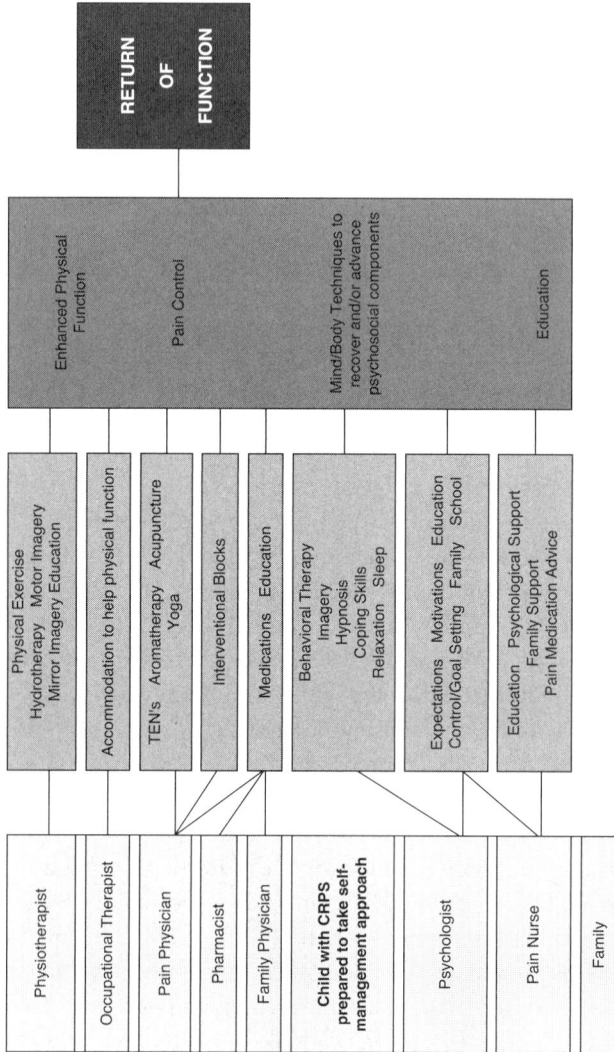

FIGURE 61.1 Biopsychosocial model of pain management, emphasizing return to function.

therefore not the correct environment to try to make any progress with appropriate therapy due to the complex nature of the condition and the time required to institute change.

3. What are the main issues for consideration in the ED?

A thorough history and examination should be performed to *confirm the diagnosis* of CRPS and *exclude an acute remediable cause* for the exacerbation of pain. During this evaluation, *acknowledge and believe* that the child has pain. Determine the factors, other than pain, that have most impact in the child's life, including altered mood or poor sleep, to plan appropriate discharge medications. Use a calm approach and explain to the child and family why severe pain continues after 3 months. Be careful to ensure that the language you use does not demean the child or convey a stigmatizing message. Outline the **interdisciplinary approach** to management of this condition. Explain that **physiotherapy** is the *principal therapy* that will improve function in the painful area. Clarify that the purpose of medications is to provide some analgesia to facilitate the initiation and maintenance of physiotherapy and not to provide a complete pain-free state. Medications used must be tailored to individual patients. A multimodal approach using simple medications first is a suitable approach. Organize follow-up for the child so that long-term interdisciplinary management can be instituted by a **CPMT**. Wherever possible avoid "medicalization" and admission. In an extremely busy ED this may not be possible, and a brief admission may be needed to provide analgesia and develop a therapeutic plan.

4. Should an interventional block be performed in the ED?

Interventional blocks should not be used as a "magic wand" to minimize pain but as a means to facilitate paced **physical therapies** and improve function. The ED is not the arena for that purpose. CRPS pathophysiology exists within the peripheral and central nervous system, so nerve blocks that target only the periphery and/or the spinal cord may not be effective in the relief of pain. Where sympathetically mediated and/or maintained

Table 61.1

PHARMACOLOGICAL OPTIONS FOR CHILDREN WITH CRPS

Drug	Characteristics
Gabapentin	*Action*: Binds the alpha-2-delta subunit of the voltage-dependent calcium channel in the CNS *Metabolism:* None; renal excretion *Drug Interactions*: None; no effect on hepatic microsomal enzymes *Side effects*: Somnolence, dizziness, peripheral edema, weight gain and mood swings (including suicidal ideation) *Comment*: Has a withdrawal syndrome; should be weaned off
Pregabalin	*Action, Metabolism, Drug Interactions, Side effects, Withdrawal syndrome*: As per gabapentin *Dosing*: Either BID or TID *Comment*: Can be titrated more rapidly than gabapentin
Amitriptyline	*Action*: Prevents the reuptake of serotonin and norepinephrine *Metabolism*: Hepatic, subject to genetic variance in enzymatic function *Drug interactions*: Multiple, especially inhibitors of CYP 2D6 (e.g., SSRIs) and those that prolong cardiac QTc interval *Side effects*: Sedation, dry mouth, blurred vision, weight gain, orthostatic hypotension, and prolonged QTc *Comment*: An ECG should be strongly considered before starting TCA therapy. Nortriptyline is less sedating, doxepin less anticholinergic. Should be weaned off.
Topical lidocaine 5% patch	*Action*: Blockade of upregulated sodium channel receptors in injured nerves *Metabolism*: NA, absorption negligible *Drug interactions*: NA, absorption negligible *Side effects*: Mild skin reactions *Comment*: Useful for very localized CRPS pain

(*continued*)

Table 61.1 (*continued*)

Drug	Characteristics
Tramadol	*Action*: Weak μ opioid receptor agonist. Also inhibits spinal cord release of serotonin and reuptake of norepinephrine. *Metabolism*: A pro-drug. Dependent on hepatic microsomal system: hence, interindividual, pharmacogenetic variability. *Drug interactions*: Multiple, especially inhibitors of hepatic P450 systems and serotonin uptake inhibitors *Side effects*: Nausea and vomiting *Comment*: Serotonin toxicity possible, especially if co-administered with SSRIs, SNRIs, MAOIs, or TCAs. Dose reduction is advised with renal impairment.
Opioids	*Action*: Mu-antagonist primarily *Metabolism*: Hepatic *Drug interactions*: Additive with sedating medications, alcohol *Side effects*: Sedation, nausea, constipation, pruritus *Comment*: Can help with doing physiotherapy. Long-term use rarely indicated.
Clonidine	*Action*: Selective α2 adrenoceptor agonist with analgesic, sedative, anxiolytic, and cardiovascular effects *Metabolism*: Hepatic and renal (roughly 50:50) *Drug interactions*: Beta blockers, tricyclic antidepressants *Side effects*: Sedation, dry mouth, hypotension *Comment*: A useful adjunct; can be used as an opioid-sparing agent

Note: Combined therapy with gabapentin/pregabalin and a TCA seems to be more efficacious than either modality given alone.

pain is evident, it may be appropriate to perform a sympathetic block. However, the ED is not the place to perform a block that requires certain expertise, preparation, equipment, and follow-up. If thought useful, referral for a sympathetic or other block can be made to a physician expert in the technique in children.

5. What are options for pharmacological treatments that could begin in the ED?

ED medications are administered to provide enough comfort to enable discharge and prevent recurrent ED attendance or hospital admission. Unfortunately, there is very little published evidence to support specific pharmacological therapies in children with CRPS. Recommendations are governed by adult studies, pediatric case reports, expert opinion, and the experience and expertise of the pain physician/team dealing with the child (Berde & Lebel, 2005). Simple medications and opioids may be useful if there is an inflammatory or traumatic element to the acute exacerbation of pain but may not be effective for CRPS pain. Table 61.1 reviews a number of medications used for CRPS treatment in children that could be started in the ED.

SUMMARY

1. As for all children with complex needs, appropriate care of CRPS requires a careful history and examination.
2. Emergency care in the ED for these patients requires titration of appropriate medication to provide comfort.
3. Patients should be discharged whenever possible, with a plan for appropriate long-term care, including enough medications to help control their symptoms until they can be seen by a CPMT.

ANNOTATED REFERENCES

- Berde CB, Lebel A. Complex regional pain syndromes in children and adolescents. *Anesthesiology* 2005; 102(2): 252–255.

  A good overview on CRPS; includes the differences between the condition in children/adolescents and adults. Also critically appraises the evidence for modalities of treatment, including intravenous regional blockade and continuous nerve blocks.

- Harden RN, Bruehl S, Stanton-Hicks M, Wilson PR. Proposed new diagnostic criteria for complex regional pain syndrome. *Pain Med* 2007; 8: 326–331.

  Clarifies the diagnostic criteria for CRPS.

- Lauder GR, Massey R. *Complex Regional Pain Syndrome (CRPS) Explained. For Teenagers by Teenagers*. Bloomington, IL: Xlibris Publishing, 2010.

  Book recently written for teenagers with CRPS. A good source of education specifically intended for these patients.

Further Reading

Eccleston C, Malleson PN, Clinch J, Connell Sourbut C. Chronic pain in adolescents: evaluation of a program of interdisciplinary cognitive behavior therapy (ICBT). *Arch Dis Child* 2003; 88: 881–885.

Gilron I, Bailey JM, Tu D, Holden RR, Jackson AC, Houlden RL. Nortriptyline and gabapentin, alone and in combination for neuropathic pain: a double-blind, randomised controlled crossover trial. *Lancet* 2009; 374(9697): 1252–1261.

Hoebert M, van der Heijden KB, van Geijlswijk IM, Smits MG. Long-term follow-up of melatonin treatment in children with ADHD and chronic sleep onset insomnia. *J Pineal Res* 2009; 47(1): 1–7.

Khaliq W, Alam S, Puri N. Topical lidocaine for treatment of postherpetic neuralgia, *Cochrane Database Syst Rev* 2007; 18:CD004846.

Lee BH, Scharff L, Sethna NF, et al. Physical therapy and cognitive behavioral treatment for complex regional pain syndromes. *J Pediat* 2002; 140: 135–140.

Maynard CS, Amari A, Wieczorek B, Christensen JR, Slifer KJ. Interdisciplinary behavioral rehabilitation of pediatric pain-associated disability: a retrospective review of an inpatient treatment protocol. *J Pediatr Psychol* 2010; 35(2): 128–137.

Perry TL. *Neurontin: Clinical pharmacologic opinion of Dr. Thomas L. Perry.* Accessed Feb. 10, 2011. http://dida.library.ucsf.edu/pdf/oxx18p10.

Sherry DD, Wallace CA, Kelley C, Kidder M, Sapp L. Short- and long-term outcomes of children with CRPS type 1 treated with exercise therapy. *Clin J Pain* 1999; 15: 218–223.

PART 13

CHALLENGES IN PEDIATRIC

SYNDROMES

62

Down Syndrome

ERICA P. LIN AND JAMES P. SPAETH

INTRODUCTION

Trisomy 21, or Down syndrome, is the most common human chromosomal syndrome, with an overall incidence of 1:700 live births. Because of its association with other congenital anomalies, children with this syndrome often present for surgical procedures that require general anesthesia. Anesthesiologists caring for these patients must be familiar with the implications of Down syndrome on perioperative care.

LEARNING OBJECTIVES

1. Be familiar with the clinical presentation of Down syndrome.
2. Consider the following challenges that are commonly associated with Down syndrome: airway difficulties, cervical spine instability, congenital heart disease.
3. Understand the implications of general anesthesia for these patients, beginning with preoperative evaluation and extending into postoperative care.

CASE PRESENTATION

A 2-year-old boy with Down syndrome presents for bilateral myringotomies with pressure-equalization tube placement and adenotonsillectomy. His medical history is significant for an uncomplicated delivery at term and corrective cardiac surgery in infancy for an **atrio-ventricular canal** defect. He completed a course of antibiotics 4 days ago for otitis media. Parents note that he is a noisy breather who regularly snores when sleeping and has self-resolving pauses lasting 5 to 10 seconds. The patient has the typical **Down's facies** and breathes with an open mouth and his tongue slightly protruded. Physical exam is otherwise normal. He has not had any cervical spine x-rays.

He undergoes inhalational induction with oxygen, nitrous oxide, and sevoflurane. Airway obstruction occurs on induction but resolves with a jaw thrust and placement of an oral airway. His heart rate, however, decreases to the 40s. Sevoflurane and nitrous oxide are discontinued, chest compressions (CPR) are commenced, and the emergency call system is activated. His blood pressure is 48/24. Atropine 10 mcg/kg is administered intramuscularly. An IV catheter is secured in the right wrist with difficulty. **Bradycardia** and hypotension (SBP now in the 30s) persist and femoral pulses remain diminished, despite an additional dose of IV atropine. Epinephrine (adrenaline) (1 mcg/kg) is given IV with prompt correction of hemodynamics.

Hyperextension of the neck is carefully avoided during laryngoscopy, and the patient's airway is secured with a 3.5-mm endotracheal tube (ETT). Anesthesia is maintained with oxygen, air, and sevoflurane. The otolaryngologist forgoes suspension for the adenotonsillectomy, and the surgery proceeds uneventfully. Rectal acetaminophen (paracetamol) 30 mg/kg and fentanyl 1 mcg/kg IV is administered for analgesia. The patient is extubated awake, but recovery in the PACU is complicated by **airway obstruction, apneic pauses**, and persistent **oxygen desaturation**. He is **admitted to the intensive care unit** for continued close monitoring.

DISCUSSION

1. What are the characteristic physical features of a patient with Down syndrome?

Children with Down syndrome are easily recognized by their **typical facial features**, which include brachycephaly, flat nasal bridge, epicanthal folds with upslanting palpebral fissures, and Brushfield spots on the iris. Their hands have a single palmar crease (simian crease) and a hypoplastic middle phalanx of the fifth finger, while their feet have a larger-than-normal gap between the large and second toes. The joints are hypermobile, and muscle tone may be decreased. Developmental delays are common, as are short stature and obesity.

Table 62.1 lists anesthesia considerations in Down syndrome patients by system.

2. How is the airway altered in these children? How does this affect what size ETT is used?

In the upper airway, the nasopharynx is often narrow, and the midface is hypoplastic. Micrognathia, large tonsils and adenoids, and a large tongue all contribute to airway obstruction at both the oropharyngeal and hypopharyngeal level, and to an increased prevalence (as high as 63–79%) of obstructive sleep apnea. Furthermore, even among those patients whose parents deny sleep problems, a considerable percentage have evidence of obstructive sleep apnea on polysomnography (Marcus et al., 1991).

Subglottic stenosis is more prevalent in Down syndrome patients, with the majority of cases being acquired. Because children with Down syndrome are more likely to require surgery and intubation at a young age, these patients are predisposed to develop subglottic narrowing. Gastroesophageal reflux disease, common in children with Down syndrome, may also contribute to the development of subglottic stenosis. In the face of previous mucosal injury, acid reflux encourages scar formation in the glottis.

In addition to anatomically narrow airways and the presence of subglottic stenosis, Down syndrome patients are often smaller and weigh less than children without Down syndrome, which can further contribute to smaller airway size. In general, initial intubation of Down syndrome patients should be performed with an ETT at least two sizes smaller than would be used in a child of the same age without Down syndrome. After intubation, it is critical

Table 62.1

CONSIDERATIONS IN DOWN SYNDROME, BY SYSTEM

System	Pathophysiology	Anesthetic Considerations
Cardiac	Congenital heart disease Pulmonary hypertension	1. Careful preoperative assessment 2. Tailor anesthetic to patient's cardiopulmonary function. 3. SBE prophylaxis when indicated
Airway/ pulmonary	Narrow nasopharynx, hypoplastic midface, large tongue, micrognathia Hypertrophic tonsils and adenoids Recurrent respiratory infections Subglottic stenosis Sleep apnea	1. Prone to airway obstruction 2. Use an appropriately sized ETT (likely a smaller size); perform a leak test as confirmation. 3. Extubate "awake" when possible. 4. Factor airway/respiratory issues into postoperative care plans.
Neurologic	Cognitive deficiencies Hypotonia	1. Cooperation and assessment limitations 2. Reduced airway tone with sedation/anesthesia
Musculoskeletal	Atlanto-axial instability Occipito-atlantal instability	1. Careful preoperative assessment 2. Avoid neck extension/flexion/rotation during laryngoscopy, intraoperative positioning.

to confirm the fit of the ETT by using a leak test to determine the leak pressure (the inspiratory pressure needed to cause an audible escape of gas around the ETT). A leak between 10 and 30 cmH_2O is desirable (Shott, 2000).

3. Should every patient with Down syndrome get cervical spine films preoperatively?

In 1983, the Special Olympics mandated routine **radiographic cervical spine screening** for all Down syndrome patients prior to participation in high-risk sports. Since then, the issue of screening for craniovertebral instability in this patient population has developed into a controversial topic, with the literature providing conflicting and confusing data. There is no doubt that patients with Down syndrome are at risk for craniovertebral joint instability that results from both abnormal joint anatomy and ligamentous laxity. In fact, evidence of atlanto-axial instability (AAI) can be found in 10% to 30% of patients with Down syndrome (Brockmeyer, 1999). AAI can be asymptomatic; symptoms occur when subluxation is severe enough to compress the spinal cord. It is not clear whether asymptomatic AAI progresses to symptomatic AAI. In addition, patients with Down syndrome may have rotatory instability stemming from occipito-atlantal instability, a concept that is relatively overlooked.

Although difficult in uncooperative and developmentally delayed children, a thorough history and physical exam is the most important step to identify patients who may have cervical spine instability. Neurologic manifestations of symptomatic instability include the preference for a sitting position, difficulty walking, abnormal gait, including falling and/or staggering, neck pain, limited neck mobility, torticollis, incoordination and clumsiness, sensory deficits, spasticity, and hyperreflexia.

Primary physicians screen most of these patients radiologically during the preschool years. Standard cervical spine screening consists of plain lateral radiographs in the neutral, flexion, and extension positions to measure the atlanto-dens interval (ADI, the distance between the posterior surface of the anterior arch of C1 and the anterior surface of the dens) and the neural canal width (NCW, the distance between the posterior surface of the dens and the anterior surface of the posterior arch of C1). If the ADI is greater than 4.5 mm or the NCW less than 14 mm, then an MRI should be obtained. When screening uncovers atlanto-axial and/or occipito-atlantal instability, the patient should be referred for evaluation by a qualified physician with experience in evaluating and treating pediatric spine disorders. The weight of evidence suggests that patients with Down syndrome undergo little to no change in the degree of their subluxation over time. Therefore, if no significant instability is discovered by the age of 10 years, screening may be stopped. Obviously, any patient who presents with new symptoms concerning for myelopathy should be immediately referred for evaluation. Elective procedures should be postponed and urgent/emergent surgical patients should be treated with cervical spine precautions.

The American Academy of Pediatrics recommends that all children with Down syndrome have cervical spine radiographs between the ages of 3 and 5 (American Academy of Pediatrics, 2001). If a patient older than this presents for anesthesia without previous cervical spine films, it may be prudent to obtain radiographs to screen for gross abnormalities and bony deformities and to provide a baseline study. If films were taken prior to 3 years of age, bony ossification may have been incomplete and repeat radiography may show better bony definition. When difficult laryngoscopy is anticipated, or extreme and/or prolonged non-neutral head/neck positioning for surgery is necessary, one may want radiographic evidence of cervical spine stability. In any case, when intubating and positioning these patients, the anesthesiologist should always be mindful to avoid extensive, forceful neck movements.

4. How does a history of congenital heart disease (CHD) affect the anesthetic management?

Anesthetic risk in these patients increases in the presence of cardiac disease, particularly when associated with pulmonary hypertension. Approximately 40% to 60% of patients with Down syndrome have cardiac malformations. **Atrioventriculoseptal** defects are the most common, followed by ventricular septal defects, patent ductus arteriosus, and tetralogy of Fallot (Weijerman et al., 2010). Screening infants with echocardiography facilitates early identification of CHD and optimal management. Compared to patients without Down syndrome, surgical correction in these patients is associated with increased morbidity and mortality secondary to coexisting pulmonary hypertension and to increased susceptibility to recurrent infections, including pneumonia. Post-cardiac surgery patients may have residual defects, including conduction disturbances. Depending on the type of cardiac lesion and the procedure to be performed, antibiotic prophylaxis for subacute bacterial endocarditis may be required. Anesthetic technique should be tailored to each patient's cardiopulmonary function. See also Chapter 32.

5. Does pulmonary hypertension occur in patients with Down syndrome who do not have CHD?

Down syndrome patients are at increased risk of developing pulmonary hypertension. This may be due to several factors other than the presence of CHD with persistent left-to-right shunting. It may be due to chronic upper airway obstruction, hypoventilation, obstructive sleep apnea, and chronic hypoxemia from recurrent pulmonary infections. Patients with Down syndrome appear to develop pulmonary hypertension at a faster rate and have persistent pulmonary hypertension after cardiac surgery. Although damage to the pulmonary vasculature occurs over time, patients with Down syndrome also have a higher incidence of idiopathic pulmonary hypertension of the neonate (PPHN), suggesting that these patients may have an intrinsic cause for the development of pulmonary vascular disease (Cua et al., 2007).

6. What anesthesia-related complications should one anticipate?

The most frequent complication is **bradycardia**, specifically **during induction**. This may occur in the absence of heart disease.

Since cardiac output is partly dependent on heart rate, especially in younger children, bradycardia can have a profound effect on a patient's hemodynamic stability. Neonates and infants in particular exhibit decreased sympathetic activity and may benefit from vagal blockade with atropine preoperatively. While atropine can help maintain the heart rate, it will not prevent or reverse the negative inotropic effects of volatile anesthetics. Gradually increasing the concentration of inspired sevoflurane during inhalation induction (as opposed to a rapid induction with 8% sevoflurane) will help prevent, but may not completely eliminate, hypotension and bradycardia. Close observation of heart rate and blood pressure during induction is imperative. If bradycardia occurs, immediately decrease the concentration of sevoflurane and administer atropine. Atropine should be given intramuscularly if an IV is not already in place. The extreme example in this case is a reminder that if bradycardia does not resolve or if hemodynamic compromise persists, then epinephrine (adrenaline) should be given. Other significant anesthesia-related complications include airway obstruction and post-intubation stridor (Borland et al., 2004).

7. What are common concerns in the early postoperative period?

Patients with Down syndrome are prone to airway complications, specifically **airway obstruction**, **oxygen desaturation**, and post-intubation stridor. They have a higher incidence of upper and lower respiratory tract infections, which can contribute to perioperative respiratory compromise. Younger patients with a known history of **obstructive sleep apnea** and/or other medical comorbidities may be candidates for **ICU admission** postoperatively, especially after airway procedures. For patients with a known history of airway obstruction, consider placing either an oropharyngeal or nasopharyngeal airway prior to extubation. Patients with Down syndrome should generally be extubated awake, not deep. Post-intubation stridor can result from subglottic edema due to the use of too large an ETT or the incorrect use of a cuffed ETT. Once identified, stridor can be treated with humidified oxygen, nebulized racemic epinephrine, and IV dexamethasone (see Chapter 30).

Pain management in the postoperative period can be challenging. While patients with Down syndrome clearly experience pain, they may express pain and discomfort more slowly and less precisely due to their developmental delay. Parents may be less able to recognize the level of pain experienced by their child with Down syndrome compared to that experienced by normal siblings. Therefore, to accurately assess pain, observe both behavioral and objective measures of pain, such as heart rate. Opioids must be administered carefully and incrementally to avoid respiratory compromise in patients who already have an at-risk airway. When appropriate, regional anesthesia techniques offer excellent long-lasting pain relief without the respiratory depression of opioids.

SUMMARY

1. Patients with Down syndrome can have multisystem abnormalities including airway obstruction, sleep apnea, an increased incidence of CHD, cervical spine instability, developmental delay, and obesity.
2. Risks on the induction of anesthesia include airway obstruction, bradycardia, and hypotension.
3. A smaller-than-normal ETT should be used and the head should be kept in neutral position for intubation.
4. Close postoperative observation for airway obstruction and desaturation is critical.

ANNOTATED REFERENCES

- Borland LM, Colligan J, Brandom BW. Frequency of anesthesia-related complications in children with Down syndrome under general anesthesia for noncardiac procedures. *Pediatr Anesth* 2004; 14: 733–738.

This retrospective chart review encompasses ~74,000 anesthetic encounters of Down syndrome patients undergoing non-cardiac surgeries and identifies the most prominent anesthesia-related complications.

- **Brockmeyer D. Down syndrome and craniovertebral instability.** *Pediatr Neurosurg* 1999; 31: 71–77.

    This article provides a thorough topic review, summarizing much of the data previously presented. Based on a literature review and study of the biomechanics of the craniovertebral junction, it makes recommendations for both screening and clinical management algorithms when instability is detected.

- **Shott SR. Down syndrome: analysis of airway size and guide for appropriate intubation.** *Laryngoscope* 2000; 110: 585–592.

    This study prospectively evaluated the airway size in children with and without Down syndrome and makes recommendations for choosing the proper ETT size.

Further Reading

American Academy of Pediatrics. Committee on Genetics. American Academy of Pediatrics: Health supervision for children with Down syndrome. *Pediatrics* 2001; 107(2): 442–449.

Cua CL, Blankenship A, North AL, Hayes J, Nelin LD. Increased incidence of idiopathic persistent pulmonary hypertension in Down syndrome neonates. *Pediatr Cardiol* 2007; 28: 250–254.

Dyken ME, Lin-Dyken DC, Poulton S, Zimmerman MB, Sedars E. Prospective polysomnographic analysis of obstructive sleep apnea in Down syndrome. *Arch Pediatr Adolesc Med* 2003; 157: 655–660.

Hata T, Todd MM. Cervical spine considerations when anesthetizing patients with Down syndrome. *Anesthesiology* 2005; 102: 680–685.

Kobel M, Creighton RE, Steward DJ. Anaesthetic considerations in Down's syndrome: experience with 100 patients and a review of the literature. *Can J Anaesth* 1982; 29: 593–599.

Marcus CL, Keens TG, Bautista DB, von Pechmann WS, Ward SLD. Obstructive sleep apnea in children with Down syndrome. *Pediatrics* 1991; 88: 132–139.

Weijerman ME, van Furth AM, van der Mooren MD, van Weissenbruch MM, Rammeloo L, Broers CJM, Gemke RJBJ. Prevalence of congenital heart defects and persistent pulmonary hypertension of the neonate with Down syndrome. *Eur J Pediatr* 2010; 169: 1195–1199.

63

Muscular Dystrophy

**RENEE NIERMAN KREEGER AND
JAMES P. SPAETH**

INTRODUCTION

Gastrostomy tube placement is typically a routine surgical procedure with little concern for morbidity and mortality. However, in patients with Duchenne muscular dystrophy (DMD), this is not the case. Patients with DMD present a unique clinical dilemma since they often do not require gastrostomy tube placement until their physical status has deteriorated to the point that they have respiratory insufficiency or failure and clinically significant cardiomyopathy. An understanding of the pathophysiology of this disorder and a proactive approach to perioperative management are important to ensure a positive patient outcome.

LEARNING OBJECTIVES

1. Appreciate the natural history of DMD.
2. Become familiar with the American College of Chest Physicians Consensus Statement for anesthetic management of patients with DMD.
3. Identify management strategies for perioperative care of patients with advanced DMD.
4. Understand the importance of a proactive approach to the care of patients with advanced DMD.

CASE PRESENTATION

A 17-year-old boy with DMD presents for percutaneous endoscopic ***gastrostomy*** *tube placement for nutritional support due to significant weight loss. A preoperative anesthesia consultation has been requested prior to the day of surgery secondary to the advanced nature of his disease. The patient is* ***wheelchair bound*** *with minimal independent movement. His airway exam shows a Mallampati II with mildly decreased neck range of motion and mouth opening. His lungs are clear, and heart sounds are normal. The patient reports a significant increase in his respiratory efforts and in respiratory illnesses in the past year. His most recent* ***pulmonary function tests (PFTs)*** *demonstrate a significant decrease from previous measurements, with a forced vital capacity (FVC) of 38% predicted with a peak cough flow (PCF) of 240 L/min and a maximum expiratory pressure (MEP) of 55 cmH$_2$O. His room air oxygen saturation is 98%. A postoperative pediatric intensive care unit (PICU) admission is recommended for extubation to* ***nasal positive pressure ventilation*** *(NPPV).*

Cardiac evaluations from a week ago include an echocardiogram that demonstrates evidence of stable ***dilated cardiomyopathy (DCM)*** *with a shortening fraction (SF) of 20%. The electrocardiogram (ECG) shows normal sinus rhythm (NSR) with occasional premature ventricular contractions (PVCs). The cardiologist states that the patient is in optimal condition this time and that she will be available postoperatively to assist as needed.*

In the operating room, standard American Society of Anesthesiologists (ASA) monitors are applied and the patient undergoes an IV induction with etomidate and fentanyl after preoxygenation. Mask ventilation is somewhat difficult and improves with insertion of an oropharyngeal airway. Direct laryngoscopy with a Macintosh blade reveals only the epiglottis. With significant cricoid pressure and the use of a straight blade, the posterior arytenoids are visualized and the patient is intubated successfully with a styletted endotracheal tube (ETT). Infusions of propofol and remifentanil are initiated for maintenance of anesthesia. A ***dopamine infusion*** *is set up on a pump but held in reserve. The surgeon begins the gastrostomy* *tube insertion, and the patient's oxygen saturation is noted to decrease to 88%. Gastric insufflation is reduced and a few distending breaths are given, with increase of positive end-expiratory pressure (PEEP) from 5 to 8 cmH₂O, leading to a quick return to baseline. PVCs are noted to increase in frequency, but the patient's hemodynamics are unaffected. The procedure is completed without incident and the patient is transferred to the PICU intubated. The patient is* **extubated to NPPV** *later that afternoon and is weaned to room air with spontaneous ventilation and cough assist by the next day.*

DISCUSSION

1. What is the definition and natural history of DMD?

DMD is a progressive, X-linked neuromuscular disorder with an incidence of 1 in 3,500 male live births. It is estimated that approximately 8% to 10% of female carriers have some mild manifestations of the disease, such as minor muscle weakness. The hallmarks of the disease are abnormal motor development, including lack of independent walking by 18 months of age, an inability to run, jump, or climb stairs, and pseudohypertrophy of the calf muscles. The classic Gower's sign, involving the use of a wide-based stance and the aid of hands on the thighs to rise from the floor, is often seen. Approximately 30% of these patients have some degree of developmental delay. These clinical signs are the manifestations of a deletion or mutation in the dystrophin gene, resulting in muscular necrosis and replacement with connective or adipose tissue. For two thirds of children with DMD, no family history of the disease exists; the mean age at diagnosis for these children is 4.5 years. The disease is relentless; patients are **wheelchair bound** by the age of 12 years and have progressive involvement of respiratory muscles concomitant with the development of a dilated cardiomyopathy. One third of patients have dilated cardiomyopathy by age 14, with nearly all patients developing cardiomyopathy by age 18. If untreated, the mean age at death is 19 years. With corticosteroid treatment and close attention to pulmonary support and toilet, patients can survive into the third decade.

2. What are the perioperative concerns for patients with DMD?
The main concerns for the anesthesiologist are the patient's cardiopulmonary status, potential difficult airway, and the possibility of malignant hyperthermia-like reactions. One should be alert to the significant risk of airway difficulty, given the known association of DMD with a combination of macroglossia, weak upper airway muscles, limited cervical spine movement, and limited mandibular mobility. From a respiratory standpoint, these patients are often quite debilitated, with many requiring the use of NPPV. In addition, they have a diminished cough reflex, increasing the baseline and postoperative risk of respiratory infection. Preoperative **pulmonary function testing** can guide both intraoperative and postoperative respiratory care. Postoperatively, elective admission to the ICU is prudent and allows the patient to be extubated at an appropriate time to **NPPV** or similar noninvasive ventilator support.

Patients with DMD develop a **dilated cardiomyopathy**, which predisposes them to hemodynamic instability and **dysrhythmias** as well as fulminant cardiac failure. Depending on the extent of the cardiomyopathy, the patient may require a high-dose opioid-based anesthetic to ensure hemodynamic stability. An alternative anesthetic is ketamine, when clinically appropriate. Medications such as propofol, which may cause significant hypotension when used in induction doses, should be used with great care in severely affected patients. Careful fluid management and optimization of electrolytes are important. In cases where blood loss is more prominent than in this gastrostomy case, boys with DMD seem to lose more blood than average; blood transfusion should be anticipated. It is prudent to have **inotropic support** readily available, as many patients will require such support, even for "minor" procedures.

Traditional teaching outlines an increased risk of malignant hyperthermia in patients with muscular dystrophies (see Chapter 8).

However, a 2009 review of the anesthesia literature by a group at Children's Hospital of Philadelphia (CHOP) instead cites an increased risk of a *malignant hyperthermia-like syndrome* with associated rhabdomyolysis in patients who receive inhaled anesthetics (Gurnaney et al., 2009). Therefore, inhalational anesthetics should be avoided unless specifically indicated. There is a life-threatening hyperkalemia risk associated with succinylcholine (suxamethonium) administration in these patients, making succinylcholine contraindicated for patients with DMD.

3. What are perioperative guidelines for care of DMD patients?

Patients with DMD have a number of body systems about which the anesthesiologist must be concerned. While it is important to pursue preoperative testing and optimization, patients can develop complications intra- and postoperatively even if the results of those tests seem reassuring. It is prudent to prepare an ICU bed, for instance, and to be prepared to support cardiac and pulmonary function both intra- and postoperatively. Table 63.1 summarizes guidelines for the perioperative care of these patients, based on recommendations from the American College of Chest Physicians.

4. Are there alternatives to placement of an ETT?

There are case reports in the literature outlining the use of alternative airway devices and methods of ventilation. These options have been explored for a variety of reasons, including the preference of some patients with end-stage disease not to be intubated (see Chapter 6). There are reports of the use of NPPV with bilevel positive airway pressure (BiPAP), laryngeal mask airways (LMAs), and mouthpieces or nasal masks (Birnkrant et al., 2006). These devices have been used successfully but have inherent risks. The patient using NPPV may have difficulty once sedation is given and may cease spontaneous ventilation. With LMA use, there can be issues with proper fit as well as with an inability to pass the endoscope to allow for percutaneous endoscopic gastrostomy (PEG) tube placement.

Table 63.1

PERIOPERATIVE CARE OF PATIENTS WITH DMD

Preoperative

Multidisciplinary approach:
Pulmonary consultation and evaluation: include FVC, maximum inspiratory pressure (MIP), MEP, PCF, and room air oxygen saturation via pulse oximetry.

i) FVC: <50% predicted = increased risk of respiratory complications; <30% predicted = high risk. Recommend possible preoperative training for NPPV.

ii) PCF and MEP: <270 L/min or < 60 cmH_2O respectively = high risk of ineffective cough. Recommend preoperative training in manual and mechanically assisted cough devices.

Cardiology referral: clinical evaluation and optimization

Note: *normal ECG and echocardiogram results are only modestly reassuring.*

Nutritional assessment with optimization and dysphagia management

Discuss advanced directives, DNR status, anesthesia risks and benefits.

ICU admission planned ahead

Intraoperative

TIVA

Maximize medical personnel available.

Explore options for respiratory support, such as mechanical ventilation with ETT, NPPV, BiPAP, LMA.

Support ventilation via an assisted or controlled mode for patients with FVC <50%.

Monitoring: standard ASA monitors at minimum

Table 63.1 (*continued*)

Postoperative

Consider extubating to NPPV in patients with FVC <50%.

Consider delaying extubation if respiratory secretions are poorly controlled or oxygenation is below baseline.

Use supplemental oxygen with caution while investigating an etiology for decreased oxygen saturation.

Use manual and cough assist devices.

Optimize pain control, delaying extubation if necessary.

Consult cardiology to maximize cardiac function.

Begin a bowel regimen.

If enteral feeding will be delayed >24 to 48 hours, begin parenteral feeding.

Source: Birnkrant DJ, Panitch HB, Benditt JO, et al. American College of Chest Physicians Consensus statement on the respiratory and related management of patients with Duchenne muscular dystrophy undergoing anesthesia or sedation. *Chest* 2007; 132(6): 1977–1986.

SUMMARY

1. The natural history of DMD is characterized by progressive muscle weakness beginning in the preschool years and progressing to loss of ambulation by age 12, and progressive dilated cardiomyopathy and respiratory insufficiency/failure by the teenage years, often requiring assisted ventilation. Aggressive treatment with high-dose steroids helps increase the life expectancy into the 20s.

2. The American College of Chest Physicians 2007 Consensus statement is an excellent resource for perioperative care.

3. Multidisciplinary preoperative evaluation is essential to identify and optimize the patient's medical problems and to design the best perioperative care.
4. Key intraoperative principles include avoiding succinylcholine and inhaled anesthetics. Total intravenous anesthesia (TIVA), careful monitoring, and management of the dilated cardiomyopathy is required.
5. Postoperative care should occur in the ICU, with careful attention to maximizing respiratory function.

ANNOTATED REFERENCES

- Birnkrant DJ, Ferguson RD, Martin JE, Gordon GJ. Noninvasive ventilation during gastrostomy tube placement in patients with severe Duchenne muscular dystrophy: Case reports and review of the literature. *Pediatr Pulmonol* 2006; 41: 188–193.
    This paper offers alternative methods for airway management in patients with DMD, including LMA and NPPV.
- Birnkrant DJ, Panitch HB, Benditt JO, et al. American College of Chest Physicians Consensus statement on the respiratory and related management of patients with Duchenne muscular dystrophy undergoing anesthesia or sedation. *Chest* 2007; 132(6): 1977–1986.
    This is the best summary of the vital components of the perioperative care of patients with DMD. It provides parameters for assessing risk for complications as well as a proactive multidisciplinary approach to management. It is a must-read for any anesthesiologist who may encounter these patients.
- Brambrink AM, Kirsch JR. Perioperative care of patients with neuromuscular disease and dysfunction. *Anesthesiol Clin North Am* 2007; 25: 483–509.

A good overview of the most common neuromuscular disorders. It highlights the specific anesthetic challenges that are most commonly encountered with each disorder and offers suggestions for patient management.

Further Reading

Bushby K, Bourke J, Bullock R, Eagle M, Gibson M, Quinby J. The multidisciplinary management of Duchenne muscular dystrophy. *Current Pediatrics* 2005; 15: 292–300.

Gurnaney H, Brown A, Litman RS. Malignant hyperthermia and muscular dystrophies. *Anesth Analg* 2009; 109(4): 1043–1048.

Ihmsen H, Schmidt J, Schwilden H, Schmitt HJ, Muenster T. Influence of disease progression on the neuromuscular blocking effect of mivacurium in children and adolescents with Duchenne muscular dystrophy. *Anesthesiology* 2009; 110(5): 1016–1019.

64

Mucopolysaccharidoses

GEOFF FRAWLEY

INTRODUCTION

The mucopolysaccharidoses (MPS) are a group of seven chronic progressive diseases caused by deficiencies of 11 different lysosomal enzymes required for the catabolism of glycosaminoglycans (GAGs). Hurler syndrome (MPS IH) is an autosomal recessive storage disorder caused by a deficiency of α-L-iduronidase. Hunter syndrome (MPS II) is an X-linked recessive disorder of metabolism involving the enzyme iduronate-2-sulfatase. Many of the MPS clinical manifestations have potential anesthetic implications. Significant airway issues are particularly common due to thickening of the soft tissues, enlarged tongue, short immobile neck, and limited mobility of the cervical spine and temporomandibular joints. Spinal deformities, hepatosplenomegaly, airway granulomatous tissue, and recurrent lung infections may inhibit pulmonary function. Odontoid dysplasia and radiographic subluxation of C1 on C2 is common and may cause anterior dislocation of the atlas and spinal cord compression.

LEARNING OBJECTIVES

1. Review the anesthetic issues related to Hurler syndrome.
2. Develop the ability to recognize and manage the difficult pediatric airway.
3. Discuss the management of anticipated difficult intubation in children with MPS.

CASE PRESENTATION

A 16-kg, 5-year-old girl with classical features of **Hurler syndrome** *presents with an irreducible umbilical hernia. She was assessed to be unsuitable for* **bone marrow transplantation** *as an infant due to neurologic involvement but has been receiving intravenous* **enzyme replacement** *since the age of 3. She has moderate* **developmental delay***. Her general health is good but her parents report that she* **snores** *a lot at night and sometimes has pauses in her breathing. She is currently being assessed for a* **nocturnal CPAP device***. Her past history includes a* **carpal tunnel release** *12 months ago; the anesthesia chart records moderate difficulty in visualizing the larynx. On examination the child is short (height 98 cm). Cardiac auscultation demonstrates a grade III systolic murmur. Echocardiogram shows normal LV function, moderate symmetrical* **left ventricular hypertrophy***, a thickened tricuspid aortic valve with* **mild aortic stenosis***, and a thickened,* **dysplastic mitral valve***. She was not able to comply with a lung function test. Sleep studies demonstrate moderate* **obstructive sleep apnea** *with three episodes of saturation less than 85% during periods of REM sleep. The child is anxious and tearful in the preoperative area, so a midazolam premedication is given.*

Specialized airway devices are prepared. After a sevoflurane induction, almost complete **airway obstruction** *occurs and the patient's SpO_2 drops to 80%; attempted mask ventilation is inadequate. Direct laryngoscopy is performed and no laryngeal structures are recognizable. Rapid desaturation is partially corrected by successful placement of a LMA; some resolution of hypoxia is observed, although partial obstruction with rocking chest movements is still seen and tidal volumes are small. Intubation is attempted using a 2.8-mm fiberoptic bronchoscope. It is passed through the laryngeal mask and reveals a partial occlusion of the laryngeal inlet by* **supraglottic tissue** *and a down-folded epiglottis. Endotracheal intubation is accomplished only after downsizing to size 3.5-mm uncuffed ETT. Surgery for the hernia was uneventful, but the postoperative period was complicated by repeated failure of extubation and development of post-obstructive pulmonary edema. She is reintubated in the same* *manner as previously and transferred to the PICU. She is given IV dexamethasone and is extubated 24 hours later; she requires mask CPAP for a further 24 hours.*

DISCUSSION

1. **What treatment options are available to ameliorate the long-term clinical course of Hurler (MPS IH) and Hunter (MPS II) syndrome?**

Treatment options include palliative care, **hematopoietic stem cell transplantation** (HSCT) from bone marrow or umbilical cord blood, or recombinant human **enzyme replacement therapy** (ERT). Hurler syndrome patients receive recombinant human alpha-L-iduronidase (Aldurazyme®, laronidase), whereas Hunter syndrome patients receive idursulfase (Elaprase®).

a) Hurler Syndrome (MPS IH)

The best clinical outcome of HSCT has been observed in children who receive transplants before they are 2 years old and have a developmental quotient above 70 at the time of transplant (Meunzer et al., 2009). Successful HSCT in patients with MPS I modifies disease progression with increases in life expectancy, resolution of hepatosplenomegaly, stabilization of cardiac disease, and improvement in airway obstruction. The procedure, however, is not curative, and neurologic outcomes are variable. ERT with alpha-L-iduronidase (laronidase) infusion has recently been approved by the FDA for patients with the milder or attenuated forms of MPS type IH and for patients with neurologic impairment. The enzyme is not expected to cross the blood–brain barrier and affect central nervous system disease.

b) Hunter Syndrome (MPS II)

As with Hurler syndrome, HSCT is currently not recommended for the severe form of MPS type II, since neurologic preservation has not been observed. Bone marrow transplantation has been used to treat some symptoms in milder forms of Hunter syndrome. Recombinant ERT with idursulfase (Elaprase®) infusion improves exercise tolerance but has produced severe allergic reactions in some patients. ERT improves OSA pulmonary function tests in patients with a similar condition called Hurler Scheie disease (MPS I H/S). There are no data to suggest a reduction in airway complications after HSCT, but the reduction in upper airway soft tissues following transplant and to a lesser extent ERT in children should improve the airway management and the ease of intubation.

2. For MPS IH and MPS II, what are the key features of a pre-operative assessment?

Airway Assessment: Ideally, one would review a recent anesthetic chart describing the intubation and possible ventilation difficulties (along with techniques used to overcome those difficulties). The case described had these on record from 12 months ago. Before ERT, one could predict this child's airway would become more difficult with time; a careful history of obstructive symptoms gives a surrogate marker as to how the disease has progressed. The alpha-L-iduronidase may have attenuated the disease progression since the last anesthetic. Special investigations could include sleep studies, nasoendoscopy, and cervical spine x-ray (demonstrating the atlanto-axial joint and odontoid process). Upper airway imaging techniques such as MRI and CT are not routinely used to assess the airway preoperatively but can be performed in cooperative older children (or recreated from previous CT scans of the cervical spine). Clinically significant upper airway obstruction has been reported in 70% of patients with MPS due to enlarged tongue, tonsils, and adenoids, narrowed trachea, redundant airway tissue, and thickened vocal cords (Yeung et al., 2009). Most severe MPS I patients develop obstructive upper airway disease by 2 or 3 years of age.

Respiratory Assessment: All MPS patients are at risk of severe respiratory compromise from restrictive lung disease and recurrent infection. Exercise tolerance compared to their peers is a useful index of cardiorespiratory function; formal respiratory function testing is difficult in children under 7 years of age and may be impossible with developmental delay.

Cardiology Assessment: All patients with Hurler and Hunter syndrome should undergo a cardiology evaluation at diagnosis and every 1 to 2 years thereafter (Meunzer et al., 2009). Cardiac manifestations are common and worsen with age. In patients with severe MPS I, valvular disease, arrhythmia, cardiomyopathy, congestive heart failure, coronary artery disease, and pulmonary and systemic hypertension may occur. Moderate to severe narrowing of the coronary arteries can occur within the first year of life, and complete coronary occlusion has been reported within the first 5 years of life. In MPS II, valvular heart disease is common (prevalence 50%); cardiomyopathy is less common but can be associated with dysrhythmias.

3. What are clues to a potentially difficult airway in young infants with MPS?

The overall incidence of difficult airway in children with MPS in the era of HSCT and ERT is unknown. Before these therapies were available, the incidence of difficult intubation was 25% overall, with much higher rates in Hurler (54%) and Morquio syndrome (50%). Prediction of difficult intubation is more an art than a science; features that would raise suspicion are listed in Table 64.1. A recent previous anesthetic record would of course be of most practical use.

4. What airway devices and techniques are appropriate in managing the airway?

Most published series report the need for experienced anesthetists and multiple airway devices. Most authors recommend inhalational induction prior to airway management. As opposed to the steps in an adult difficult airway algorithm, awake fiberoptic intubation is usually not feasible in children with MPS, and emergency tracheostomy is likely to be extremely difficult and

Table 64.1
SOMATIC MANIFESTATIONS OF MPS ASSOCIATED WITH DIFFICULT AIRWAY MANAGEMENT
Hurler or Morquio syndrome (higher incidence than Hunter syndrome)
Older children or teenagers not suitable for stem cell transplantation
Previous difficult intubation
Enlarged tongue, adenoids, or tonsils
Obstructive sleep apnea (particularly if the child requires a nocturnal home CPAP machine)
Radiologic evidence of tracheal narrowing or tracheal collapse on neck flexion
Cardiac disease (cardiomyopathy, septal hypertrophy, infiltration of coronary artery with ischemia, mitral or tricuspid valve incompetence)
Short or immobile neck
Atlanto-axial subluxation
Obstructive lung disease
Kyphoscoliosis and/or lumbar lordosis

prolonged. The most common forms of airway management in patients with MPS involve the use of a supraglottic airway device; these can be used alone or as a conduit to fiberoptic intubation. To maintain airway and anesthesia for the purpose of fiberoptic intubation, various devices have been used, including LMAs, a modified intubating facemask (VBM Medizintechnik, Sulz, Germany), and a contralateral nasopharyngeal airway. The devices currently available to help difficult intubation in adults are well described (Niforopolou et al., 2010), and many should be considered for intubating children with MPS.

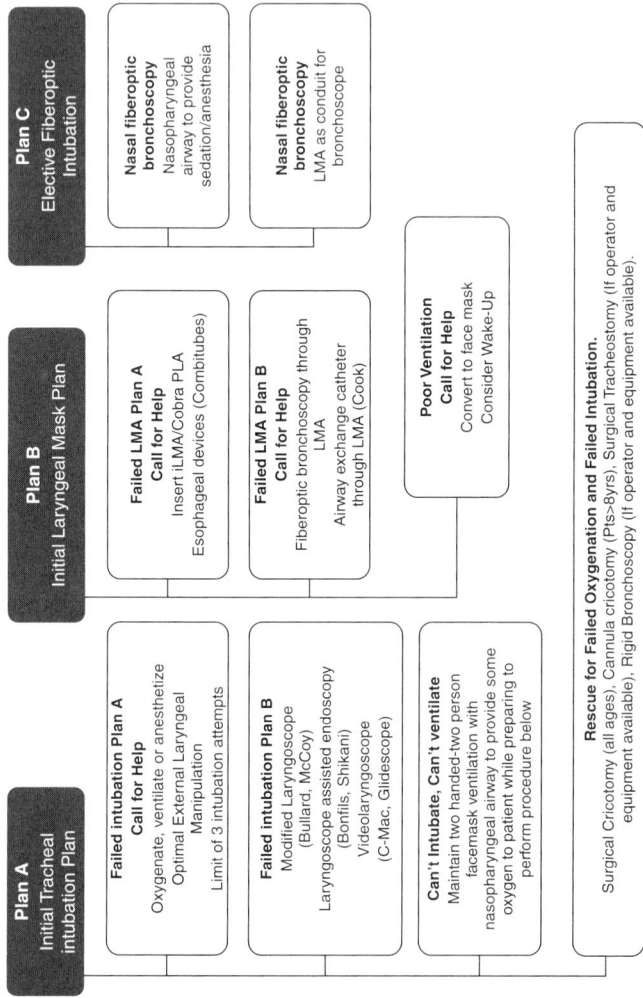

FIGURE 64.1 Suggested difficult airway management in children with mucopolysaccharidoses.

5. What maneuvers can rescue a compromised airway in patients with MPS?

Of all the devices available for anticipated difficult pediatric airway management, only seven have been reported in MPS patients. Although the successful use of the LMA is well described in these patients (Walker, 2000), it is not universally successful. The other LMA derivatives (including Flexible LMA and LMA ProSeal) have not been described in patients with MPS. The I-Gel LMA has been described in an adult with Hunter syndrome. Emergency tracheostomy in the "can't intubate, can't ventilate" situation is much less of an option for MPS children due to short neck, impalpable tracheal rings, and pretracheal GAG deposits and could take up to an hour. In the emergency situation, it may make more sense to try to wake the patient than to struggle with that airway and wait for the tracheostomy. A suggested difficult airway algorithm is seen in Fig. 64.1.

6. Is awake regional anesthesia appropriate in this patient?

Neurologic problems due to MPS deposition are recognized in MPS IH and II, which may represent a relative contraindication to regional anesthesia. There have only been a few successful reports of neuraxial blockade in children. An epidural failed to work in a 9-year-old Hurler syndrome boy; it is thought the deposition of GAGs in either the epidural space or the nerve fiber sheath may have prevented the direct access of local anesthetic to the nerve (Vas & Naregal, 2000).

SUMMARY

1. Most children with MPS have significant airway anomalies that predispose to difficult airway management. Anesthesia requires meticulous assessment and planning and the help of an expert team.

2. Sedation should be avoided if the patient has significant obstructive sleep apnea or upper airway obstruction.
3. Spontaneous respiration should be maintained until the airway is either secured or fully assessed.
4. Ongoing training and regular practice of advanced airway techniques are essential.

ANNOTATED REFERENCES

- Muenzer J, Wraith J, Clarke L. Mucopolysaccharidosis 1: Management and treatment guidelines. *Pediatrics* 2009; 123: 19–29.

    This is a consensus paper from a MPS working party that outlines all aspects of disease presentation and management but has minimal anesthetic input.

- Walker R, Darowski M, Wraith J. Anaesthesia and mucopolysaccaridoses. *Anaesthesia* 1994; 49: 1078–1084.

    A paper from the leading authority on the anesthetic management of MPS details techniques in use prior to the widespread availability of HSCT and enzyme replacement.

Further Reading

Aucoin S, Vlatten A, Hackmann T. Difficult airway management with the Bonfils fiberscope in a child with Hurler syndrome. *Pediatr Anesth* 2009; 19: 421–422.

Crocker K, Black A. Assessment and management of the predicted difficult airway in babies and children. *Anaesth Int Care Med* 2009; 10(4): 200–205.

Difficult Airway Society. *Simple Composite Chart*, 2001. Accessed Jan. 28, 2011. http://www.das.uk.com/guidelines/downloads.html.

Mahoney A, Soni N, Vellodi A. Anesthesia and the mucopolysaccaridoses: a review of patients treated by bone marrow transplantation. *Pediatr Anesth* 1992; 2: 317–324.

Niforopolou P, Pantazopoulos I, Demestiha T, et al. Video-laryngoscopes in the adult airway management: a topical review of the literature. *Acta Anaesthesiol Scand* 2010; 54: 1050–1061.

Vas L, Naregal F. Failed epidural anesthesia in a patient with Hurler's disease. *Pediatr Anesth* 2000; 10(1): 95–98.

Walker R. The laryngeal mask airway in the difficult pediatric airway: an assessment of positioning and use in fiberoptic intubation. *Pediatr Anesth* 2000; 10: 53–58.

Yeung A, Cowan M, Rosbe K. Airway management in children with mucopolysaccharidoses. *Arch Otolaryngol Head Neck Surg* 2009; 135(1): 73–79.

65

Epidermolysis Bullosa

NANCY B. SAMOL AND ERIC P. WITTKUGEL

INTRODUCTION

Epidermolysis bullosa (EB) is a genetic skin disorder with multiple modes of inheritance that causes blister formation from shear injury and results in extensive scarring. Children with EB provide an array of unique challenges when presenting for anesthetic care. Anticipation and management of a potentially difficult airway as well as the protection of fragile skin and mucous membranes are high priorities during anesthetic planning. Complications can arise with use of even the most routine anesthesia monitors and placement of a simple peripheral IV line. Thorough preoperative planning and meticulous perioperative care will reduce complications and result in a smooth anesthetic for both patient and clinician.

LEARNING OBJECTIVES

1. Review the pathology and clinical presentation of EB with special focus on anesthetic challenges.
2. Discuss principles of preoperative evaluation and perioperative management of EB patients.
3. Develop an anesthetic plan for EB patients, including induction, monitoring, airway management, and postoperative care.

CASE PRESENTATION

*A 12-year-old white boy with recessive dystrophic EB and **esophageal strictures** presents for esophageal dilation. He has been having progressive difficulty swallowing solids for the past year to the point of eating only thinly puréed foods. His past medical history is significant for chronic sinusitis, asthma that is well controlled, and dental caries. Parents report **difficult intubation** with a prior anesthetic performed 1 year ago for dental rehabilitation at an outside hospital. On physical examination, the patient is a cooperative but anxious 25-kg boy who has the characteristic features of recessive dystrophic EB: extensive **skin blistering** in various stages of healing, all extremities wrapped in dressings, **pseudosyndactyly** of hands and feet, partial alopecia, and flexion contractures of elbows and knees. His airway exam is significant for **microstomia** with only 1.4 cm of mouth opening, multiple caps on his teeth, **ankyloglossia**, and **bullae of the oral mucosal surfaces**. Chest exam demonstrates occasional rhonchi but no wheezing.*

*After the OR is prepared (the difficult airway cart and fiberoptic bronchoscope are available), the patient and his parents are brought to the induction room. A **well-lubricated mask** is gently applied to the face for inhalational induction with oxygen, nitrous oxide, and sevoflurane. Oxygen saturation is measured with a **clip pulse oximeter probe** rather than an adhesive-style probe. The blood pressure cuff is applied over several layers of cotton gauze wrapping the extremity and cycled sparingly. ECG leads are placed with the adhesive portion removed and secured to the patient with nonadhesive wraps. A tourniquet is placed gently over layers of gauze and an IV catheter is placed in the antecubital fossa. The IV is then secured with **nonadhesive dressing**, wrapped gently with gauze, and then covered with an elastic wrap. After the administration of IV muscle relaxant and opioid, gentle direct laryngoscopy is performed with a lubricated blade, and a styletted 5.0 cuffed ETT is placed with some difficulty under limited visualization. The tube is secured loosely behind the neck with cotton ties. The eyes are lubricated with preservative-free eye drops and covered with gauze pads moistened with saline. Using a hydrostatic* *balloon technique and fluoroscopy, the pediatric surgeon performs esophageal dilation. The patient is **extubated fully awake** and transported to the PACU, where his recovery is uncomplicated with no evidence of airway obstruction from **new bullae formation**. After a period of close observation, he is discharged home with the understanding that he will return yearly for esophageal dilation.*

DISCUSSION

1. What is the basic pathophysiology and clinical presentation of EB?

EB is a group of rare, genetically determined diseases in which blister formation and subsequent scarring occur with even minor skin trauma. The pathophysiology involves abnormalities in the attachment complexes anchoring the epidermis to the underlying dermis and below. There are three main categories of EB based on the skin layer in which **blistering** occurs, with 20 subtypes described. EB simplex (92% prevalence) with autosomal dominant inheritance is the mildest variant. It results from an abnormality in the basement membrane of the epidermis and causes generalized bullae, but overall the lesions heal without scarring. Junctional EB (1% prevalence) has an autosomal recessive inheritance pattern and manifests as an abnormality in the basement membrane of the dermis. With its extensive mucosal involvement, this variant can result in death from respiratory distress or sepsis before the age of 2 years. Dystrophic EB (5% prevalence) may be either autosomal recessive or dominant and results from abnormalities below the layer of the basement membrane. This incapacitating, disfiguring variant results in extensive scarring, often with oral and esophageal involvement.

Patients with recessive dystrophic EB typically have limited mouth opening (**microstomia**) due to scarring and contractures at the corners of the mouth, scarring of the tongue to the floor of the mouth (**ankyloglossia**), and erosions and **bullae of the oral mucosa**. The teeth are often angled inward, and extensive dental caries may be present. Due to eyelid scarring, EB patients often have difficulty closing their eyes and develop recurrent corneal abrasions. **Extreme skin fragility** is evidenced by extensive blisters and erosions along with scars from healing wounds. **Strictures** may be very proximal in the esophagus. Contractures of the extremities are present, along with fusion of the digits resulting in mitten deformities (**pseudosyndactyly**). Growth retardation and failure to thrive due to the high caloric demand of the constant healing process is common. Malnutrition can result in impaired immunity and may lead to chronic infection in the face of compromised skin integrity. Anemia due to iron deficiency and chronic disease is often present. Finally, from a cardiorespiratory standpoint, these patients may exhibit aspiration with frequent respiratory infections as well as decreased pulmonary function due to the mechanical restriction created by scarring of the chest wall. Recessive dystrophic patients may develop a dilated cardiomyopathy.

2. What issues deserve attention during preoperative evaluation?

Management of a potentially **difficult airway** and the **fragility of the skin and mucous membranes** are of the highest priority during anesthesia. Mask ventilation is usually not difficult, but special attention must be given to airway evaluation in order to avoid unanticipated difficulties with intubation. During childhood, direct laryngoscopy is generally straightforward. As patients approach adolescence and the microstomia becomes more severe, intubation becomes difficult, often requiring **fiberoptic intubation**. A complete blood count and echocardiogram are helpful preoperative tests. Many EB centers have started to obtain annual echocardiograms to screen for cardiomyopathy.

Regional anesthesia can be offered to patients with EB. In the absence of contraindications, caudal, spinal, or epidural anesthesia for procedures involving the abdomen, pelvis, or lower extremities as well as peripheral nerve blockade for procedures on the extremities are all viable complements or alternatives to general anesthesia. Care in applying nonadhesive dressings is important.

Table 65.1 summarizes perioperative anesthetic care for patients with EB.

3. What procedures are commonly performed in children with EB?

Although patients with EB may present for any type of surgery, certain procedures are commonly performed. These include hand surgery for correction of **pseudosyndactyly**, endoscopy or balloon esophageal dilation with fluoroscopy to diagnose and manage esophageal strictures, percutaneous endoscopic gastrostomy (PEG) or open gastrostomy for nutritional supplementation, skin biopsies to rule out squamous cell carcinoma, and subsequent excision of squamous cell carcinoma with skin grafting. Dental rehabilitation is often performed to correct extensive decay and to maintain oral hygiene that may otherwise be impossible for the patient due to microstomia and delicate oral mucosa. Finally, anesthesia may be required to provide comfort during wound care such as dressing changes or whirlpool bath treatments for skin débridement.

4. What precautions should be taken in the operating room?

Operating room preparation should include a warm room, a padded operating table, and an egg crate or other soft foam mattress that stays under the patient throughout the perioperative period. Despite the potential for difficult intubation, general endotracheal anesthesia is often the safest and most effective technique for many surgical cases. The airway is protected against aspiration and optimal surgical conditions are provided for the procedure.

The skin and mucous membranes are very fragile, so minimizing trauma is of the utmost importance. Premedication with oral midazolam helps promote a calm anesthetic induction with minimal anxiety, movement, and restlessness. To minimize patient anxiety, parental presence may be allowed during anesthesia

Table 65.1

BASICS OF PERIOPERATIVE ANESTHETIC CARE FOR PATIENTS WITH EB

General Principles

- Avoid shearing forces to minimize bulla formation.
- Compressive forces to the skin are tolerated.
- Lift, do not slide, patient during transfer.
- Avoid all adhesive tape, ECG leads, adhesive pulse oximeter probes.
- If patient dressings are in place and not in the way, leave them in place.
- Columnar mucosa of nares, larynx, trachea distal to vocal cords are not affected.
- Tracheal intubation is acceptable.

OR Preparation

- Warm OR
- Padded OR table
- Gentle transfer of patient
- Egg crate mattress that stays under patient throughout perioperative period
- Lubricate eyes with preservative-free, non-lanolin lubricant (Refresh®) and cover eyes with moistened gauze pads or nonadhesive tape (Mepitel® or Mepiform®).
- Assemble all necessary supplies ahead of time.
- Check IV site frequently as IVs tend to become dislodged more easily.

Airway Management

- Mask lubricated with ointment (e.g., Aquaphor®)
- Avoid oral airway if possible as it may cause blistering.
- Gentle intubation with well-lubricated laryngoscope and small ETT
- Anticipate difficult intubation.
- Oral fiberoptic intubation if needed; avoid nasal intubation unless necessary
- Laryngeal mask airway (LMA) may cause mucosal trauma and pharyngeal bullae.
- Secure ETT with nonadhesive cotton tape or suture to teeth.

(continued)

Table 65.1 (continued)

Anesthetic Techniques

- General endotracheal anesthesia is advisable for esophageal dilation, dental rehabilitation, or major abdominal procedures.
- Mask anesthesia for brief procedures as appropriate
- Total intravenous anesthesia (TIVA) for whirlpool treatments or peripheral surgery using ketamine, propofol, remifentanil
- Regional anesthesia is acceptable: peripheral blocks, spinal, epidural, caudal
- Muscle relaxants including succinylcholine are acceptable.

Emergence/Postoperative Care

- Smooth emergence to avoid airway and skin trauma
- Suction gently when needed with lubricated suction catheter.
- Awake extubation to minimize airway obstruction and need for mask pressure
- Appropriate analgesia with avoidance of histamine-releasing medications
- Care for new skin lesions
- Preemptively treat postoperative nausea and vomiting.
- Monitor for airway compromise.

induction. Due to difficulties in establishing venous access, anesthesia is usually induced by mask with inhalational anesthetics. The **anesthesia mask** is **lubricated** with Aquaphor® or similar ointment to minimize skin trauma and must be handled gently. Using another approach, nonadhesive dressings (Mepilex®) may be placed on the face where the anesthesia mask and the anesthetist's hands contact the face. Alternately, a peripheral IV line may be placed in an awake patient for IV induction of anesthesia.

The tourniquet is placed gently over layers of gauze. IV lines are secured with a nonadhesive dressing (Mepitel® or Mepitac®) and then wrapped gently with gauze and Coflex® wrap. Gentle laryngoscopy with a lubricated blade is important to minimize oral trauma. The ETT is secured with cotton ties secured loosely behind the neck. The eyes should be lubricated with eye lubricant containing no lanolin, closed, and covered with saline-moistened gauze pads or nonadhesive tape. *No adhesive tape* of any kind may be used (Figs. 65.1a and 65.1b).

Extreme skin fragility poses challenges to the use of routine anesthesia monitors. A **clip pulse oximeter probe** is preferable to adhesive-style probes. The blood pressure cuff is applied over several layers of cotton gauze wrapped around the extremity. Electrocardiogram leads, if used, must have the adhesive portions removed and are secured to the patient with gauze or other non-adhesive wraps. A precordial stethoscope may simply be placed on the chest without adhesive.

Muscle relaxants may help facilitate intubation after adequate mask ventilation is demonstrated, and antiemetics are

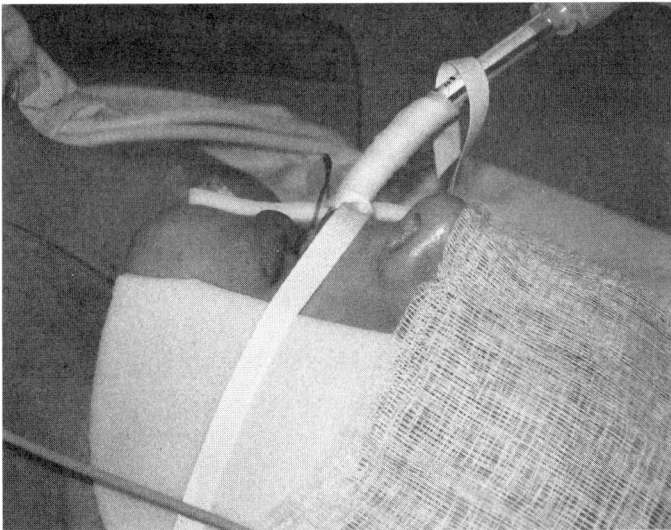

FIGURE 65.1a Airway secured without adhesives, eyes protected with moist gauze.

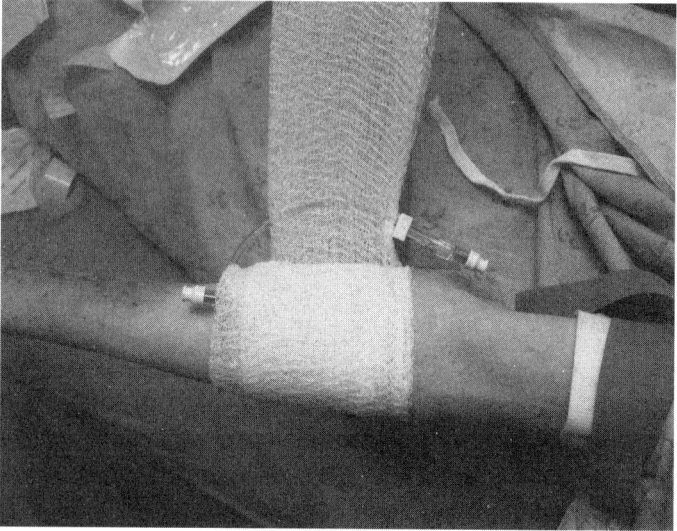

FIGURE 65.1b Peripheral venous catheter, secured without adhesives.

given to prevent postoperative nausea and vomiting. Medications that cause histamine release should be avoided to decrease the risk of postoperative pruritus. Although **awake extubation** at the conclusion of the procedure may be associated with coughing and patient movement, it minimizes the risk of aspiration and the need for continued mask pressure to the face after extubation. Although there is a risk of **postoperative airway obstruction from bullae formation**, significant airway obstruction in the recovery period is uncommon. After a period of close observation, many patients may be discharged home the same day.

5. **What supplies are necessary?**
   - Nonadhesive dressing: e.g. Mepitel®, Mepiform®, Mepilex®, Mepitac tape® (Molnlycke Healthcare, Goteburg, Sweden, www.molnlycke.com) or Vaseline gauze/Telfa®
   - Nonadhesive wrap: e.g. Coflex® (Andover) wrap or Coban® (3M), Kling® (J&J), Webril® (Kendall)

- Methylcellulose eye lubricant
- Cotton tape to secure the ETT
- Aquaphor® ointment (or similar) to lubricate anesthesia mask, water-based lubricant (e.g. Surgilube®) to lubricate oral airways and laryngoscope blade
- Clip pulse oximeter probe
- Silicone-based adhesive remover

SUMMARY

1. EB is a genetically determined, blistering disorder that affects multiple organ systems and can have profound effects on anesthetic care.
2. OR preparation must account for delicate positioning and movement of the patient, as well as difficult airway and IV access.
3. Intraoperative monitoring needs modest adjustments to be done safely, and postoperative pain management may proceed as for other patients.

ANNOTATED REFERENCES

- Bissonnette B. Epidermolysis bullosa. In Bissonnette B, ed. *Syndromes: Rapid Recognition and Perioperative Implications*. New York: McGraw-Hill, 2006: 272–275.

  An excellent overview of the disease and perioperative anesthetic management.
- Herod J, Denyer J, Goldman A, Howard R. Epidermolysis bullosa in children: pathophysiology, anaesthesia and pain management. *Paediatr Anaesth* 2002; 12: 388–397.

  This comprehensive review article provides a multidisciplinary approach to EB management with an overview of pathophysiology, complications, and practical recommendations for anesthetic care.

Further Reading

Ames WA, Mayou BJ, Williams K. Anaesthetic management of epidermolysis bullosa. *Br J Anaesth* 1999; 82: 746–751.

Azizkhan RG, Stehra W, Cohen AP, Wittkugel E, Farrell MK, Lucky AW, Hammelmane BD, Johnson ND, Racadio JM. Esophageal strictures in children with recessive dystrophic epidermolysis bullosa: an 11-year experience with fluoroscopically guided balloon dilation. *J Pediatr Surg* 2006; 41(1): 55–60.

Baum VC, O'Flaherty JE. Epidermolysis bullosa. In *Anesthesia for Genetic, Metabolic and Dysmorphic Syndromes of Childhood*. Philadelphia: Lippincott Williams & Wilkins, 2007: 122–124.

Goldschneider KR, Lucky AW, Mellerio JE, Palisson F, Vinuela Miranda MDC, Azizkhan RG. Perioperative care of patients with epidermolysis bullosa: proceedings of the 5th International Symposium on Epidermolysis Bullosa, Santiago, Chile, Dec. 4–6, 2008. *Pediatr Anesth* 2010; 20: 797–804.

Iohom G, Lyons B. Anaesthesia for children with epidermolysis bullosa: a review of 20 years' experience. *Eur J Anaesthesiol* 2001; 18: 745–754.

Mellerio JE, Weiner M, Denyer JE, Pillay EI, Lucky AW, Bruckner A, Palisson F. Medical management of epidermolysis bullosa: Proceedings of the IInd International Symposium on Epidermolysis Bullosa, Santiago, Chile, 2005. *Int J Dermatol* 2007; 46(8): 795–800.

Spielman F, Mann E. Subarachnoid and epidural anesthesia for patients with epidermolysis bullosa. *Can Anaes Soc J* 1984; 31(5): 549–551.

66

Osteogenesis Imperfecta

MARIO PATINO AND ANNA M. VARUGHESE

INTRODUCTION

Osteogenesis imperfecta (OI) is a heterogeneous inherited disorder of type I collagen. Although it is most commonly known for the "brittle bones" that lead to multiple and recurrent fractures, OI has manifestations in other tissues where type I collagen is present. Moreover, the brain stem, cervical spine, and lungs can be affected indirectly due to the resultant bone abnormalities. A pre-anesthetic evaluation must review all systems and specific anesthetic considerations are necessary to reduce complications and improve outcomes of patients with OI.

LEARNING OBJECTIVES

1. Recognize the most common clinical manifestations of OI.
2. Differentiate the types of OI.
3. Identify the important anesthetic issues during the preoperative evaluation of a patient with OI.
4. Develop a specific plan for the perioperative care of a patient with OI to minimize complications and improve outcomes.

CASE PRESENTATION

*An 8-year-old, 17-kg girl is undergoing bilateral femoral osteotomies and intramedullary rod placement to correct severe, bilateral bowing of the femurs due to type III OI. She has had multiple procedures in the past secondary to **fractures of long bones**, as well as an anterior and posterior thoracolumbar spinal fusion to correct severe scoliosis. She is currently receiving intravenous pamidronate to enhance bone density. The patient has a **history of** a poor glottic exposure leading to **difficult intubation**, requiring fiberoptic intubation. She had progressive **restrictive lung disease** secondary to scoliosis. However, after the anterior and posterior spinal fusion her respiratory status has stabilized. She has bilateral **hearing loss**. There is no history of abnormal bleeding, although her parents report she received two units of blood during her spinal fusion. The parents are concerned about the use of a blood pressure cuff because she has had previous fractures from noninvasive blood pressure monitoring. Her physical exam is notable for short stature, a cast on her right arm, **limited mouth opening**, severe restriction of neck mobility, 60-degree **scoliosis with thoracic cage deformity**, and femoral bowing. Preoperative complete blood count, renal panel, PT, and PTT are normal.*

*In the operating room, the patient is moved with extreme care to the operating room table to avoid any further injuries. Standard monitors are applied with a well-padded blood pressure cuff placed on the left upper extremity, which is set to cycle every 10 minutes. An inhalation induction is performed with nitrous oxide, oxygen, and sevoflurane. Two 22-gauge IV catheters are placed for access in the left arm. A **fiberoptic intubation** with a 4.5 cuffed endotracheal tube is performed. The patient is positioned with the upper extremities well padded. During the procedure, the surgeon complains of excessive oozing at the surgical site. A type and screen is sent and one unit of blood is requested. Two hours after the start of the procedure, the estimated blood loss is 500 mL, the systolic BP is 60 mmHg, and hematocrit is 20%. One unit of packed red blood cells is transfused intraoperatively. The patient's condition stabilizes, with a final hematocrit of 27%. At the end of the procedure the patient is extubated* *awake and an IV patient-controlled analgesia (PCA) pump with morphine is started. Once in the post-anesthesia care unit (PACU), the patient complains of pain in the left upper extremity where the blood pressure cuff was placed. A recent left humeral fracture is noted on x-ray and a cast is placed on this extremity. The patient is discharged on the third postoperative day.*

DISCUSSION

1. What is OI?

OI is a heterogeneous inherited disorder of type I collagen. Collagen, the most abundant protein in the human body, is the main protein in connective tissue and is also an important component of osteoid (the organic matrix that helps to form bone). The structure of collagen is formed by three polypeptide chains, two alpha-1 and one alpha-2, that form a triple helix structure. Alteration in type I collagen leads to a connective tissue disorder with osteopenia. Type I collagen is found in bone, skin, tendon, sclera, ears, teeth, chordae tendinae, blood vessels, and scar tissue. Two genes are involved in the synthesis of type I collagen: COL1A1 and COL1A2. The most common cause of OI is an inherited mutation on one of these genes that codify the information to synthesize collagen type I. Less commonly, a spontaneous mutation can cause the disease. In the most severe forms, the mutation leads to an abnormal synthesis of polypeptide chains that are unable to form the characteristic triple helix of the collagen and are enzymatically degraded. In the less severe forms, the mutation leads to a decreased synthesis of type I collagen but the protein is normal.

OI was originally classified into four types according to the clinical characteristics manifested (Table 66.1), although a more recent classification includes up to eight genetic types.

Type I is the most common and mildest form, with an incidence of 1 in 30,000 live births (Benca et al., 2009; Karabiyik et al., 2004). These patients have normal type I collagen but it is

		Table 66.1	
		MAJOR TYPES OF OSTEOGENESIS IMPERFECTA	
OI Type	*Inheritance*	*Manifestations*	*Life Span*
I	Autosomal dominant	Fragile bones, blue sclera, hearing impairment, normal stature	Normal
II	Autosomal dominant, sporadic new mutations	Intrauterine fractures, pulmonary function and swallowing compromised from birth	Lethal as neonate
III	Autosomal dominant, sporadic new mutations	Fragile bones, progressive bowing of long bones, short stature, kyphoscoliosis, poor dentition, triangular facies	Decreased
IV	Autosomal dominant	Moderate skeletal fragility, short stature, early blue sclera becoming white with age, dental involvement variable	Normal

present in low quantities. Type I is usually a nondeforming type of OI and the patient's susceptibility to fractures decreases after puberty. Type III is the most severe of the nonlethal forms. It is associated with severe deformities due to the **multiple fractures** that occur with minimal stress, growth retardation, **kyphoscoliosis, hearing impairment**, and abnormal dentition. Kyphoscoliosis is due to vertebral compression fractures, spondylolisthesis, and ligament instability. Ocular manifestations include a thin cornea and a thin, blue-appearing sclera. The life span is decreased to the second to fourth decade of life. The most common cause of death is respiratory failure secondary to **thoracic cage deformities** and scoliosis.

2. Why does this patient have a difficult airway, and is this common in patients with OI?

Patients with the most severe form of OI have a greater incidence of airway abnormalities, and this can make airway management difficult. In this patient, previous facial and mandibular fractures limit the mouth opening, and remodeled bone as a result of previous cervical fractures may restrict neck flexion and extension. Mask ventilation must be gentle since new facial and mandibular fractures can occur. Positioning can be challenging in patients with severe kyphoscoliosis and can make intubation even more difficult. Neck movement during direct laryngoscopy must be limited because excessive cervical extension can lead to cervical fractures and spinal cord injury. Abnormal dentition is also commonly present in many patients with OI; therefore, a dental guard can be used during the perioperative period to protect the teeth from injury. **Fiberoptic intubation** is often a prudent choice. In case of a difficult airway, a laryngeal mask airway can be a useful alternative to intubation.

3. What other considerations are important in the preoperative evaluation of patients with OI?

During the preoperative evaluation, it is important to *include the caregivers* in the discussion. They care for these patients on a daily basis and can make suggestions as to the *handling and positioning* of the patient in order to minimize the risk of fractures. Questions regarding the kind of forces that have induced fractures in the past can be helpful in avoiding similar injuries. It is important during the preoperative evaluation to document both previous and recent fractures.

Varying degrees of **restrictive lung disease** due to the kyphoscoliosis and chest wall abnormalities can be seen in these patients. It is important to evaluate the respiratory status preoperatively, including a history of an oxygen requirement, spirometry findings, and evaluations by pulmonary medicine.

Patients with OI can also have cardiovascular abnormalities. Associated cardiac anomalies such as atrial septal defects, ventricular septal defects, and valvular anomalies have been found. Alterations in the chordae tendinae due to abnormal collagen type I can lead to aortic insufficiency (the most common manifestation), mitral valve prolapse, and mitral insufficiency. As with other disorders of the connective tissue, some degree of aortic dilation can be present. These cardiovascular abnormalities usually occur during the second to fourth decades of life. In patients with thoracic cage deformities, there is a risk of cor pulmonale. A preoperative echocardiogram is indicated in patients with suspected associated cardiac anomalies and thoracic cage deformities and after the second decade of life (Stynowick et al., 2007).

Central nervous system manifestations are usually due to effects of the abnormal bone formation. Brain stem compression can occur due to invagination of the cervical spine into the foramen magnum as result of abnormalities of the clivus and the occipital bone. This usually occurs after the first decade of life. OI patients should be evaluated for signs and symptoms of upper cervical cord compression, such as arm pain and paresthesias with neck movement, progressive weakness of the extremities, and bowel and bladder dysfunction. These patients are susceptible to develop atlanto-axial instability and hydrocephalus due to bone abnormalities that can obstruct the normal flow of cerebrospinal fluid.

Bleeding abnormalities occur in 10% to 30% of patients with OI due to alterations in type I collagen present in blood vessels that result in problems with platelet adhesion, aggregation, and blood vessel constriction. Routine coagulation studies are usually normal (Stynowick et al., 2007; Keegan et al., 2002).

4. What are the intraoperative considerations and potential pitfalls for patients with OI?

When there is a history of previous fractures with the use of a blood pressure cuff, it is desirable to minimize the use of a cuff. An arterial line placement after induction, avoiding excessive extension on the wrist, is an alternative to noninvasive blood pressure monitoring. Preoperative evaluation should include a discussion with parents about the risks and benefits of invasive versus noninvasive blood pressure measurement. The placement of tourniquets for hemostasis can result in fractures and should be used with caution. OI is an absolute contraindication for the placement of intraosseous needles for vascular access, barring lack of alternatives in a life-threatening emergency.

In this case scenario, a detailed history regarding the severity of bleeding should have been elicited to identify the need for a type and cross-match preoperatively. Desmopressin and factor VII have been used for excessive bleeding with improvement of the coagulation status. Given the platelet dysfunction found in OI patients, NSAIDs should only be used with caution. If NSAID therapy is used, cyclooxygenase-2 selective inhibitors may be preferable in the perioperative period because they have less platelet inhibition.

Another common phenomenon in patients with OI is a hypermetabolic state with increased temperature and metabolic acidosis. This phenomenon is not related to malignant hyperthermia (MH). Respiratory acidosis and muscle rigidity are not present. The hyperthermia usually responds well to a cooling blanket. OI patients are not considered at higher risk for MH than the general population. Anticholinergics should be used cautiously since they can interfere with heat dissipation and thereby contribute to fever. Succinylcholine is relatively contraindicated because muscle fasciculations can induce bone fractures.

Fragile skin is common in patients with OI, and careful positioning with appropriate padding is critical to avoiding injury. Positioning and movement of the patient should be done extremely gently since injuries to the ligaments and tendons as well as fractures can occur. Type I collagen is also present in scar tissue, and delayed wound healing can occur.

Emergence from anesthesia has to be controlled since coughing, bucking, and a restless patient can lead to multiple fractures. Because communication can be limited due to hearing impairment, it is important to plan ahead so that effective communication with the child can occur in the PACU, allowing for a calmer emergence.

5. What is the role for regional anesthesia in OI patients?
Regional anesthesia has been used in patients with OI to provide intraoperative and postoperative analgesia. However, patients with OI, especially those with bleeding abnormalities, may have a higher risk of an epidural hematoma. Also, positioning for regional anesthesia can be a challenge and can lead to new fractures. Needle puncture can also injure abnormal bone and predispose to vertebral fractures. If regional anesthesia is considered, a peripheral nerve block or a single-shot caudal would seem to have less overall risk of complications than the placement of an epidural catheter.

SUMMARY

1. OI is a collagen deficiency that results in bone weakness. It can compromise multiple organ systems, which must, therefore, be carefully managed throughout the perioperative period.
2. Airway management can be difficult, due to both inherent airway issues and restriction on manipulation of the head and cervical spine
3. Bleeding risk can be elevated and hard to predict. Careful observation is required.

ANNOTATED REFERENCES

• Baum VC, O'Flaherty JE. Osteogenesis imperfecta. In *Anesthesia for Genetic, Metabolic and Dysmorphic Syndromes of Childhood*, 2nd ed. Philadelphia: Lippincott Williams & Wilkins, 2007: 283–285.

This chapter about OI is in an outstanding textbook that offers concise and practical recommendations for the anesthetic management of many different pediatric disorders.

- **Benca J, Hogan K. Malignant hyperthermia, coexisting disorders and enzymopathies: risks and management options.** *Anesth Analg* 2009; 109: 1049–1053.

  A review article about the association (or lack thereof) of different disorders with MH.

- **Stynowick GA, Tobias JD. Perioperative care of the patient with osteogenesis imperfecta.** *Orthopedics* 2007; 30: 1043–1049.

  An excellent review of the perioperative care of patients with OI.

Further Reading

Cunliffe M, Sarginson R. Osteogenesis imperfecta. In Bissonnete B, Dalens B, eds. *Pediatric Anesthesia: Principles and Practice*. New York: McGraw-Hill, 2002: 1096.

Ghert M, Allen B, Davids J, Stasikelis P, Nicholas D. Increased postoperative febrile response in children with osteogenesis imperfecta. *J Pediatr Orthop* 2003; 23: 261–264.

Karabiyik L, Capan Z. Osteogenesis imperfecta: different anaesthetic approaches to two paediatric cases. *Pediatr Anesth* 2004; 14: 524–525.

Kastrup M, von Heymann C, Hotz H, Konertz WF, Ziemer S, Kox WJ, Spies C. Recombinant factor VIIa after aortic valve replacement in a patient with osteogenesis imperfecta. *Ann Thorac Surg* 2002; 74: 910–912.

Keegan M, Whatcott B, Harrison B. Osteogenesis imperfecta, perioperative bleeding and desmopressin. *Anesthesiology* 2002; 97: 1011–1013.

Porsborg P, Astrup G, Bendixen D, Lund AM, Ording H. Osteogenesis imperfecta and malignant hyperthermia: Is there a relationship? *Anaesthesia* 1996; 51: 863–865.

Tetzlaff J. Osteogenesis imperfecta. In Fleisher L, ed. *Anesthesia and Uncommon Diseases*. Philadelphia: Elsevier, 2005: 341–343.

67

Cerebral Palsy

GEORGE CHALKIADIS

INTRODUCTION

Cerebral palsy (CP) is the most common cause of childhood disability. Children with CP have a number of problems, resulting in frequent need for surgery and anesthesia. They present a series of added challenges to the anesthetist that may have an impact on perioperative anesthesia and pain management. Theses include spasticity and other movement disorders, cognitive impairment, seizure management, behavioral disturbances, malnutrition, and difficulties in communication and swallowing. An understanding of these issues will help the anesthetist formulate a management plan that is tailored to the individual child's needs.

LEARNING OBJECTIVES

1. Know what to look for in the preoperative assessment of a child with CP presenting for surgery.
2. Appreciate the anesthetic issues in a child with CP.
3. Know the issues in providing postoperative analgesia to children with CP.

CASE PRESENTATION

*A 12-year-old **nonverbal** boy with **spastic quadriplegic** CP presents for single-event multilevel orthopedic surgery that will include bilateral femoral derotational osteotomies and hamstring and calf lengthening. He takes topiramate for **seizure** management, omeprazole for **gastroesophageal reflux**, and baclofen for management of spasticity via a percutaneous gastrostomy. He is thin and has contractures of his knees and elbows. His parents are uncertain of his level of understanding, but he looks at people when they are speaking to him. The parents mention that he took a **long time to wake** following anesthesia for a magnetic resonance imaging scan recently. They have questions about how he will be kept comfortable after surgery and how nurses will **assess** his **pain**.*

DISCUSSION

1. **What is CP?**

CP is the most common cause of childhood disability, occurring in 2 to 3 per 1,000 live births in developed countries. It is a non-progressive disorder of motion and posture that results from damage to the central nervous system that may have occurred antenatally, perinatally, or postnatally during the period of early brain growth and development. The motor disorder is often manifest by spasticity and contractures that lead to a progressive deformity that can be treated with orthopedic surgery. Depending on the extent of the initial brain insult, other disabilities may coexist, including sensory loss (hearing and vision), seizures, communication and behavioral disturbances, cognitive impairment, and intellectual disability. The likelihood of such deficits and associated disabilities is increased in those with a greater degree of spasticity involving a greater number of limbs.

The clinical picture of CP, unlike the cerebral lesion, evolves over time. In its mildest form only mild spastic monoplegia or diplegia may be evident. At its most severe, in addition to the problems listed above, **gastroesophageal reflux** and bulbar palsy may predispose to recurrent aspiration, and over time scoliosis may develop.

2. **What are specific functional conditions to look for preoperatively?**

Previous anesthesia issues: Severely affected children with CP often have **prolonged emergence** from anesthesia, as in this scenario. Delayed emergence may be even more likely in the setting of major surgery, hypothermia, and the administration of opioid analgesia or clonidine.

Seizures: It is important to ask if the child has had **seizures**, if they are still occurring, and if they are well managed. In this case, the child is on anticonvulsant therapy. The parents should be instructed to administer his usual dose of topiramate on the morning of surgery. Postoperatively, the usual dose of topiramate should be prescribed. It is also prudent to have a plan for what anticonvulsant to administer and by which route should the child experience protracted postoperative nausea and vomiting.

Cognitive impairment and intellectual disability: It may be difficult to ascertain a child's **ability to understand** what is said to him or her and the child's ability to take in what is happening around him or her. Although in this case the child attends to people when spoken to, a lack of eye contact may be due to cortical blindness. One should always assume that the child does have some capacity to understand. Addressing the child by name and explaining things to him or her is often appreciated by the parents, and possibly even more so by the child. It is also important to ask the parents how they might know if their child is experiencing pain. **Pain assessment** in children with cognitive impairment may be difficult, and having an idea of the child's usual behavior and sleep pattern is helpful. A parent is often the best-placed person to distinguish between pain and other causes of distress.

Spasticity: Children with severe **spasticity** may startle easily. In this case, it is important to approach them gently and quietly to avoid this. They may also be on treatment to reduce spasticity, such as in this case, where the child is receiving **baclofen**. It is important to continue this medication in the perioperative period, as baclofen withdrawal can be severe, even fatal. Other oral antispasticity medications include diazepam, dantrolene, and tizanidine. Parents sometimes forget to mention that their child is receiving continuous intrathecal (IT) baclofen. Presence of an IT catheter is a relative contraindication to an epidural; contaminating or severing the IT catheter would be disastrous.

Gastroesophageal reflux and swallowing problems and aspiration: By the age of 12 years, most children with significant reflux and swallowing problems secondary to bulbar palsy will have undergone fundoplication and will be fed via gastrostomy, as in this case. It is important to ask if the child has a history of recurrent chest infections; this may indicate that he or she is experiencing silent or overt recurrent aspiration.

Temperature: Parents of children with severe CP often describe that their child has cold extremities. These children are more likely to be hypothermic intraoperatively.

3. What are key physical traits of CP to look for preoperatively?

Microcephaly: This condition reflects the severity of the cerebral insult. These children are likely to have more disability and sensitivity to anesthesia. Intraoperative hypothermia and prolonged emergence from anesthesia are more common in this group.

Contractures: There may be fixed contractures that may make positioning on the operating table difficult. In this case it may be problematic placing his arms securely and safely away from the surgical field, particularly as good access to his hips will be needed when performing femoral osteotomies.

Nutritional status: Children with severe CP are often thin and malnourished. They may have osteopenia that predisposes them to pathological fractures. Careful and gentle handling is required in the operating room.

Scoliosis: Older children with severe CP often develop scoliosis, which can restrict pulmonary function and make it difficult to insert an epidural catheter.

Venous access: Contractures and relative dehydration sometimes make venous access difficult to find. Inhalational induction of anesthesia may be preferable in this instance to avoid multiple attempts at venous cannulation.

4. What are intraoperative considerations?

Hypothermia: Children with CP undergoing single-event multi-level surgery are prone to hypothermia. This is contributed to by many factors, including temperature dysregulation, the child's nutritional status, exposure of the child prior to surgery for epidural and urinary catheter insertion, and extensive exposure and prepping for surgery. Warm intravenous fluids and a forced-air warmer should also be used, but these are often insufficient to warm the child once hypothermic. There is anecdotal evidence that preoperative warming of the child reduces the degree of hypothermia that occurs.

Logistical issues: Inserting intravenous cannulas in the mid-forearm allows this to be used as a natural splint. This facilitates wrist and elbow movement if contractures are not present. Careful positioning, pressure area care, and transfers are required due to contractures, thinness of the child, and osteopenia. Children undergoing bilateral derotational femoral osteotomies often require blood transfusion either during or after surgery. Blood should be available for transfusion if required.

Maintenance of anesthesia: There is evidence to suggest that **nonverbal** children with CP and cognitive impairment require less propofol than normal children to obtain similar bispectral index values. Children with CP and intellectual disability also seem to have lower minimum alveolar concentration values for halothane compared to normal children.

Analgesia: While children with CP seem to receive less intra-operative opioid analgesia than normal children (e.g., Long et al., 2009), there is no evidence to suggest that their analgesic requirements are less. The most effective analgesia is achieved using epidural analgesia. In this case the dermatomes to be covered are T12–S2. It is often difficult to achieve good analgesia bilaterally over this extent. The most painful parts of the planned surgery for this case are the femoral osteotomies, and hence careful consideration should be given to achieving good analgesia to cover the dermatomes for the osteotomies (T12–L2). The epidural catheter should thus be inserted at L1-2 or L2-3.

Given the **difficulty in assessing** children with CP, it is important to assess the functionality of an epidural intraoperatively so that a catheter of doubtful function can be replaced or repositioned prior to emergence. The epidural catheter should be inserted and the block established prior to incision in the anesthetized child. Increases in heart rate or blood pressure in response to surgery suggest that the epidural block is inadequate. If the epidural block remains inadequate after a further bolus of local anesthetic agent, an epidurogram can be performed to visualize the nature of the problem. The catheter can be pulled back if inserted too far or replaced, depending on the results. Should there be persistent doubt regarding the effectiveness of the epidural, plans should be made for alternate analgesic treatment.

5. What are postoperative considerations?
The most common problem after orthopedic surgery is painful muscle spasm, which may occur even in the mildest CP cases. This is a result of postoperative pain and is most likely an exaggerated reflex response to postoperative pain that is secondary to pre-existing spasticity.

Muscle spasm can often be observed and results in sudden, severe, and prolonged distress, often described as coming in waves. Muscle spasm can often be avoided in the early postoperative phase by optimizing epidural analgesia. No pain usually means no spasm. Liberal use of antispasticity agents may also be needed. Oral diazepam should be given as required. Intravenous diazepam should be available until the patient is ready for enteral medication. It is important to think ahead and include this in the postoperative drug prescription to facilitate timely administration. Although he presents on a baseline dose of baclofen, the child in this scenario should still have diazepam as required for breakthrough spasm. In children with an IT baclofen pump *in situ*, consideration should be given to increasing the rate of baclofen infusion in the postoperative period.

Patients with CP can benefit from the same range of adjunct medications as other patients. Patient-controlled analgesia may have to be carried out by trained nurses or well-educated parents, and opioid or ketamine infusions, nonsteroidal anti-inflammatory agents, and acetaminophen can be used as well. Tramadol can also be used if there is no history of seizures. Neuropathic pain should be sought following multilevel surgery if there are difficulties in achieving adequate postoperative analgesia (Lauder & White, 2005). Allodynia is often a giveaway sign. Neuropathic pain is often the result of a nerve stretch injury, which is more likely to occur after soft tissue surgery such as hamstring lengthening, particularly when knee contractures were present preoperatively.

Postoperative epidural care should include inspection of the insertion site, pressure areas (sacrum and heels), and checks of the dermatomes covered during each nursing shift. In the **nonverbal** child, pressure over the osteotomy wounds and the child's reaction to the application of ice over the relevant dermatomes can help establish if the extent of epidural block is adequate. Postoperative fever is common for up to 48 hours after major orthopedic surgery. If the epidural infusion is providing adequate analgesia and there are no signs of epidural infection at the insertion site (redness, pus, or tenderness), the benefits of maintaining epidural analgesia in this situation outweigh the risks or effects of premature removal. Postoperative epidural analgesia is maintained for 48 to 96 hours.

Adequate discharge analgesia must be prescribed. Diazepam is often necessary following discharge because muscle spasms remain troublesome for some time. Constipation is often problematic in these children, and hence aperients should also be prescribed, particularly if opioid analgesia is prescribed.

SUMMARY

1. Preoperative assessment issues in these patients include seizures, cognitive impairment, intellectual disability, microcephaly, spasticity and its management, venous access, gastroesophageal reflux, swallowing difficulties, temperature dysregulation, contractures, nutritional status, and scoliosis.
2. Anesthetic issues include hypothermia, difficult intravenous cannulation, positioning and transfers, potential for reduced anesthetic agent, epidural analgesia, and blood loss.
3. Postoperative issues include analgesia, muscle spasm, fever, and neuropathic pain.

ANNOTATED REFERENCES

- Lauder GR, White MC. Neuropathic pain following multilevel surgery in children with cerebral palsy: a case series and review. *Pediatr Anesth* 2005; 15: 412–420.

This case series describes six children who experienced neuropathic pain following multilevel surgery and includes a comprehensive review of potential etiology and treatment options.

- Nolan J, Chalkiadis GA, Low J, Olesch C, Brown TCK. Anaesthesia and pain management in cerebral palsy. *Anaesthesia* 2000; 55: 32–41.

This comprehensive review article highlights the etiology, one classification, and the anesthetic implications for children with CP and their management. It includes pain assessment and the management of chronic pain problems in this patient population.

Further Reading

Frei FJ, Haemmerle MH, Brunner R, Kern C. Minimum alveolar concentration for halothane in children with cerebral palsy and severe mental retardation. *Anaesthesia* 1997; 52: 1056–1060.

Long LS, Ved S, Koh JL. Intraoperative opioid dosing in children with and without cerebral palsy. *Pediatr Anesth* 2009; 19: 513–520.

Saricaoglu F, Celebi N, Celik M, Aypar U. The evaluation of propofol dosage for anesthesia induction in children with cerebral palsy with bispectral index (BIS) monitoring. *Pediatr Anesth* 2005; 15: 1048–1052.

PART 14

CHALLENGES IN THE

POST-ANESTHESIA CARE UNIT

68

Emergence Agitation

CHARLES B. EASTWOOD AND
PAUL J. SAMUELS

INTRODUCTION

Emergence delirium is a common and challenging post-anesthetic complication in children characterized by a brief period of inconsolability, disorientation, and combativeness. Emergence delirium threatens patient safety due to potential self-injurious behavior or by untimely removal of intravenous lines, urinary catheters, and surgical drains. The economic impact of emergence delirium is a consequence of delayed post-anesthesia care unit (PACU) discharge and the need for additional medication administration and increased PACU staffing. In addition, despite the short duration of emergence delirium, its dramatic and frightening presentation can diminish parental satisfaction. Although no consistently effective treatment for emergence delirium has been described, familiarity with this clinical entity and approaches to its management and prevention are important to those who provide pediatric anesthesia care. This chapter will focus on our present understanding of emergence delirium in children.

LEARNING OBJECTIVES

1. Review the characteristics, incidence, and risk factors for emergence delirium.
2. Identify anesthetic plans that may affect the incidence of emergence delirium.
3. Discuss management of emergence delirium.

CASE PRESENTATION

An otherwise healthy **4-year-old** boy presents for myringotomy with pressure-equalization tubes for recurrent otitis media. He is on preventive antibiotics and has been asymptomatic for several weeks. He has no allergies and has had **no previous surgery**. His physical examination is unremarkable.

Anesthesia is induced via mask inhalation with **sevoflurane** in 60% nitrous oxide/40% oxygen. Following induction, rectal acetaminophen (paracetamol) (40 mg/kg) is administered and the fraction of inhaled sevoflurane is reduced to 3%. Anesthesia is administered throughout the procedure via mask. No intravenous access is obtained, given the brevity of the surgical procedure.

Shortly after arrival in the PACU, the patient emerges from anesthesia **crying**, **thrashing**, and **confused**. Two nurses and his mother are required to restrain his flailing arms and legs and hold him in his bed. He **does not seem to recognize his mother** and appears very **frightened**, screaming over and over, "No! No! No!"

After 10 minutes he begins to calm down. Twenty minutes later he is alert, cradled in his mother's arms, and requesting a red Popsicle. Within an hour, he has met PACU discharge criteria and shortly thereafter leaves the hospital with his mother.

DISCUSSION

1. How does emergence delirium present?

Emergence delirium occurs following a general anesthetic and is characterized by **wild or poorly controlled motor activity and disorientation**, and an altered response to individuals, stimuli, or comfort measures. These behaviors are unrelated to pain but may be difficult to differentiate from pain. The phenomenon is also known as "emergence agitation." Emergence delirium is typically observed within 30 minutes of emergence from general anesthesia. Episodes last an average of 5 to 15 minutes, though rarely they may be more prolonged. In the pediatric population, emergence delirium is a common perioperative complication, occurring after 10% to 50% of general anesthetics (Vlajkovic & Sindjelic, 2007).

Emergence delirium was first described in the early 1960s following exposure to ether or cyclopropane. From the 1960s to the early 1990s, when halothane and isoflurane were the predominant vapor anesthetics used in pediatrics, emergence delirium was seldom reported in the anesthesia literature. Renewed interest in emergence delirium occurred in the late 1990s, when **sevoflurane** and desflurane were introduced into anesthesiology practice and clinicians began to observe emergence delirium with greater frequency.

2. What causes emergence delirium?

The etiology of emergence delirium is poorly understood. Inadequate analgesia may result in many of the behaviors associated with emergence delirium. However, pain and emergence delirium are distinct entities, reflected by the observation that patients who have complete local anesthetic-induced sensory blockade of their surgical sites, or have undergone nonpainful procedures such as MRIs, are also susceptible to emergence delirium. Preoperative patient anxiety has been inconsistently associated with the development of emergence delirium. A recent study in rats exposed to sevoflurane demonstrated increased norepinephrine concentrations in the locus ceruleus, a neural structure responsible for generalized CNS arousal (Yasui et al., 2007). Further work will determine if this finding represents a possible cellular mechanism underlying the excitation seen in emergence delirium.

Sevoflurane and desflurane are commonly believed to result in emergence delirium more frequently than halothane or isoflurane due to their lower blood-gas solubility coefficients and associated rapid emergence. However, studies comparing rates of emergence delirium in children have not conclusively demonstrated one volatile anesthetic causing more emergence delirium than another. Halothane is no longer commercially available in the United States, and arguments comparing contemporary anesthetic agents to halothane are no longer clinically relevant.

3. How can emergence delirium be identified?

The dramatic presentation of emergence delirium can be difficult to differentiate from other common pediatric PACU behaviors secondary to pain, fear, anxiety, or anger. A variety of scales have been described in the literature to measure emergence delirium in children, but they lack appropriate psychometric power to accurately distinguish emergence delirium from other similar entities. To address this gap, Sikich and Lerman published the Pediatric Anesthesia Emergence Delirium (PAED) scale (Table 68.1) in 2004, and confirmed its reliability and validity (Sikich & Lerman, 2004). While the scale assists in measuring the severity of emergence delirium, it does not clearly differentiate between its presence or absence, nor does it indicate when intervention should occur.

Table 68.1
PEDIATRIC ANESTHESIA EMERGENCE DELIRIUM (PAED) SCALE

1. The child makes eye contact with the caregiver. 2. The child's actions are purposeful. 3. The child is aware of his/her surroundings.	4 = not at all 3 = just a little 2 = quite a bit 1 = very much 0 = extremely
1. The child is restless. 2. The child is inconsolable.	0 = not at all 1 = just a little 2 = quite a bit 3 = very much 4 = extremely

Maximum total score = 20.

4. What are the risk factors for emergence delirium?

There are many potential risk factors for emergence delirium. These include pain, rapid awakening from anesthesia, inhalational anesthetics, **preschool age**, **lack of previous surgery**, poor adaptability, preoperative anxiety, and head and neck surgery. Unfortunately, many studies contradict one another, an observation that may be due to study design or differences in power (Vlajkovic & Sindjelic, 2007). The most powerful predictor of emergence delirium seems to be a short time to emergence from anesthesia (Voepel-Lewis et al., 2003).

5. How can emergence delirium be prevented?

While no single anesthetic technique has eliminated emergence delirium, many options have been suggested to reduce the chance that a child will get emergence delirium. For children who appear to be at high risk, one can consider relying on anesthetic agents associated with slower emergence, or using a variety of other medications, including opioids, benzodiazepines, boluses and infusions of propofol, alpha-agonists, and NMDA receptor antagonists such as ketamine.

In considering the options, one should bear in mind that cumulative data suggest that administration of benzodiazepines and 5HT-3 receptor antagonists (such as ondansetron) at any point in the perioperative period does not alter the risk of developing emergence delirium. Conversely, intraoperative administration of ketamine, α-agonists, or intranasal fentanyl reduces the incidence of emergence delirium. Oddly, intravenous fentanyl seems to increase the incidence of emergence delirium (Dahmani et al., 2010). Propofol, given as an intraoperative infusion or as a bolus at the end of a surgical case, is protective but bolus administration at the beginning of an operation is not. Both intravenous and epidural administration of clonidine are associated with a lower frequency of emergence delirium. Dexmedetomidine, a highly selective alpha-2 agonist with sedative and analgesic properties, reduces the incidence of emergence delirium when administered as a single intraoperative dose (Ibacache et al., 2004) or as a continuous infusion (Shukry et al., 2005).

6. How can emergence delirium be treated?

The most important element of emergence delirium management is the prevention of patient injury, so for a patient who appears to be at higher risk, several steps should be considered. Surgical incisions and dressings, vascular lines, and drains must be protected. Padding and gentle restraint may be required to safeguard the patient from self-injury or from injuring healthcare providers. It is imperative to quickly rule out serious medical causes of agitation or altered mental status, such as airway compromise, hypoxia, impaired ventilation, or bleeding. Pain, if present, should be adequately treated. The presence of emergence delirium frequently requires an escalation of nursing coverage,

---

Table 68.2

TREATMENT OPTIONS FOR EMERGENCE DELIRIUM PREVENTION AND MANAGEMENT

Agent	Emergence Delirium Prevention	Emergence Delirium Treatment
Desflurane	−	NA
Sevoflurane	−	NA
Bolus propofol	+/−	+
Propofol infusion	++	NA
Ondansetron	+/−	+/−
Clonidine or Dexmedetomidine	+	+
Fentanyl	+	+
Ketamine	+/−	−
Midazolam	+	+

++ very effective, + effective, +/− neutral, − ineffective, NA not applicable

and given the frequency of emergence delirium in the PACU, some degree of flexibility should be incorporated into PACU staffing models. In some circumstances, sedation or re-induction of anesthesia (following appropriate equipment and personnel preparation) with either propofol, an opioid, or an alpha-2 agonist may be required to prevent patient injury. Table 68.2 lists options for the prevention and treatment of emergence delirium. Resedation will delay emergence, ideally providing a more stable and secure return to consciousness. Although emergence delirium is usually of short duration, it can be dramatic and disconcerting; reassurance of parents and healthcare providers should not be forgotten.

SUMMARY

1. Emergence delirium is a poorly understood clinical phenomenon characterized by a brief period of disorientation and combativeness following general anesthesia.
2. The cause of emergence delirium is likely multifactorial, with no single medication or anesthetic technique responsible.
3. The most successful approach to reducing the incidence of emergence delirium is employing a balanced anesthetic technique whose objective is a smooth and pain-free recovery.

ANNOTATED REFERENCES

- Dahmani S, Stanly I, Brasher C, Lejeune C, Bruneau B, Wood C, Nivoche Y. Pharmacological prevention of sevoflurane- and desflurane-related emergence agitation in children: a meta-analysis of published studies. *Br J Anaesth* 2010; 104(2): 216–223.

A meta-analysis of studies, combining over 1,600 patients, focused on reducing the incidence of emergence delirium. Although no single treatment is demonstrated as being superior, multiple options, including propofol, NMDA receptor antagonists, alpha agonists, and narcotics, may be helpful. The timing and route of medication administration influence the effectiveness of the intervention.

- **Voepel-Lewis T, Malviya S, Tait R. A prospective cohort study of emergence agitation in the pediatric postanesthesia care unit.** *Anesth Analg* **2003; 96: 1625–1630.**

  A cohort analysis of 571 patients identifying factors associated with the development of emergence delirium, its incidence, and impact.

- **Wells L, Rasch DK. Emergence "delirium" after sevoflurane anesthesia: paranoid delusion?** *Anesth Analg* **1999; 88: 1308–1310.**

  A series of brief case reports detailing observations of patients who experienced emergence delirium. Also contains self-reports from patients who were able to recall what they experienced during these episodes. No emergence delirium episode was characterized as painful. Varying degrees of disorientation, paranoia, and terror appear as common themes.

Further Reading

Cravero JP, Beach M, Thyr B, Whalen K. The effect of small-dose fentanyl on the emergence characteristics of pediatric patients after sevoflurane anesthesia without surgery. *Anesth Analg* 2003; 97: 364–367.

Galinkin JL, Fazi LM, Cuy RM, Chiavacci RM, Kurth CD, Shah UK, Jacobs IN, Watcha MF. Use of intranasal fentanyl in children undergoing myringotomy and tube placement during halothane and sevoflurane Anesthesia. *Anesthesiology* 2000; 93: 1378–1383.

Ibacache ME, Munoz HR, Brandes V, Morales AL. Single-dose dexmedetomidine reduces agitation after sevoflurane anesthesia in children. *Anesth Analg* 2004; 98: 60–63.

Sikich N, Lerman J. Development and psychometric evaluation of the Pediatric Emergence Delirium Scale. *Anesthesiology* 2004; 100(5): 1138–1145.

Shukry M, Mathison CC, Kalarickal PL, Ramadhyani U. Does dexmedetomidine prevent emergence delirium in children after sevoflurane-based general anesthesia? *Pediatr Anesth* 2005; 15: 1098–1104.

Vlajkovic GP, Sindjelic RP. Emergence delirium in children: Many questions, few answers. *Anesth Analg* 2007; 104(1): 84–91.

Yasui Y, Masaki E, Kato, F. Sevoflurane directly excites locus coeruleus neurons of rats. *Anesthesiology* 2007; 107(6): 992–1002.

69

Stridor After Extubation

JUNZHENG WU AND C. DEAN KURTH

INTRODUCTION

Infants and young children who were intubated and mechanically ventilated occasionally present with stridor in the post-anesthesia care unit (PACU) after extubation. In severe cases, respiratory distress and oxygen desaturation accompany the stridor. Prophylactic measures and prompt management help to prevent post-extubation stridor and ameliorate the signs and symptoms should it occur.

LEARNING OBJECTIVES

1. List the contributing risk factors for post-extubation stridor.
2. Describe the prophylactic techniques to reduce the risk of post-extubation stridor.
3. Describe the management of stridor to prevent re-intubation and subglottic stenosis.

CASE PRESENTATION

An infant develops a high-pitched squeaking sound and difficulty breathing 30 minutes after extubation in the operating room. The previously healthy, 7.2-kg, full-term 10-month-old boy had just had an *inguinal hernia repair. The baby appears irritable and has a sporadic dry cough and **inspiratory stridor,** along with **retractions** at the suprasternal notch. Vital signs are heart rate 155, respiratory rate 48, blood pressure 87/46, and temperature 37.5°C. SpO_2 is 95% with blow-by cool humidified oxygen mist at 10 L/min. The mother states that her baby frequently has noisy breathing at home, especially when upset. For the past 2 weeks, he had a stuffy nose and an intermittent dry cough. The anesthesia record reveals that the patient had a moderately difficult view of the airway. He had been **intubated** by a resident with a 3.5 cuffed ETT **after three attempts**. **No air leak around the ETT** had been detected with positive inspiratory airway pressure up to* **35 cmH_2O**. *The patient received sevoflurane, 5 mcg fentanyl, and 150 mL of lactated Ringer's solution during surgery.*

*A diagnosis of post-extubation stridor is made. The infant receives nebulized **racemic epinephrine (adrenaline)** (0.3 mL of 2.25%, diluted in 5 mL normal saline) and 3.5 mg IV **dexamethasone**. The patient's condition gradually deteriorates in the ensuing 20 minutes, evidenced by labored breathing, worsening **stridor**, and intercostal **retractions**. SpO_2 slowly drifts below 90%, and breath sounds are barely audible. Positive-pressure ventilation via facemask provides no improvement. After IV atropine (0.1 mg), propofol (20 mg), and succinylcholine (suxamethonium) (10 mg) are administered, a 2.5-mm ETT is inserted into the trachea with some resistance. The air leak is heard at 35 cmH_2O. The baby is sedated with an IV infusion of fentanyl and midazolam and is transported to the pediatric intensive care unit (PICU).*

*In the PICU, the baby remains sedated with a continuous infusion of IV fentanyl and midazolam and is mechanically ventilated using a pressure support mode. Pulmonary edema is not evident on chest x-ray. **Dexamethasone** is administered every 6 hours. 24 hours after **reintubation**, SpO_2 remains above 98%, the tidal volume is 50 to 70 mL, and his spontaneous respiration rate is 30/min with the assistance of pressure support. The air leak around the ETT is now 12 cmH_2O. The patient is extubated successfully with no further respiratory distress. The baby is transferred to the regular ward and is* *discharged home the next day. Mild **congenital subglottic stenosis** is diagnosed 2 months later.*

DISCUSSION

1. What are the contributing risk factors for post-extubation stridor?

Post-extubation croup, also known as post-intubation croup, is defined as **inspiratory stridor** developing after extubation. The condition usually presents within 1 hour after extubation, though sometimes it develops as late as the first 24 hours. Post-extubation stridor arises from glottic and subglottic edema caused by ischemia of the tracheal mucosa from pressure by the ETT. The symptoms appear after extubation because compression by the ETT prevents narrowing of the tracheal lumen; upon its removal, the edema develops to narrow the lumen. Symptoms include **inspiratory stridor, hoarseness,** and **chest retractions**. If the airway obstruction becomes severe, arterial desaturation occurs and **re-intubation** can be required to maintain a patent airway.

The following factors increase the risk of post-extubation stridor: (1) *ETT:* tightly fitting in trachea with a **leak** pressure **above 25 cmH₂O**; (2) *Age:* children younger than 4 years, due to their disproportionately smaller airway lumen; (3) *Intubation maneuver:* **multiple** and/or traumatic **attempts**; (4) *Duration of endotracheal intubation:* risk for trauma or ischemia increases with prolonged intubation; (5) *Head or neck surgery:* frequent position changes of the head and neck, common with this type of surgery, increase the risk for trauma or ischemia of tracheal mucosa; (6) *Ongoing upper airway infection:* tracheal mucosa is already inflamed or edematous; (7) *Airway trauma or reactivity:* inhalation and burn injury, history of spasmodic croup or reactive airway disease; (8) *Extubation:* coughing vigorously when ETT is present; and (9) *Subglottic stenosis:* congenital or acquired lesions or syndromes associated with a disproportionately narrow airway for age, such as Down syndrome (Suominen et al., 2006; Cohen et al., 2011).

2. What techniques might reduce the risk of post-extubation stridor?

To reduce the risk of post-extubation stridor, it is necessary to address each risk factor. *Appropriate ETT*: An old and common practice was to use an uncuffed ETT in children under 8 years old, and the size was determined by the equation (age in years + 16)/4. Accumulating data reveal no difference between uncuffed versus cuffed ETTs in the incidence of post-extubation stridor. In children, a cuffed ETT, 0.5 mm outer diameter smaller than the equation, may be used without increasing the risk of post-extubation stridor. Cuffed tubes carry advantages over uncuffed tubes, including less anesthetic gas contamination, better mechanical ventilation, and decreased risk of aspiration and infection in mechanically ventilated children. Better mechanical ventilation is especially advantageous when high inflation pressure is required to ventilate the lungs during an acute or chronic lung disease. After intubation, a leak test should be performed. The uncuffed ETT should leak between 10 and 30 cmH$_2$O to permit ventilation and to maintain perfusion of the tracheal mucosa. With a cuffed ETT, the leak should be the same as for the uncuffed ETT when the cuff is fully deflated. If the leak is less than 20 cmH$_2$O, the cuff should be inflated meticulously until the air leak is "just sealed" at 20 cmH$_2$O. *Atraumatic intubation with a high success rate*: Multiple and traumatic intubations should be avoided. A skilled anesthetist should perform the intubation if the potential for difficult airway exists, especially in an infant. *Smooth extubation:* Vigorous movement and forceful coughing during extubation increases the risk of subglottic injury and swelling. A good technique during the extubation process minimizes or eliminates these risk factors. *Elective procedure and URI:* Surgery should be postponed if the patient has a recent viral URI and prolonged intubation is required for the procedure. *Dexamethasone:* IV administration of **dexamethasone** prior to extubation helps to reduce airway swelling if the patient is undergoing airway surgery or has experienced multiple and traumatic attempts at intubation. *Air leak test:* Prior to extubation after prolonged intubation, a repeat leak test may predict the occurrence of post-extubation stridor. Infants should remain intubated as short a time as possible.

3. What is the management of established post-extubation stridor?

The incidence of post-extubation stridor has decreased significantly during the past 20 years as the pathogenesis was better understood and preventive measures were instituted. Although the effectiveness of some treatments for post-extubation stridor is still debatable, the following are widely advocated to treat it: (1) *Postoperative agitation management:* Crying and agitation in the PACU exacerbates stridor and difficulty breathing. Sedation with dexmedetomidine or other agents and control of pain with opioids have the goal of preventing crying and agitation and promoting smooth respiration; (2) *Cool and humidified mist* ameliorates post-extubation stridor by reducing mucosal edema and is recommended for use during mild cases when only stridor is present; (3) *Racemic epinephrine* is recommended for moderate post-extubation stridor, such as when **retractions** and dyspnea occur. In theory, it reduces mucosal swelling through vasoconstriction. Both in the PACU and in the PICU, the dose is 0.2 to 0.5 mL of 2.25% racemic epinephrine diluted into 3 to 5 mL of normal saline, administered by nebulizer over 5 to 10 minutes. The patient should be observed for 4 hours after administration for potential "rebound effect"—that is, the stridor could recur as the drug's effect dissipates; (4) *Heliox (helium–oxygen mixture):* Heliox, a gas that is less dense than air, increases laminar flow and reduces turbulent flow. A recent study demonstrated its successful use in the PICU in the treatment of post-extubation croup not responding to racemic epinephrine. Heliox works temporarily to alleviate symptoms of upper airway obstruction and to prevent re-intubation until other therapies become effective or the disease process naturally resolves; (5) *Corticosteroids:* Recent data suggest that prophylactic corticosteroids may reduce the incidence of post-extubation stridor and the subsequent need for re-intubation in patients who had prolonged mechanical ventilation or in patients who underwent an airway operation (Markowitz & Randolph, 2002). It decreases airway swelling putatively by interrupting inflammation resulting from intubation-induced airway injury. **Dexamethasone** can be given as follows: 0.5 mg/kg, every 4 to 6 hours, for a maximum of 40 mg/day, for 2 days in patients at high risk before extubation. Alternatively, aerosolized budesonide may be administered; (6) *Re-intubation*: In patients with severe stridor and impending ventilatory failure that is unresponsive to the above-mentioned treatments, re-intubation should be performed before post-obstructive pulmonary edema, hypoxemia, and acidosis ensue. The ETT should be smaller than the one originally placed. An ETT 0.5 sizes smaller than predicted should be used, with size confirmed by the leak test. The ETT should be left in place for 24 to 48 hours to allow swelling to recede. It is important to provide sedation to avoid further airway trauma. Propofol and a nondepolarizing muscle relaxant are appropriate to facilitate re-intubation, followed by an infusion of sedatives, titrated to effect. The patient may be extubated when an appropriate air leak is observed.

Table 69.1 provides an overview of post-intubation stridor.

4. What are the guidelines for discharge in patients who develop post-extubation stridor?

In a mild case, defined by inspiratory stridor only with minimal agitation, cool mist, sedation, and pain management are sufficient. Patients still can be discharged after surgery if the situation is improving or has not worsened after an extra hour of observation. The parents should receive appropriate instruction prior to discharge. For a moderate case, defined by stridor, moderate dyspnea, and suprasternal retractions during inspiration, nebulized racemic epinephrine and dexamethasone are added to the treatment. The patient may be discharged home after the

Table 69.1

OVERVIEW OF POST-INTUBATION STRIDOR

Risk Factors	Preventive Options
Air leak >30 cmH$_2$O	Maintain air leak around ETT < 30 cmH$_2$O
Age <4 years	
Multiple attempts at intubation, or traumatic intubation	Atraumatic intubation
Prolonged intubation	Shortest possible intubation time
Head/neck surgery	
URI	Delay elective surgery if intubation is required if child has an URI
Airway trauma, inhalation injury (e.g., burn), or spasmodic croup, asthma	
Coughing vigorously prior to extubation	Smooth emergence (avoid coughing)
Subglottic stenosis	Dexamethasone
Signs	*Treatment*
Inspiratory stridor	Manage agitation
Agitation	Cool mist oxygen
Retractions	Inhaled racemic epinephrine
Hoarseness	Dexamethasone IV or inhaled budesonide
Oxygen desaturation	Helium–oxygen mixture
	Re-intubation

symptoms have dramatically improved and the window for potential "rebound effect" from racemic epinephrine has passed with no further stridor. The patient should be admitted if symptoms are not improving significantly and additional doses of nebulized racemic epinephrine are administered, especially in infants. In patients who develop severe post-extubation stridor presenting with severe difficulty breathing, intercostal retractions, inability to maintain oxygen saturation, and lethargy, the patient should be re-intubated with a smaller ETT and admitted to the ICU.

SUMMARY

1. Post-extubation stridor is most often seen in children under 4 years of age; other risk factors include ongoing URI, history of narrow airway, prolonged intubation, and traumatic intubation.
2. Anticipation and prophylactic treatment of risk factors, followed by prompt recognition and treatment of symptoms, may prevent re-intubation.
3. The decision to discharge a patient home depends on the severity of symptoms and their clinical course.

ANNOTATED REFERENCES

- Markovitz BP, Randolph AG. Corticosteroids for the prevention of reintubation and postextubation stridor in pediatric patients: A meta-analysis. *Pediatr Crit Care Med* 2002; 3(3): 223–226.

  Data analysis from six controlled clinical trials showed convincing evidence that IV steroids reduce the risk of post-extubation stridor and re-intubation.
- Newth CJ, Rachman B, Patel N. The use of cuffed versus uncuffed endotracheal tubes in pediatric intensive care. *J Pediatr* 2004; 144: 333–337.

  The study results demonstrate the significant advantages using cuffed ETTs in pediatric patients as opposed to the traditional textbook teaching that cuffed tubes should not be used in children younger than 8 years of age.

Further Reading

Cohen T, Deutsch N, Motoyama EK. Induction, Maintenance and Recovery. In Davis PJ, Cladis FP and Motoyama EK, eds. *Anesthesia for Infants and Children*. Mosby-Elsevier, 2011: 365–394.

Metha R, Hariprakash SP, Cox PN, Wheeler DS. Diseases of the upper respiratory tract. In Wheeler DS, Wong HR, eds. *Pediatric Critical Care Medicine: Basic Science and Clinical Evidence*. London: Springer, 2007: 480–505.

Sinha A, Jayashree M, Singhi S. Aerosolized L-epinephrine vs. budesonide for postextubation stridor: A randomized controlled trial. *Indian Pediatr* 2010; 47: 317–322.

Suominen P, Taivainen T, Tuoninen N, et al. Optimally fitted tracheal tubes decrease the probability of postextubation adverse events in children undergoing general anesthesia. *Pediatr Anesth* 2006; 16: 641–647.

Postoperative Nausea and Vomiting in Patients with Prolonged QTc

SHILPA RAO AND JERROLD LERMAN

INTRODUCTION

A panoply of pharmacological and nonpharmacological strategies are currently employed to attenuate the risk of postoperative nausea and vomiting (PONV) in children, including 5-hydroxytryptamine type 3 (5-HT$_3$) receptor antagonists. 5-HT$_3$ receptor antagonists can prolong the QT interval, which can be a precursor of torsades de pointes (TdP), particularly in children with congenital or acquired prolonged QT interval. This chapter summarizes the causes of prolonged QT interval, the potential interactions of prolonged QT interval with antiemetics and anesthetics, and strategies to prevent PONV.

> ## LEARNING OBJECTIVES
>
> 1. Understand the nature and risks of prolonged QT intervals.
> 2. Explain the potential effects of 5-HT$_3$ receptor antagonists on cardiac repolarization.
> 3. Review current and future antiemetics.
> 4. Manage children with prolonged QT interval and PONV.

CASE PRESENTATION

A 6-year-old, 21-kg **boy** *is scheduled for adenotonsillectomy for chronic throat infections, as an outpatient. His past medical history is unremarkable except for a vague history of a single episode of* **syncope** *that physicians suggested may have been due to a "***prolonged QT interval.***" There was no cardiology follow-up. Physical examination on the day of surgery is unremarkable. The child is taking no medications. After premedication with 15 mg oral midazolam, anesthesia is induced with 70% nitrous oxide in oxygen and 8% inspired sevoflurane. After tracheal intubation, spontaneous ventilation resumes while the child breathes 3% sevoflurane in 70% nitrous oxide. Towards the end of surgery, the child receives a single IV dose of morphine 1.8 mg, a rectal dose of acetaminophen (paracetamol) 650 mg, a single IV dose of the* **5HT-3 receptor** *antagonist* **ondansetron** *2 mg, and a single IV dose of dexamethasone 8 mg. Within 1 minute of administering the ondansetron, the ECG displays* **premature ventricular contractions** *that deteriorate into* **ventricular tachycardia***. IV lidocaine 20 mg is administered with conversion to sinus rhythm within 20 seconds. Surgery is concluded hastily, the airway extubated, and the child transferred to the PACU breathing spontaneously, saturating 100%, and in normal sinus rhythm. In the PACU, a 12-lead ECG was normal except for a* **prolonged QT interval, 480 msec***. The child recovers uneventfully.*

DISCUSSION

1. What is the QT interval, and which factors affect it?

The **QT interval** is a measure of the time required for ventricular myocardial cells to repolarize to their resting membrane potential, approximately −90 mV. Electrophysiologically, this interval extends from the beginning of phase 1 of the action potential (AP) until the end of phase 3. Repolarization is regulated by the opening and closing of several transmembrane ion channels that facilitate movement of cations and anions in and out of the myocardial cell. Specifically, during the action potential there is a brief and early influx of Na^+ with a contemporaneous efflux of K^+, the latter being the dominant factor in moderating repolarization. Electrocardiographically, the **QT interval** is the time interval between the initiation of the QRS complex and the end of the T wave.

The **QTc interval** is the QT interval corrected for heart rate. In adults, the normal **QTc interval** is less than 450 msec in men and less than 470 msec in women. In children (beyond the neonatal and early infancy period), the normal **QTc interval** is less than 450 msec for both sexes. Several factors affect the duration of the **QT interval**, including congenital causes of long QT syndrome (cLQTS) and drugs. The incidence of cLQTS in the population ranges from 1 in 2,500 to 1 in 6,500. Five genes (LQT1, 2, 3, 5, 6) code for more than 200 mutations in three ion channels: slow and rapid delayed K^+ channel and the slow Na^+ channel. These ion channels are formed by the products of one or more of these genes; for example, the slowly activating delayed rectifier potassium channel, I_{Ks}, comprises the products from the KCNQ1 and KCNE1 genes. Of the cLQTS mutations, 95% involve the K^+ channel (outward flux of potassium during repolarization) and 5% involve the Na^+ channel (slow inward flux of sodium). In terms of the genes, LQT1 and LQT5 account for 60% of the cLQTS cases, LQT2 and LQT6 account for 35% of the cases, LQT3 accounts for 4%, and individually, the LQT5 and LQT6 account for 1%. cLQT4 is extremely rare and not a channelopathy. The most common phenotype of cLQTS is the Romano-Ward syndrome, an autosomal dominant defect representing 99% of cases, which involves mutations in LQT1 to LQT7. Jervill and Lange-Nielson syndrome is another defect that occurs in less than 1% of patients with cLQTS on an autosomal recessive basis that is associated with deafness (Chiang & Roden, 2000).

A number of acquired conditions prolong the **QTc interval**. The **QTc interval** may be prolonged in the presence of electrolyte abnormalities such as hypokalemia, hypomagnesemia, and hypocalcemia, with hypothyroidism, and with other assorted conditions such as coronary artery disease, cardiomyopathy, hypertension, bradycardia, hypothyroidism, female gender, and stroke. Anorexia nervosa, liquid protein diet, gastroplasty, and celiac disease may also prolong the **QTc interval**. Certain medications can also affect the QTc interval (see Table 70.1 and discussions below).

Isolated prolonged **QT interval** is usually a silent disorder, rarely manifesting arrhythmias. The risk of arrhythmias increases if the uncorrected **QT interval** exceeds 500 msec or the QTc exceeds 470 msec. Children with undiagnosed syncope or who have a family history of sudden death or unexplained death under

---

Table 70.1

DRUGS THAT CAN PROLONG THE QT INTERVAL

Class I and III antiarrhythmics
Inhalational anesthetics
5-HT$_3$ receptor antagonists (except palonosetron)
Droperidol
Phenothiazines
Tricyclic antidepressants
Linezolid
Chloral hydrate
Lithium
Diphenhydramine
Erythromycin
Cocaine
Diuretics
Doxorubicin
Ionic contrast media
Prednisone
Tacrolimus
Vasopressin

---

anesthesia should have a 12-lead EGG preoperatively to determine their risk for arrhythmias.

The genesis of malignant arrhythmias such as **premature ventricular contractions**, **ventricular tachycardia**, and TdP (Fig. 70.1) from defects in repolarization requires the presence of two preconditions: prolonged QT interval and increased dispersion of repolarization. Although **prolonged QT interval** is well described, *dispersion of repolarization* is an unfamiliar expression. The dispersion of repolarization is a measure of the variance or heterogeneity of the QT interval across the ventricular cardiac muscle. As the dispersion of repolarization increases, the risk of malignant arrhythmias increases. The optimal ECG metric to estimate the dispersion of repolarization is unclear.

2. What are the ECG effects of the 5-HT$_3$ receptor antagonists?
5-HT$_3$ receptor antagonists affect the ECG by prolonging the PR, QRS complex, and **QT interval**. They block the rapid potassium efflux during repolarization (via the HERG receptor) in the cardiac myocyte, widening the QT interval. The order of potency of these antagonists to inhibit the K$^+$ efflux via the HERG channel is ondansetron > granisetron > dolasetron. The active metabolites of dolasetron may block the sodium channels, independent of their effects on 5-HT$_3$ receptor-blocking activity.

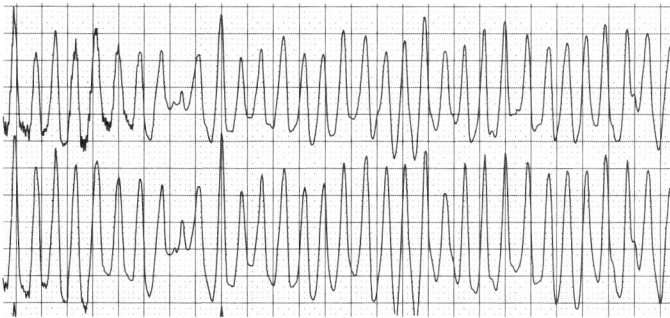

FIGURE 70.1 Torsades de pointes, ECG leads I and II.

5-HT$_3$ receptor antagonists are given routinely to asymptomatic children without a preoperative screening ECG. To date, there have been only a handful of reports of polymorphic ventricular arrhythmias including **ventricular tachycardia** and **TdP** in children after ondansetron, tropisetron, and dolasetron, with the vast majority returning spontaneously to normal sinus rhythm (e.g., McKechnie & Froese, 2010). In healthy children, recent evidence demonstrated that 0.1 mg/kg ondansetron had no clinical effect on the **QT interval**, and in no cases did it exceed 500 msec. Furthermore, the dispersion of repolarization was unchanged (Mehta et al., 2010). Nonetheless, it would seem imprudent and ill advised to administer a medication that prolongs the QT interval to a child with a known **prolonged QT interval,** especially when alternative strategies are available to prevent perioperative nausea and vomiting.

The new 5-HT$_3$ receptor antagonist palonosetron differs from the current 5-HT$_3$ receptor antagonists in at least three ways: (1) it does not bind to 5-HT$_3$ receptors; (2) it does not prolong the **QT interval**; and (3) it is resistant to polymorphisms in the drug transporter channel P glycol and to isoforms of CYP450 2D6.

The current **5-HT$_3$ receptor antagonists** bind to 5-HT$_3$ receptors via their indole rings; however, the new 5-HT$_3$ receptor antagonist palonosetron lacks an indole ring. As a result, palonosetron distorts the conformational structure of the receptor, rendering it inactive. This conformational change, combined with evidence that palonosetron causes internalization of the 5-HT$_3$ receptor, explains in part the markedly prolonged elimination half-life of palonosetron. The net effect of these properties of palonosetron is an antiemetic with a 30- to 40-hour half-life after a single dose IV.

3. What about droperidol and the QT interval?

It is inadvisable to use droperidol in children with prolonged **QT interval**. The U.S. Food and Drug Administration issued a black-box warning in 2004 against its use as a routine antiemetic out of concern for several cases of malignant arrhythmias and TdP.

Recent evidence demonstrated that a single dose of droperidol 0.02 mg/kg IV significantly increased the **QT interval** in healthy children, although the increase was clinically irrelevant. Moreover, none of the children developed **QT intervals** of more than 500 msec. The dispersion of repolarization did not change significantly after droperidol (Mehta et al., 2010).

4. How should one manage ventricular tachycardia or TdP?

Managing polymorphic ventricular contractions, ventricular tachycardia, and TdP requires specific interventions while eschewing others. Key treatments include increasing the heart rate, cardiac shock (1–2 joules/kg), IV magnesium (50 mg/kg), and IV lidocaine (1 mg/kg). Class III antiarrhythmics such as amiodarone as well as class I antiarrhythmics (quinidine) must be avoided as they are likely to exacerbate the already prolonged QT interval.

5. How effective and safe is dexamethasone?

Numerous studies have established the antiemetic effect of dexamethasone in the perioperative period. Dexamethasone has no effect on the **QT interval**. A single dose of dexamethasone very rarely causes side effects. It has precipitated several cases of tumor lysis syndrome, which has resulted in at least one death in a child with an undiagnosed acute leukemia.

6. What are the NK1 antiemetics?

Substance P, the dominant peptide in the neuropeptide family, is believed to mediate emetogenic activity. It acts primarily on the G-protein receptor subtype NK1 (neurokinin 1). This receptor subtype is present in the central and peripheral nervous systems as well as in the gastrointestinal tract. The current NK1 receptor antagonists are very effective antiemetics that cause no sedation. Several prototypical compounds (e.g., aprepitant) have been developed, but only for oral administration. Phosphorylating aprepitant resulted in fosaprepitant, a water-soluble compound that is an effective IV antiemetic. No data are available in children.

In adults, doses up to 3 mg/kg do not prolong the **QT interval** (Marbury et al., 2009). Fosaprepitant has a 30-minute onset of action and causes pain when administered IV.

7. Are there effective antiemetics for the PACU?

Few studies have addressed the efficacy of secondary treatments for emesis in the PACU after prophylactic therapy failed in a child with a prolonged **QT interval**. Metoclopramide is a moderately effective antiemetic, although dystonia has been reported rarely as a side effect. Dimenhydrinate is also moderately effective but produces sedation as a side effect (Vener et al., 1996).

8. What other antiemetic therapies are available?

There are a number of strategies apart from antiemetic therapy to reduce PONV in children. Other interventions include keeping the fasting interval to a minimum (as per American Society of Anesthesiologists' guidelines) and postoperatively providing oral fluids only when the child requests them. Intraoperative strategies include avoiding inflating the stomach during mask ventilation, using total intravenous anesthesia with propofol, and avoiding nitrous oxide. Regional anesthesia may reduce the need for opioid analgesia, along with the use of other non-opioid analgesics. Superhydration with IV fluids may also reduce PONV.

SUMMARY

1. Nausea and vomiting in children with prolonged QT interval should be managed with dexamethasone and dimenhydrinate and/or metoclopramide.
2. In children with prolonged QT interval, care must be taken to limit exposure to all factors (including medications) that prolong the QT interval.
3. In the near future, the ideal triad for prophylactic antiemetics may include palonosetron, dexamethasone,

and an NK-1 agonist, none of which should interfere with ventricular repolarization and cause ventricular dysrhythmias.

ANNOTATED REFERENCES

- Chiang C-E, Roden DM. The long QT syndromes: genetic basis and clinical implications. *J Am Coll Cardiol* 2000; 36: 1–12.

This review introduces the genetics and the clinical presentation of channelopathies of the ventricular muscle for the uninitiated.

- McKechnie K, Froese A. Ventricular tachycardia after ondansetron administration in a child with undiagnosed long QT syndrome. *Can J Anesth* 2010; 57: 453–457.

An 11-year-old with a recognized long QT interval has ventricular tachycardia after a single dose of ondansetron. After IV lidocaine, the ECG converted to sinus rhythm.

- Mehta D, Sanatani S, Whyte SD. The effects of droperidol and ondansetron on dispersion of myocardial repolarization in children. *Pediatr Anesth* 2010; 20: 905–912.

This is the first study to measure the QT interval and dispersion of repolarization in children undergoing elective anesthesia after ondansetron, droperidol, both drugs, and neither drug. Although the QT interval increased statistically, the increase was clinically irrelevant, 10 msec. The dispersion of repolarization did not differ before and after the study medications.

Further Reading

Apfel CC, Malhotra A, Leslie JB. The role of neurokininin-1 receptor antagonists for the management of postoperative nausea and vomiting. *Curr Opin Anaesthesiol* 2008; 21: 427–432.

Choi EM, Lee MG, Lee SH, Choi KW, Choi SH. Association of ABCB1 polymorphisms with the efficacy of ondansetron for postoperative nausea and vomiting. *Anaesthesia* 2010; 65: 996–1000.

Ho K-Y, Gan TJ. Pharmacology, pharmacogenetics, and clinical efficacy of 5-hydroxytryptamine type 3 receptor antagonists for postoperative nausea and vomiting. *Curr Opin Anaesthesiol* 2006; 19: 606–611.

Marbury TC, Jin B, Panebianco D, Murphy MG, Sun H, Evans JK, Han TH, Constanzer ML, Dru J, Shadle CR. Lack of effect of aprepitant or its prodrug fosaprepitant on QTc intervals in healthy subjects. *Anesth Analg* 2009; 109: 418–425.

Rojas C, Stathis M, Thomas AG, Massuda EB, Alt J, Zhang J, Rubenstein E, Sebastiani S, Cantoreggi S, Snyder SH, Slusher B. Palonosetron exhibits unique molecular interactions with the 5-HT$_3$ receptor. *Anesth Analg* 2008; 107: 469–478.

Towbin JA, Wang Z, Li H. Genotype and severity of long QT syndrome. *Drug Metabolism and Disposition* 2001; 29: 574–579.

Vener DF, Carr AS, Sikich N, Bissonnette B, Lerman J. Dimenhydrinate decreases vomiting after strabismus surgery in children. *Anesth Analg* 1996; 82: 728–731.

Vincent GM. The long QT syndrome. *Indian Pacing Electrophysiol J* 2002; 2: 127–146.

Disclosure After Complication in the OR

MARK J. MEYER AND NORBERT J. WEIDNER

INTRODUCTION

In matters of medical error and complications, patients and families overwhelmingly want to be informed. Most patients want providers to disclose if a complication or an error has occurred, and want to be informed of any possible adverse outcomes from the event. Most want to be informed immediately following an event and expect an investigation when the cause is not readily identified. When the event is due to an error, patients and families want honest disclosure and a sincere apology from those responsible. Afterward, they want continued emotional and psychological support, and they expect efforts to identify and correct the cause. Historically, physicians and institutions have been slow to fully disclose errors, especially if they were preventable. Patients have frequently not been provided with the support they require and often have felt frightened and alienated. The immediate effects of medical mistakes can be devastating, but the subsequent emotional, personal, and relational consequences can be very distressing. Silence, shame, guilt, and fractured trust disrupt the therapeutic relationship and leave patients, families, and caregivers to suffer alone.

LEARNING OBJECTIVES

1. Distinguish between medical error and adverse event.
2. Identify the key elements for the safe disclosure of unanticipated outcomes to patients and families.
3. Understand the components of an institutional policy for the management of patients after an adverse event that caused harm.

CASE PRESENTATION

A 9-month-old boy presents for surgical excision of a large nevus under general anesthesia. He was born full term and is healthy. Following mask induction of general anesthesia, IV access is established and a laryngeal mask airway is placed and secured. The surgeon requests that cefazolin 40 mg/kg is given prior to incision.

Several minutes after administration of the antibiotic, the patient becomes tachycardic and hypotensive. The pulse oximeter waveform and capnograph trace are lost. There are no palpable pulses. The surgical site is covered, the surgical drapes are removed, chest compressions age begun, and the patient is intubated. After two doses of epinephrine and 40 mL/kg of lactated Ringer's, faint pulses are felt. The patient stabilizes with an infusion of dopamine. The surgical site is rapidly closed and the patient is transferred to the intensive care unit for further management.

Several hours later, the patient is weaned off the dopamine and is extubated. Workup is consistent with an anaphylactic reaction, and the suspected cause is the antibiotic. It is later discovered that the patient had a known allergy to cephalosporins. His records indicate a previous hospital admission for wheezing and edema after a course of cephalexin was started for treatment of otitis media. This information is clearly included on his preoperative history and examination. His allergy bracelet reads, "cephalosporins." The anesthesiologist and surgeon involved request to meet with the parents.

DISCUSSION

1. What are adverse events? What type of event was this?

An injury or complication attributable to the medical management of a patient is considered an adverse event. This is in distinction to an injury or complication that results directly from an underlying disease process. An adverse event can be caused by a medical error or other causes such as medication side effects. Medical *error* is a failure in the delivery of medical care to be completed as intended or the use of the wrong plan to achieve an aim. Examples of medical error include misdiagnoses, using the wrong medication, or giving the wrong dose. In this case, the failure of the doctors, nurses, and pharmacists involved in this patient's care to prevent the administration of a harmful medication is an error. Medical errors are classified as *serious errors, minor errors,* and *near-misses. Serious errors* have the potential to cause permanent injury or transient but potentially life-threatening harm. *Sentinel events* are serious errors that demand immediate intervention. These are unanticipated, not related to the patient's illness, and result in serious physical or psychological injury. Examples of sentinel events include wrong-site surgery and cardiac arrest. *Minor errors* do not cause harm but have the potential to do so. A *near-miss* is an error that could have caused harm but did not reach the patient. This case is an example of a preventable adverse event that is caused by serious medical error (Massachusetts Coalition for the Prevention of Medical Errors, 2006).

2. Is there an obligation to disclose an error if the patient is not harmed?

Disclosure should be provided following sentinel events, serious events, and other unanticipated outcomes involving harm that requires escalation of care, including increased length of stay, additional diagnostic tests, and therapeutic interventions. In cases of near-misses or harmless errors, it is not appropriate to inform the patient and family. However, harmless errors and near-misses may require an institutional response to address failures in quality and safety. Under these guidelines, the case presented qualifies for disclosure, as this is a serious error with the potential to cause harm.

3. Once the patient is stabilized, what are the next steps?

Timing of the response should be prompt, typically within the first 24 hours. The first discussion with the patient and/or family should focus on what happened, how it will affect the patient, and the prognosis. Often the outcomes cannot be known immediately following an event. If this is the case, this uncertainty should be clearly stated. If the cause is understood at this time, then an explanation is offered. If there is obvious error, an admission is made and an expression of regret and an apology are offered. However, when the mechanism of injury is unclear, disclosure of causes should be reserved until more information is available.

Medical providers with a primary relationship to the family should be involved. This is usually the attending doctor. If consulting specialists were involved, they may be present as well. Whether the result of an error or not, someone with an established relationship with the patient—usually the patient's physician—should take responsibility for the event. In this case, the attending surgeon and the anesthesiologist should be present.

The setting should be a quiet area of the institution with suitable seating for all. Interruptions must be eliminated, including those from pagers and cell phones. While the setting is important, so is the manner of communication. Eye contact, empathetic and sincere gestures, and receptive body language are paramount. Simple, straightforward language is best. Families are encouraged to ask questions and have complexities clarified with straightforward explanations. The delivery should be unhurried.

If the cause of the event requires additional information, the physician should commit to investigate the etiology. In the event of serious injury, ongoing communication with the patient and family is important. Measures taken to determine the severity of the injury, such as imaging and consultation with specialists, can be mentioned. However, not all families are able to absorb complex medical information while under duress. If this is the case, then delivery of the plan can be delayed until later. Delivering complex information in small packets can be more effective. In reality, disclosures are complex, and subtle discussions should be tailored to the nature of the event, the clinical context, and the patient–provider relationship.

Table 71.1 lists components for safe practice for disclosing unanticipated outcomes to patients.

4. Would one proceed differently if the child was recognized to have an allergy to the antibiotic but had no adverse reaction to its administration?

Even if the child came to no harm immediately following the administration of the antibiotic, a serious, preventable adverse

---

Table 71.1

COMPONENTS FOR SAFE PRACTICE FOR DISCLOSING UNANTICIPATED OUTCOMES TO PATIENTS

Provide a timely and explicit explanation about what happened and how the patient's health will be affected.

Explain the cause of the event and measures being taken to prevent future events.

Provide an empathic expression of regret and an apology when medical error is the cause.

Demonstrate a commitment to investigate to prevent future events.

Follow up with the patient and family to provide information and support.

Provide emotional support for patients and their families by trained caregivers after an event.

Reprinted with permission from National Quality Forum (NQF). *Safe Practices for Better Healthcare—2010 Update: A Consensus Report.* Washington DC: NQF, 2010.

event could have occurred. An explanation and an apology should still be offered to the parents. An institutional response is required in the form of an investigation and improvements to eliminate this preventable problem. Further follow-up is owed to the family, apprising them of institutional interventions and changes made.

5. Does disclosure affect liability in cases of serious error?

Avoiding admissions of fault in cases of medical error has long been a strategy used by risk managers to reduce legal liability. There is a commonly held belief that admissions of error can later be used during legal proceedings against doctors and hospitals. To the contrary, most states in the United States have enacted "apology laws" that allow for a disclosure while still protecting defendants in the event of liability. Eight states have laws that protect an admission of fault. This permits disclosure and apologies in the cases of medical error, but does not allow those statements to be used later in legal proceedings. Many other states protect only "expressions of sympathy" but not admissions of error (McDonnell et al., 2008).

Some institutions and health systems have adopted an open disclosure policy and are demonstrating that effective disclosure can reduce legal liability. Health systems that have implemented an open disclosure policy have reduced the number of suits, the value of awards paid, and attorney's fees. For example, the University of Michigan adopted an open disclosure policy in which doctors admit mistakes and apologize in cases of medical error. Since this policy was started the university has reduced the time to resolve complaints, attorney's fees have been reduced by more than two thirds, and the number of suits has decreased (Kachalia et al., 2010). The overall effect of "apology laws" and open disclosure policies on litigation is encouraging.

As healthcare compensation for third-party payers becomes based on measured quality and safety, providers and institutions may be driven to pursue open disclosure policies. It is through accurate reporting of safety events and outcomes that improvements in the quality of healthcare can be made. Institutions will rely on accurate reporting of adverse events and safety and quality failures to demonstrate competitiveness as this shift continues. This trend is occurring among healthcare consumers as well, as they become responsible for a larger portion of their healthcare costs.

6. What is meant by an "institutional response," and what obligation does the institution have when medical errors occur?

Following an adverse event, the institutional response begins with notification of the hospital clinical and administrative leadership. This includes safety officers, risk managers, and the ombudsman. Immediately, any medications, devices, and documentation that are relevant should be secured for analysis.

As the cause of the event becomes understood, the institution's leaders and attending doctor should devise a plan to support the patient and the care providers. Patients often feel alienated, anxious, and fearful, while providers may feel shame and remorse. The relationships between providers and patients frequently become complicated following an event; a demonstration of support from the institution and the attending doctor can buttress these challenged relationships.

Support for the patient can take many forms. The emotional and psychological trauma can be intense. Therapy and counseling may be needed immediately and in the long term. The institution may waive fees and provide compensation for additional expenses that the patient incurs. In contrast, the individual doctor should not offer to waive fees or otherwise discuss finances with the family. Addressing the additional expenses that a patient incurs following such events may be justified, especially when the event is an error. This is a means to demonstrate respect and empathy for patients at a time when it matters most to them.

Besides supporting the patient, the institution needs to support the analysis of the event. Once the analysis is complete and conclusions are made, the process for improvement must be developed and implemented.

SUMMARY

1. Families want and expect open, honest communication in case of an untoward event.
2. Open disclosure has numerous benefits, including repair of fractured trust, reduction in liability, and reduction in moral distress.
3. An apology, with a commitment to investigate and make improvements for the future, is crucial.
4. Future improvements in safety and quality are dependent upon the accurate disclosure and reporting of poor outcomes and errors. This will result in a safer system of care.

ANNOTATED REFERENCES

- Delbanco T, Bell SK. Guilty, afraid and alone—struggling with medical error. *N Engl J Med* 2007; 357: 1682–1683.

  This article reveals the strong negative emotions felt by those involved in a medical error. Patients are fearful of retribution and further mistreatment. Family members feel guilty they did not do more. Physicians involved feel ashamed and alone.
- Gallagher TH, Studdert D, Levinson W. Disclosing harmful medical errors to patients. *N Engl J Med* 2007; 356: 2713–2719.

  This article discusses the current state of disclosure of medical errors as a safe practice to improve the delivery of high-quality healthcare.
- Massachusetts Coalition for the Prevention of Medical Errors. *When Things Go Wrong: Responding to Adverse Events: A Consensus Statement of the Harvard Hospitals, 2006.* Accessed Jan. 23, 2011. http://www.ihi.org/NR/rdonlyres/

A4CE6C77-F65C-4F34-B323–20AA4E41 DC79/0/Responding
AdverseEvents.pdf

This effort provides thorough recommendations for the
management of medical error, including guidance on open disclosure and the appropriate institutional response. Well worth
reading.

- **National Quality Forum (NQF).** *Safe Practices for Better
  Healthcare—2010 Update: A Consensus Report.* **Washington
  DC: NQF, 2010. Accessed Dec. 12, 2010.** http://www.quality-
  forum.org/Publications/2010/04/Safe_Practices_for_Better_
  Healthcare_%e2%80%93_ 2010_Update.aspx.

The 2010 update presents 34 practices that have been demonstrated to be effective in reducing the occurrence of adverse
healthcare events.

Further Reading

Bell SK, Moorman DW, Delbanco T. Improving the patient, family, and
clinician experience after harmful events: the "When Things Go Wrong"
curriculum. *Acad Med* 2010; 85: 1010–1017.

Gallagher TH, Waterman AD, Ebers AG. Patients' and Physicians'
attitudes regarding disclosure of medical errors. *JAMA* 2003; 289(8):
1001–1007.

Hickson GB, Federspiel CF, Pichert JW, Miller CS, Gauld-Jaeger J, Bost P.
Patient complaints and malpractice risk. *JAMA* 2002; 287: 2951–2957.

Hobgood C, Peck CR, Gilbert B, Chappell K, Zou B. Medical errors—what
and when: what do patients want to know? *Acad Emerg Med* 2002; 9: 1156–
1161.

Kachalia A, Kaufman SR, Boothman R, Anderson S, Welch K, Saint S,
Rogers MA. Liability claims and costs before and after implementation of a
medical error disclosure program. *Ann Intern Med* 2010; 153(4): 213–221.

Matlow AG, Moody L, Laxer R, Stevens P, Goia C, Friedman JN. Disclosure
of medical error to parents and pediatric patients: assessment of parent's
attitudes and influencing factors. *Arch Dis Child* 2010; 95: 286–290.

McDonnell WM, Guenther E. Do state laws make it easier to say "I'm
sorry?" *Ann Intern Med* 2008; 149: 811–815.

INDEX

Note: Page numbers followed by *f* and *t* indicate content found in figures and tables, respectively.